DICTIONARY OF VETERINARY NURSING

DICTIONARY OF VETERINARY NURSING

D. R. LANE BSc(Vet Sci), FRCVS, FRAgS
Former Senior Examiner in Veterinary Nursing

S. GUTHRIE PhD, BA, BVetMed, MRCVS
Former Chief Examiner RCVS Veterinary Nursing Scheme

BUTTERWORTH
HEINEMANN

OXFORD AUCKLAND BOSTON JOHANNESBURG MELBOURNE NEW DELHI

Butterworth-Heinemann
Linacre House, Jordan Hill, Oxford OX2 8DP
225 Wildwood Avenue, Woburn, MA 01801-2041
A division of Reed Educational and Professional Publishing Ltd

A member of the Reed Elsevier plc group

First published 1999

British Library Cataloguing in Publication Data
A catalogue record for this book is available from the British Library

Library of Congress Cataloguing in Publication Data
A catalogue record for this book is available from the Library of Congress

ISBN 0 7506 3615 7

Typeset by BC Typesetting, Bristol BS31 1NZ
Printed and bound in Great Britain by Biddles Ltd,
Guildford and King's Lynn

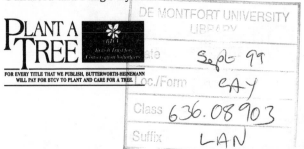

Contents

Preface

The need for a dictionary of terms used in veterinary nursing has been apparent for many years. The first book on animal nursing was published by the BSAVA as long ago as 1966 but until now student nurses have had to use the veterinary dictionaries of a traditional nature designed for agricultural students or the more specific veterinary dictionaries containing every word that the practising veterinarian or veterinary student might encounter in the course of his or her work. A revised syllabus for the RCVS Certificate in Veterinary Nursing and a change in the examination system requires individual study by the student nurses sitting the Level 2 and Level 3 examinations. The age of the graduate veterinary nurse arrived when a BSc Honours course in veterinary nursing commenced in 1998. This *Dictionary of Veterinary Nursing*, co-authored by two veterinary surgeons with long experience in the examination system for veterinary nursing, has been written with concise definitions of words relative to the nursing care of small animals. Various sources were used in the lists prepared by the authors and veterinary nurses have assisted in compiling the tables and helping with the line drawings. The assistance of Hannah Riches VN and Sarah Richards VN is acknowledged for their help and criticism during the preparation of the text.

The choice of words was at times difficult and was based on a search of the veterinary nursing literature but it does not go deeply into the specialist fields. Dictionaries may have their shortcomings and the authors would welcome notification of corrections or suggestions for additional words that may present problems. We hope that this contribution to the understanding of nursing terms will be a new source of information and, with the tables added, will collect together all the frequently required information used by veterinary nurses. The dictionary is also commended to veterinary practice managers, veterinary office and reception staff.

D.R. Lane
S. Guthrie

A

aardvark A rare burrowing animal also known as an earth pig. Favoured by veterinary practices that wish their name to head alphabetic directory lists.

abaxial Away from the centre plane or axis.

abdomen The area between the diaphragm and the pelvis that contains the abdominal viscera.

abdominocentesis A technique for the collection of fluid from the abdomen, by using sterile procedures fluid can be aspirated from the most prominent part of the abdomen, usually in the midline.

abducens nerve (VI) The sixth cranial nerve that supplies the lateral rectus eye muscle and the retractor muscle of the eyeball.

abduct To move away from the median plane or axis of the body; the word is used for abductor muscles, the process of limb abduction, etc., *see also* ADDUCTION.

Aberdeen suture A method used for stitching small domestic mammals where the suture knot is buried under the skin so that the animal cannot bite at it with its teeth.

abiotrophy Progressive reduction in nervous or ocular function.

ablate To remove totally, a term used in the surgical correction of diseases of the external ear canal.

abortion Termination of pregnancy; the loss of viable fetuses through infection, hormonal failure or mechanical damage, as with a traumatic injury involving fetal membranes, *see also* PREGNANCY.

abrasion An open wound, usually with extensive loss of epithelial tissue, often painful due to exposed nerve endings.

abscess A focus of pus surrounded by inflamed or damaged tissue.

absorbtion The process of transfer across a membrane – taking in nutrients or reclaiming substances in the kidney being examples.

academic Term used to describe university level instruction or knowledge; the opposite of practical or applied, *see also* VOCATIONAL.

acanthosis A skin disorder where there is an increased thickness of epithelial cells, sometimes pigmented with melanin. The increase of pigmented cell layers may be found in the axillae then it is known as acanthosis nigricans.

acapnia Decrease in the carbon dioxide content of the blood, *see also* HYPOCAPNIA.

acaracide Medical substance used to kill off surface parasites.

acariasis Infestation with surface parasites such as ticks or mites, does not include flea infestation.

accommodation Process to focus the image on the retina, the ciliary muscles can flatten or swell the lens at will.

acetabulum Part of the hip joint structure, the recess in the pelvic bone to receive the femur head. The depth of the socket of the hip joint affects the radiographic interpretation, *see also* VALGUS, HIP DYSPLASIA.

acetylcholine Chemical neurotransmitter synonymous with parasympathetic nerve activity; excess is destroyed by cholinesterase, *see also* ORGANOPHOSPHATE.

acetylcholinesterase Enzyme produced in nerve endings, muscle and erythrocytes that breaks down acetylcholine in nerve tissue to choline and water.

acetylpromazine A premedicant from the phenothiazine group.

acetylsalicylic acid Pharmaceutical compound used to reduce platelet aggregation; traditional remedy for fever and pain control, commonly known as aspirin.

achalasia Condition affecting the motility of the muscles of the oesophagus; failure of relaxation of the sphincter at the entrance to the stomach, *see also* MEGAOESOPHAGUS.

Achilles tendon The group of tendons that run down to the hock connecting the muscles (gastrocnemius, semitendinosus and biceps femoris) to the point of the hock (tuber calcis).

achlorhydria Absence of hydrochloric acid in the stomach.

achondroplasia Inherited disorder where the bones of the legs fail to grow to their normal size and have a curved or twisted appearance.

achromasia Lack of normal skin pigmentation.

achromotrichia Bleached appearance of the coat due to a lack of pigment, *see also* VITILIGO.

acid Chemical substances with pH lower than 7, releasing hydrogen ions when dissolved in water.

acidaemia Condition of the blood characterised by high pH. The acid–base balance is the relative amounts of carbonic acid and bicarbonate present, normally the blood will remain slightly alkaline.

acid citrate dextrose (ACD) Anticoagulant mixture used when collecting blood for subsequent transfusion.

acid fast Term used for those bacteria with capsules that once stained with carbol fuchsin resist decolourisation by acid alcohol, usually it is mycobacteria that are identified in this way, *see also* ZIEHL–NEELSEN.

acidosis Disease condition due to depletion of alkali reserve. May be metabolic e.g. after diarrhoea due to shock. Respiratory acidosis could occur when there is decreased respiration and less carbon dioxide is removed from the blood and the normal buffering system cannot function.

acid phosphatase An enzyme usually measured to assess prostate disease, but not a satisfactory marker for the disease of prostate cancer in canines.

acinus Small cavity surrounded by secretory gland cells; in the lung it is the name for the terminal air sac of the alveoli.

acne Describes a skin condition with many micropustules extending into the dermis, hormonal changes and secondary bacteria are involved, repeat treatments may be needed.

acquired A condition that develops after birth and not attributable to a hereditary cause.

acral Relates to the limb extremities, including the carpus regions, *see also* LICK GRANULOMA.

acromegaly Growth hormone abnormality that causes a relative increase in the size of the extremities.

acromelanism Deposition of pigment in the body extremities possibly due to the lowered temperature at these sites, responsible for the typical Siamese cat pigmentation.

acromion The hook-like prominence at the end of the spine of the scapula bone.

acrosome (of sperm) The hat or covering of the head of the sperm, necessary to supply the enzyme for penetration of the outer wall of the ovum to permit fertilisation.

actin A protein found in muscle that plays an important part in the process of contraction, *see also* MYOSIN.

action (gait) Term used to describe the locomotion of a four-legged animal; often some slight abnormality will be detected that does not amount to lameness.

actinomycosis Bacterial infection, characterised by multiple sinuses that open on the skin.

active immunity Immunity produced by the animal in response to stimulus of an antigen brought into the body.

active principle That part of a drug that is involved in producing the therapeutic effect.

acupuncture A traditional Chinese system of healing all sorts of disorders that depends on the ability to locate acupuncture points of the body and a compliant patient.

acute Adjective used to describe a disease of rapid onset, severe and recognisable symptoms, but often a quick recovery occurs following treatment.

acute renal failure (ARF), *see* NEPHROSIS, NEPHRITIS, ANURIA.

acyclovir An antiviral substance that inhibits the formation of DNA and has been used in animal herpes infections.

acyesis An absence of pregnancy; sometimes the word is used to indicate sterility in a female.

Addison's disease (hypoadrenocorticism) Hormonal diseases caused by an underactive adrenal cortex, with various symptoms and presentations. The acute failure of hormonal secretion is termed an addisonian crisis requiring urgent treatment for the collapse and vomiting. It may be iatrogenic in animals who have long-term steroid treatment suddenly stopped.

adduction Bringing closer to the midline; adductor muscles bring the legs closer together.

adenitis Inflammation of glandular secretory tissue.

adenocarcinoma Malignant tumour involving glandular tissue – may occur in the mammary glands or the intestines.

adenohypophysis The part of the pituitary gland that is glandular; also known as the anterior hypophysis, *see also* PITUITARY.

adenoma Benign tumour of epithelial or glandular tissue, anal adenoma being a commonly occurring example.

adenosine A nucleotide, part of the structure of DNA and RNA.

adenosine triphosphatase (ATP) Enzyme used to release energy inside the cells, *see also* MITOCHONDRIA.

adenosine triphosphate An enzyme involved in the release of energy by the mitochondria within the cell.

adenovirus One of a group of viruses involved in upper respiratory tract infections in animals and birds, *see also* HEPATITIS.

adhesion Abnormal structure connecting two sites, often the result of inflammatory reaction or trauma; may consist of a fibrous band or a diffuse area of attachment.

adipose tissue Fibrous tissue containing many fat cells; fatty deposits occur after excess nutritional uptake, *see also* LIPOMA.

adjuvant Substance that intensifies an immune response, usually such vaccines have enhanced antigenicity.

adnexa The adjoining parts of a larger organ – the fallopian tubes and the ovaries being such a relationship or appendage.

adrenal Situated close to the kidneys.

adrenal cortex The outer part, principally secreting glucocorticoids and mineralocorticoids.

adrenal gland Paired endocrine glands at the proximal pole of the kidneys, secreting adrenaline and steroid hormones.

adrenal medulla The grey core of the gland that produces adrenaline and noradrenaline.

adrenalectomy Surgical operation to remove the adrenal gland.

adrenaline Hormone secreted to prolong the actions of the sympathetic nervous system.

adrenergic Applies to the nerve fibres of the sympathetic nervous system that release noradrenaline when a signal is transmitted across the synapse. Also describes an agent that acts similar to adrenaline as a neurotransmitter.

adrenocorticotropic hormone (ACTH) The hormone produced by the anterior pituitary gland that stimulates the adrenal cortex to secrete cortisol and related steroid hormones.

adrenogenital syndrome Relates to the abnormal activity of the cortex of the adrenal gland; known as adrenal sex hormone dermatosis when skin changes are present. Sexual changes or some behaviour patterns are sometimes seen in neutered animals.

adrenolytic Reverses the activity of the adrenal gland.

adsorption Process of one substance becoming attached onto the surface of another substance.

adventitious Occurring in a place other than the usual one, or something acquired in life such as the orange skin stain from saliva, *see also* ATOPY.

Aelurostrongylus abstrusus Lung-worm in the cat associated with loss of condition and a chronic cough. Intermediate hosts are the slug and the snail. Diagnosis is by looking for larvae in faecal samples.

-aemia Word ending for relating to blood.

aerobe Bacteria that grow best in culture media with plenty of oxygen present.

aerophagy (-ia) The habit of air swallowing whilst eating, *see also* GASTRIC DILATION.

aerosol A suspension of particles used as a method of delivering a liquid substance as fine particles propelled by a gas through a fine nozzle.

aetiology The cause of something, or the study of the causes of disease.

afferent Leading in, towards, usually vessels or nerves that run to the centre.

afterbirth Common-use word to describe fetal placenta; includes the placenta, umbilical cord and the ruptured fetal membranes.

aftercare Nursing attention following an operation or the convalescent attention of a medical disease.

agalactia An absence of milk, may be due to hormone failure; a febrile disease with dehydration or emotional disturbance in the over-pampered bitch whelping for the first time, *see also* MASTITIS.

agar A colloidal protein substance derived from algae and used to pour into plates for bacterial cultures and for electrophoresis.

agent A mediator or something that helps to produce a chemical, physical or biological effect. **Anaesthetic agent** Any substance used medically to produce general or regional analgesia. **Therapeutic agent** Substance with a beneficial effect in the treatment of disease, usually with a specific action to produce a cure.

agglutination Grouping together or clumping of cells, widely used in antibody antigen measurements and blood-group typing.

agglutinin Any substance causing agglutination.

aggression A sign of threatening behaviour that may go as far as a physical attack on another animal.

agonal breathing The gasping type of respiration seen in a dying animal.

agonist Drugs that stimulate normal tissue activity, *see also* ANTAGONIST.

agouti Pattern where the hairs have alternate light and dark bands, usually with black tips, controlled genetically.

agranulocytosis A condition where there is a deficiency of neutrophils or granulocytes, *see also* PANLEUKOPENIA.

AIHA Auto-immune haemolytic anaemia.

air A mixture of oxygen and nitrogen; becomes important in anaesthesia when flows of anaesthetic gases mix in with air already in the respiratory tract.

airsacs The main areas for respiratory gas exchange in birds; physiologically equivalent to the lungs.

airway Term used to describe the route of gas exchange between the exterior and the lungs; improved by the insertion of an endotracheal tube in semi- and fully unconscious animals.

alar Wing-shaped or sometimes used to describe the cartilage of the nose.

albino Animal lacking normal dark pigmentation, usually a hereditary cause.

albumin Protein compound found in the blood, in egg white and sometimes in urine.

alcohol Organic compound with a hydroxyl element; the main use in veterinary nursing is for skin sterilisation and for the preparation of medical compound extracts as tinctures, *see also* ETHANOL.

aldosterone Hormone produced by the adrenal cortex responsible for the reabsorption of sodium by the kidney tubules. Its secretion is stimulated by angiotensin.

aleukaemia Term used for shortage or deficiency of leukocytes in the blood.

algae, blue–green Micro-organisms; plant-like substances that multiply on wet surfaces or at certain times of the year on surface water. The blue–green forms produce a toxin fatal to dogs.

alginate Protein used as a foam to help blood clotting or for wound healing.

alimentary System of the body concerned with digestion and the absorption of food; the alimentary canal runs from the mouth to the anus.

aliquot part One sample that represents the whole of the matter.

alkali Substance of high pH that has the property of neutralising an acid.

alkaline phosphatase (ALP) Enzyme produced mainly by skeletal muscle and bone that is destroyed by the liver and so it is frequently estimated as a measure of liver function in animals.

alkalosis State of the body produced by acid losses such as after vomiting. Hyperventilation, by washing out carbonic acid, can produce a similar effect with weakness and loss of consciousness.

allantochorion The outer of the two fetal membranes, relatively tough, that breaks to release fluid early on in the second stage of labour.

allele One of two or more alternate forms of the gene exerting a hereditary influence, only one of which can be present in the chromosome.

allergen A substance usually protein in nature that can produce allergy in a hypersensitised subject.

allergy Hypersensitivity reaction in the body between allergens and antibodies. **Atopic allergy** Hereditary form of allergic predisposition, most commonly seen as atopic dermatosis, *see also* ATOPY.

Allis tissue forceps Surgical instrument for holding exposed tissue by toothed edge gripping blades with a ratchet handle.

allograft Skin or similar tissue graft from a member of the same species, *see also* XENOGRAFT.

alopecia Deficiency or complete loss of hair.

alphaxalone Cat anaesthetic.

ALT The enzyme alanine aminotransferase, formerly known as SGPT.

alternative medicine Various systems for healing including homeopathy, herbal remedies, aromatherapy, etc. that are not part of the veterinary profession's orthodox treatment.

alula The first part of the bird's wing; acts as a free moving digit.

alveolar Relating to the alveolus, the alveolar volume being the volume of the respiratory tract in the terminal portion of the bronchial tree.

alveolus Cavity such as the tooth socket, or in birds the sac that is the innermost part of the bronchial tree. The mammary gland may also be described as having an alveolus for gathering the milk during lactation.

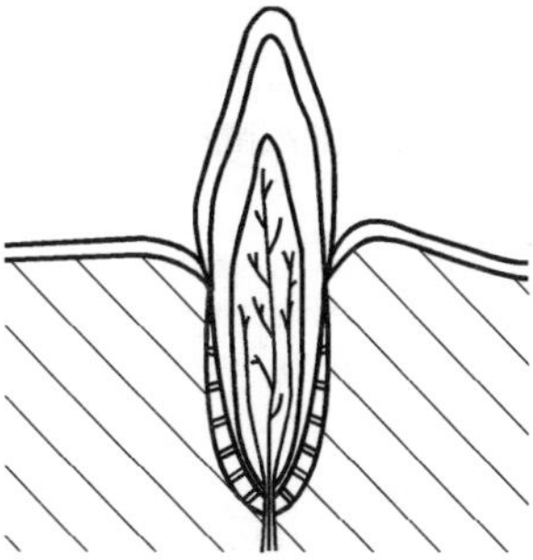

Alveolus. Cross-section of tooth to show peridontal ligament fibres, which hold the tooth in the socket

amastia Congenital absence of one or more of the mammary glands, not uncommon in the bitch where there may be an uneven distribution of teats on either side.

amaurosis Blindness, either partial or total, usually due to disease of the optic nerve or the brain.

ambylopia Poor sight not due to any visible lesion of the cornea, lens or fundus of the eye.

American Veterinary Medical Association (AVMA) which in many ways is close to the regulatory function of the RCVS in that it in the USA, it controls education including nurse technician training (AHTs). The BVA of the UK has more limited interest in veterinary nurse training and employment, other than through the BSAVA.

amine Organic nitrogen-containing substance, appears in many body compounds.

amino acid Nitrogen-containing substance produced during the breakdown of proteins, concerned with growth and repair.

aminoglycosides Group of antibiotics that includes neomycin used mainly for enteric and Gram-negative bacteria. Toxicity may restrict their use in animals to no more than 5 days' treatment.

amitraz Synthetic organic parasitic application considered safer than organophosphorus compounds.

ammonia Compound of nitrogen and hydrogen that has a specific toxic action on brain and other cells; normally it will be converted to urea by the liver. It is a colourless gas that by cooling can be turned into a liquid.

amnion Fetal membrane that forms the innermost container to protect the fetus; the amniotic fluid contained in the sac is dark and lubricant in consistency. Injury to, or puncturing, the amnion usually leads to premature birth.

amoeba Single-celled microscopic animal.

amorphous Not regularly formed in shape; of diffuse outline.

amoxycillin Antibiotic with broad spectrum activity, well absorbed from the intestine after oral administration.

amphiarthrosis A cartilagenous joint where both bone surfaces are connected but some degree of movement is possible, *see also* SYNARTHROSIS.

ampicillin Antibiotic administered by mouth or parenterally, active against urinary tract and respiratory infections.

ampoule Container, usually of glass, with a single sterile injection dose.

amputation Removal of a leg, part of a leg, dewclaw or tail. Occasionally part of some other organ is removed surgically.

amylase An enzyme that catalyses the breakdown of starch into simpler sugar compounds; traces are found in saliva but the main source of the enzyme is the pancreas.

amyloid A glycoprotein resembling starch that may be deposited in the walls of blood vessels.

anabolic Promotion of the metabolism to increase tissue growth or muscle mass by the synthesis of protein.

anaemia Defined as the decrease in the number of red blood cells below the normal range for the species of animal concerned, *see also* FELINE INFECTIOUS ANAEMIA.

anaerobe Bacterial organism that will only grow in culture with limited or no oxygen present.

anaesthesia A state of reduced perception of pain, shown as a loss of sensation or feeling in part or all of the body, *see also* ANALGESIA. **Local anaesthesia** Sensation loss induced in a part of the body where pain should not be present. **General anaesthesia** Unconsciousness of the brain induced by a chemical agent, usually implies muscle relaxation as well. **Regional anaesthesia** Loss of sensation produced by a nerve block or possibly infiltration of a whole field area; includes the injection of an anaesthetic around the spinal cord, *see also* EPIDURAL.

anaesthetic Used to describe a drug that produces anaesthesia or, when used as an adjective, such as the anaesthetic machine, it describes the use of the apparatus.

anagen Stage of the hair growth cycle equivalent to the active growth stage, *see also* TELOGEN.

anal Relates to the terminal part of the alimentary canal, *see also* PERIANAL.

anal abscess An infection within the anal sac causing a bulge in the perineum and often sudden acute pain.

anal furunculosis Infection with under-running tunnels and ulcers of the skin surrounding the anus, may be difficult to cure.

anal sacs Pair of small pockets situated venterolateral to the anus and opening by small orifice on the perineum just outside the anal sphincter.

anal sac disease Description for chronic infection associated with excessive secretion of foul smelling fluid; often seen as an inflammation of the perineum and sometimes with abscess formation.

analeptic Substance that reverses an anaesthetic state stimulating the brain and restoring consciousness.

analgesia Reduced perception of pain, without the loss of awareness.

anamnesis The taking of a history and the collection of relevant facts about a patient.

anaphase The third stage of cell division in both mitosis and meiosis.

anaphylactic shock Peracute response to an antigen in a sensitised animal characterised by collapse, difficulty in breathing and generalised permeability of the peripheral circulation, *see also* VASCULOGENIC SHOCK.

anasarca Excessive swelling of the abdomen, the legs and the prepuce due to subcutaneous oedema fluid.

anastomosis Joining together to form a functioning organ; used surgically after an intestinal obstruction. Physiologically the word is used to denote the linking of the arterial with the venous part of the circulation.

anatomic dead space The volume of air that fills the space on each inspiration without reaching the alveoli; represents the trachea, bronchii and bronchioles space.

anatomy The scientific study of the structure of the body, *see also* HISTOLOGY.

anconeal Bone process of the olecranon of the ulna in the elbow, *see also* OSTEOCHONDROSIS.

Ancylostoma Genus of parasitic worm, *A. caninum* is the commonest hookworm of dogs found in the UK; *A. duodenale* is a separate species affecting people.

androgens One of a group of steroid hormones, which includes testosterone, that stimulates the development of male sexual organs.

anechoic In ultrasound examination, a non-responsive area suggests a fluid-filled hollow organ or cyst.

aneurysm Disease of the blood vessel wall where there is a dilated area of the artery, a vein or sometimes the heart.

angiocardiography Method of studying the circulation of blood in the heart, *see also* ANGIOGRAM.

angiogenesis A situation where vascularity to an organ is created. Used in the omentalisation of prostate abscesses, *see also* PROSTATE.

angiogram Graphic depiction of the blood in circulation using a suitable dye given intravenously and a rapid series of X-rays.

Angiostongylus vasorum Lungworm of the dog, rare in the UK.

angiotensin Hormone regulating systemic and renal haemodynamics, often controlling the blood pressure. Angiotensin I and II are most common but others up to angiotensin 7 have been studied for the cause of hypertension.

angiotensin converting enzyme (ACE) inhibitor Method of treating raised blood pressure and heart failure. It works by preventing the conversion of inactive angiotensin I to the powerful vasoconstrictor angiotensin II. Administered by mouth usually as a once a day dose.

angiotribe Instrument used in the control of bleeding, similar to a strong pair of artery forceps.

angulation Refers to the carriage of the leg of the dog, especially the hind leg of breeds such as the German shepherd where over straightness or extreme flexion is a bad show point; the shoulder joint's angulation is also studied.

anhydrous Without water, used to refer to chemical substances heated to drive off the water.

anion Negatively charged particle, will move towards the positive electrode (anode) when an electric current flows.

anisocoria Unequal size of the pupils of the eye; often indicates a central (brain) injury.

anisocytosis Unequal cell size as seen in blood smears after some disturbance in the erythrocyte formation.

ankyloblepharon Disease of the eyelids where the edges stick together. Normal occurrence in the newborn kitten and puppy up to 10 days of age.

ankylosis Natural fusion together of a joint end, *see also* ARTHRODESIS.

annulus fibrosus Circular ligament surrounding the nucleus pulposus of the intervertebral disc.

anode The positive electrode to which negative ions transfer in the X-ray tube head (from the cathode) when the high-voltage current acts.

anodyne Medication reputed to dull pain, *see also* ANALGESIA.

anoestrus Cessation of reproductive activity, forms the quiet part of the oestrus cycle. The word may also be used to denote anovulatory sexual quiescence, *see also* INFERTILITY.

anogenital Refers to the perineal region; a developmental error is to have a cleft or common opening, similar to that of the bird, *see also* CLOACA.

anomaly Something that stands away from the normal, may include deformities or lethal genes.

anorchism Absence of visible testes, may be unilateral, *see also* CRYPTORCHID.

anorectal The area within the rectum and up to the external orifice, includes the para-anal sacs location.

anorexia Loss of appetite, may be used to include partial inappetence or any situation where an owner notices an animal not wolfing down its food. Pets should be weighed to ascertain how serious the problem is; rarely is it a psychological problem of the animal.

anoxaemia Reduced oxygen tension in the blood.

anoxia Absence of oxygen in the tissues; a serious condition may first be recognised by cyanosis and frequent deep respiration.

antagonist A counter-effecting agent such as the reversal of a sedative drug. The term is also used to describe a muscle that has an opposite action to an agonist muscle.

ante Before (from L.); opposite of post (e.g. mortem), *see also* DEATH.

anterior The part nearest the front of the animal, *see also* CRANIAL.

anthelminthic Medication used to kill or expel worms; may be described as broad spectrum in action or sometimes specific for cestodes only.

anthrax Bacterial infection; the cause of death in animals eating contaminated carcass meat. Zoonotic infection, but is responsive to penicillin if used early enough. Vaccination is possible using a spore vaccine.

anthropomorphism A commonly seen problem when owners equate the behaviour of animals with human reasoning and emotional responses.

anti- Indicates something against or counteracting, rather than beforehand.

anti-adrenergic Medication that opposes the effects of the sympathetic nervous system, includes beta blockers.

anti-arrhythmic Medication used in the treatment of heart disorders to stabilise the heart's rhythm. May also be used to describe substance that prevents cardiac arrhythmia.

antibacterial Substance that kills or stops the growth of bacteria.

antibiotic Substance that is produced by micro-organisms or synthesised as a derivative, to kill or inhibit the growth of bacteria or fungi.

antibody Natural substance, synthesised in the body in lymphoid tissue (B lymphocytes) in response to an antigen, that has a specific effect on antigens neutralising them or rendering them harmless. Antibody formation is much used in diagnosis and the assessment of allergies and immune status, *see also* ANTIGEN.

anticholinergic Medication that inhibits parasympathetic activity, especially acetylcholine, *see also* PARASYMPATHOLYTIC.

anticholinesterase Medication that inhibits the action of the enzyme acetylcholinesterase; allows the nerves to transmit abnormal impulses, as after nerve gas poisoning.

antidiuretic hormone (ADH) Hormone produced by the posterior pituitary gland, involved in the fluid regulation of the body, increasing water and salt resorption by the kidneys. It is produced by the pituitary gland and destroyed by the liver.

antidote Substance that reverses or neutralises a toxic substance in the body.

anti-emetic Medication to suppress or stop vomiting, may act centrally or on the stomach wall.

antifungal Destructive to fungal infections, may be a chemical agent or natural immunity by the body.

antigen Substance which, under suitable conditions, stimulates an immunological response and reacts with antibodies.

antihistamine Drug used to inhibit the effect of histamine released in the body. Used to control allergic reactions particularly skin pruritus but sometimes also used for their anti-emetic and sedation effects.

antihypertensive agents Drugs to lower blood pressure, they include angiotensin converting enzyme (ACE) inhibitors, calcium antagonists, $alpha_1$ antagonists, beta antagonists and diuretics.

antimicrobial Substance with effect against all micro-organisms including viruses, *see also* ANTIBIOTIC.

antiparasitic Substance that destroys either external or internal parasites, or both.

antiseptic Can be defined simply as a skin disinfectant. Includes any substance that inhibits the growth or spread of bacteria that is not harmful to animal tissues.

antitoxin Substance effective against specific toxins; was used to describe the serum injected to prevent tetanus after a contaminated wound was treated.

antitussive Cough suppressant; often acts centrally.

antiviral Agent effective against viruses.

antrum Describes a cavity such as the distal area of the stomach next to the pylorus. Pus in the antrum refers to an infection of the maxillary sinus of the head.

anuclear cells Those seen during vaginal cytology that indicate that the large keratinised cells are present and mating or insemination can take place with a high rate of success.

anuria Failure of the kidneys to produce urine.

anus Terminal orifice of the alimentary canal, *see also* ANAL SACS.

anvil Used to describe one of the three bones of the middle ear, *see also* INCUS, EAR, MIDDLE EAR.

anxiety Nervous state; symptoms in dogs and cats include destructive chewing, vocalisation and inappropriate defecation and urination.

anxiolytic Medication used in the treatment of animal conditions such as separation anxiety. 'Sedative' drugs such as diazepam and temazepam are used in human dentistry for patients experiencing fear and similar medication has been used for veterinary purposes in animals. Clomipramine may be effective as an alternative treatment in dogs.

aorta Major blood vessel arising from the heart's left ventricle running through the thorax and into the abdomen; arteries carry the blood on further through the body.

aortic valve Known as the semilunar valve, a valve in the proximal aorta preventing back flow of blood into the left ventricle.

APC Abbreviation for the human tablet medication of aspirin, phenacetin and caffeine that is less favoured for veterinary pain relief.

aperient Used to describe a mild laxative or one used for moderate purgation.

apex The very tip of a tooth root or the point of the heart. Apical is used also for the cranial lung lobe.

apical abscess Infection after a broken tooth may lead to a gum abscess with pain and swelling.

aphakic crescent The appearance of the eye that indicates that the lens has partially luxated; seen best with the ophthalmoscope: a 'half moon' or crescent of bright reflectivity shows where the lens has moved from and the retina reflects the light back.

aplasia Lack of development of cells or an organ, as in an aplastic anaemia being a non-regenerative condition, *see also* HYPOPLASIA.

apnoea Temporary cessation of breathing; the patient should be monitored closely.

apocrine One type of glandular tissue, found in the hair follicle as a sweat gland; equivalent to the sweat glands in the hairy parts of the human body associated with pheromones, *see also* SEBACEOUS GLAND.

aponeurosis Tendinous sheet formed where muscles join together, as in the tendinous portions of the abdominal transverse and oblique muscles that form the midline, *see also* LINEA ALBA.

apophysis Projection from a bone; also describes the pineal gland adjacent to the pituitary gland.

appendicular That part of the skeleton which is away from the spine and brain, includes all four legs.

appetite The ingestion of food is controlled by many factors including blood sugar level even in domestic animals.

apposition Placed close to, as in fracture repair, so that fragments can come into contact for better repair.

appraisal Method of monitoring an individual's progress, usually performed by the veterinary nurse's 'line manager' or next most senior person.

Approved veterinary nurse training centre (ATAC) A place for veterinary instruction of nursing students; it has to have approved facilities and may be subject to inspection by persons appointed by the Royal College of Veterinary Surgeons in the UK.

aqueous General term for a watery state.

aqueous flare Streaks or misting of the aqueous humour through an increased protein (antibody) level; may be seen after corneal ulcer repair.

aqueous humour Clear fluid that occupies the space between the cornea and the lens; loss of fluid through corneal injury can have serious consequences for vision.

aqueduct A canal containing fluid such as the aqueduct of Sylvius in the mid-brain connecting the ventricles.

arachnoid The middle of the three membranes encasing the brain and spinal cord, so named because it was thought to resemble the spiders web.

arbovirus One of a group of viruses that includes those that multiply in arthropods and then infect bitten animals.

arcus An arch shape; important in eye examination as an early stage of cataract lens degeneration.

area centralis Part of the fundus or the place on the retina first seen with the ophthalmoscope; may show the earliest signs of hyperreflectivity in a degenerative eye.

area postrema The part of the brain that is involved in vomiting reflexes, *see also* CHEMORECEPTOR TRIGGER ZONE.

areflexia Loss of reflex activity as found after major injury to the spinal cord or nerve section.

areola The different coloured part of the iris that surrounds the pupil of the eye. Also describes the brownish area surrounding the nipples of the mammary glands.

areolar connective tissue Loose spongy tissue found subcutaneously; also found between and surrounding the internal organs.

arginine Amino acid important as the cat cannot synthesise it for the hepatic urea cycle and this can lead to ammonia reaching the brain if the cat has anorexia.

aromatherapy Favoured medication in complementary medicine treatments, with essential oils being inhaled or applied direct to the skin.

arrectores pilorum Muscle used to straighten up the hair shaft, as invoked by the frightened cat or dog wishing to appear larger than normal.

arrhythmia Loss of the normal regular heart beat; the condition of sinus arrhythmia is considered a good feature on auscultation when the vagus nerve accelerates the beat on inspiration and slows or suppresses it, as on expiration.

arterial Relates to the high-pressure circulation system of the blood.

arteriole One of the smallest end vessels of the arterial circulatory system that connects to the capillary bed.

artery Elastic-walled blood vessel into which blood is propelled from the heart; contains oxygenated blood, the exception being the pulmonary artery.

artery forceps Instrument used to control small blood vessels that have been incised or damaged, especially during a surgical procedure. A versatile instrument adapted for many other uses in veterinary nursing.

arthritis Complex condition previously described as a joint inflammation. May be immune mediated, infective or the result of trauma, *see also* OSTEOARTHRITIS, DEGENERATIVE JOINT DISEASE.

arthrocentesis Aspiration of the joint by puncturing the capsule with a needle to remove fluid.

arthrodesis Surgical fusion of a joint, obliterating the joint space and removing all movement.

arthropathy Disease of a joint, often degenerative, *see also* DEGENERATIVE JOINT DISEASE.

arthroplasty Surgical remodelling of a joint as used for total hip replacement.

arthroscope Surgical equipment or endoscope to inspect the joint through a very small opening in the capsule.

articular Relating to the moving surfaces of a joint.

artificial insemination Method of introducing live sperm into the vagina, cervix or uterus of the animal to promote conception.

artificial respiration Form of life-support either by intubation and bag compression; or, less effectively, mouth-to-nose assisted breathing or thorax compression techniques.

arytenoid Word used to describe the cartilage of the larynx to which the muscles that alter the shape of the vocal cords attach.

ascarid Roundworm group that includes *Toxocara* and *Toxascaris.*

ascites Fluid accumulation in abdominal space greater in quantity and of different composition to normal peritoneal fluid.

ascorbic acid Commonly known as vitamin C; synthesised by all animals except the guinea-pig which must have a dietary source.

asepsis Usually applied to surgical procedures made without any infection present. There are rules for nurses on the maintenance of asepsis, *see also* STERILE.

ASIF Method of fracture fixation using compression plates and screws and equipment devised by the Association for the Study of Internal Fixation.

Aspartate aminotransferase (AST) An enzyme used in amino acid transamination, one of the liver enzymes; also used for muscle damage estimation as in cardiac infarction.

aspergillosis Fungal infection particularly in the nasal cavity as a chronic discharging state due to *Aspergillus fumigatus.*

asphyxia Starvation of oxygen through a restriction of inspired air reaching the lungs; suffocation.

aspiration Term used for the withdrawal of fluid to examine the contents, used for diagnosis or a temporary solution for a distended mass.

aspiration pneumonia Inflammation of the lung substance due to inhaled foreign matter, usually stomach contents, lodging in the bronchioles and alveoli.

aspirin Synthetic compound, the first of the antiprostaglandins, and used to lower cohesiveness of blood platelets. Toxicity may be a problem in cats unless very low doses are used.

assessment Used as a first-stage nursing procedure to inform the veterinary surgeon, categorize priority of treatment or plan the nursing care.

assimilation Body process for converting nutrients absorbed into the body into useful substances such as fats, protein, glucose, etc.

asteroid hyalosis Eye condition seen with the ophthalmoscope, as if there were many tiny stars shining in the vitreous; sometimes thought by the owner to be a cataract.

asthma A condition induced when narrowing of the airways produces respiratory distress accompanied by coughing and wheezing. Considered to be an allergic disorder it may also be induced by emotional stress and air pollutants such as diesel exhaust droplets. **Cardiac asthma** Term used for respiratory distress and exhaustion after minimal exercise due to advanced cardiac disease usually left ventricle dilation and failure.

astragulus One of the small bones that make up the hock joint (proximal row).

astrocyte Brain cell of ectodermal origin, in neoplasia astrocytomas may be benign or malignant.

asymmetry Unequal placing, often a congenital defect of the body but normal in the location of the kidneys. Externally, small changes of symmetry may be of great significance in identification and recognition of an individual.

asymptomatic A disorder that exists but exhibits no detectable signs.

asystole Serious heart condition when the heart beat is absent; the ECG has a 'flat line', *see also* CARDIAC ARREST.

ATAC *see* APPROVED VETERINARY NURSE TRAINING CENTRE.

ataractic Medication that produces a state of calmness and freedom of anxiety, similar to the state produced by a tranquiliser.

atavism Condition described in hereditary disorders when a very remote ancestor has exhibited a similar disorder.

ataxia Unsteady walking, shaky or unbalanced gait; may indicate a cerebellar disorder.

atelectasis Collapse or failure of part of the lung to expand.

atheroma Lipid degeneration of the walls of the arteries.

atlantoaxial joint Related to the joint between the first and second cervical vertebrae; area for subluxation with severe consequences, *see also* ODONTOID, TETRAPLEGIA.

atlas First cervical vertebra that articulates with the occipital condyles by the atlanto-occipital joint.

atonic Absence of, or diminished, muscle tone; used to describe bladder and colon dysfunction.

atopy Hereditary tendency to develop allergic signs especially skin disease, epiphora and secondary bacterial infection of abdomen and feet. Canine atopy involves IgE; such animal patients are described as atopic.

atraumatic needle Round-bodied surgical needle used for suturing soft tissue and external sites where there is the risk of the skin tearing if put under tension.

atresia The absence at birth, or the closing due to trauma, of one of the body orifices.

atresia ani Lack of a perforate anus. Seen in new-born animals that initially seem to thrive but then suck less and develop bulging of the perineum below the tail.

atresia of nasolacrimal ducts Absence of satisfactory tear drainage; leads to epiphora and face staining; sometimes only the lower of the two ducts is closed.

atrial Relates to the first chambers of the heart, *see also* FIBRILLATION.

atrioventricular Relates to both heart chambers either left or right side, or both, *see also* A–V NODE.

atrophy Condition of wasting of a normal size organ; may be due to disuse, faulty nutrition or hereditary atrophy, *see also* RETINAL ATROPHY.

atropine Natural product, now synthesised, that acts in a similar way to the sympathetic system response through its action in blocking acetylcholine. May cause long-term dilation of the pupils when applied to the cornea or reduces saliva production when injected as a premedicant.

attenuation Method of reducing virulence; the weakened organism can then be used as a vaccine.

atypical An unexpected response; pneumonia caused by *Mycoplasma* was a so-called atypical pneumonia.

auditory Relates to hearing or the ear anatomy and physiology; the ear connection with the pharynx is known as the auditory tube.

auditory brain stem response (ABR) A test to measure hearing ability, *see also* BRAINSTEM AUDITORY EVOKED RESPONSE.

aura Earliest stage of the epileptiform convulsive attack; detected in humans by some trained assistance dogs but most pet owners will not be able to discern it in their own animals if starting fits.

auricular cartilage The stiffening part of the external pinna including the funnel-shaped structure leading down to the middle ear.

auroscope Instrument for inspecting the external auditory canal.

aurotrichia Inherited disorder of miniature schnauzers where golden patches appear in the coat of the thorax and flanks.

auscultation The art of listening for noises in the thorax or abdomen, produced by gas or liquids, that leads to making a diagnosis.

autoantibody Substance produced by the body that reacts to some antigenic constituent of the body's own organs or tissues.

autoclave Vessel constructed to withstand high pressure that allows sufficient heat sterilisation to take place to destroy spores as well as bacteria.

auto-immune One of a group of disorders where the auto-antibodies destroy or damage perfectly normal functioning tissues; a mistaken protective response treating the tissue antigen as a foreign material.

autologous graft Usually a skin graft removed from one area of the body and attached to another area with a skin defect.

autonomic nervous system The often 'forgotten' part of the nervous system that controls all body functions and responses that are not under conscious control, *see also* SYMPATHETIC, PARASYMPATHETIC.

autopsy Alternative name for the post mortem examination made on a dead animal; compare this with a biopsy.

autosomal Term used in genetics for hereditary factors carried on chromosomes other than the X and Y sex chromosomes, such factors will not be sex-linked.

auto-transfusion (of blood) Technique to collect spilt blood during a procedure, filter it and transfuse it back into the animal's vein.

A–V Abbreviation for the heart valves between the atrium and the ventricle. **A–V bundle** is made of Purkinje fibres as a conductor of electrical impulses from the S–A node.

avascular Lack of blood supply; seen in the fundus at the final stage of retinal atrophy or in the normal anatomy of the cornea to assist clear vision.

avermectin Newer development of an injectable anthelminthic usually safe in very small mammals using appropriate dose rates, *see also* ANTHELMINTHIC.

avirulent Denotes a lack of ability in an infectious agent to produce disease and thus has been used to stimulate immunity as a vaccine.

A–V node Atrio-ventricular node, part of the heart's mechanism for setting off each contraction or beat, *see also* S–A NODE.

avulsion Tearing away; trauma from road-traffic accidents being the most frequent cause of such injuries.

axilla That part of the body between the thorax and the forelimb, commonly described as the armpit.

axis (1) The second cervical vertebra notable because of its weak odontoid peg structure. (2) The centre line of the body or organ, often used in anatomical descriptions.

axon A long structure of the nerve tissue that helps conduct the electrical impulse to the nerve endings. May be sheathed in myelin produced by the Schwann cells to allow quicker transit of the nerve impulse.

axonopathy, progressive Disease mainly of the boxer breed, characterised by ataxia and weakness of the hind legs.

azathioprine Cytotoxic medication used as a cortisone-sparing agent; acts as an antimetabolite and synthetic purine analogue which blocks incorporation of natural purines into DNA affecting the cell's normal metabolism.

azotaemia Presence of excess nitrogen-containing compounds in the blood (a more correct description than URAEMIA).

azygos Unequal; the word is used for the vein that drains the cranial abdomen skin across the thorax to join the right vena cava or empty directly into the right atrium.

B

B lymphocyte Lymphocytes that develop from stem cells in haemopoietic tissue – fetal liver and spleen, and the bone marrow. B lymphocytes are involved in the production of antibodies and secrete immunoglobulin (Ig) molecules. They are independent of the thymus gland lymphocytes, *see also* T LYMPHOCYTES.

Babesia Parasite that lives for part of its life cycle in the erythrocytes. There are separate species for the dog and the cat, as well as cattle. Usually spread by tick bites, the disease babesiosis in dogs is characterised by fever, haemolysis and jaundice.

bacillary typhlitis *see* TYZZER'S DISEASE.

Bacillus Gram-positive rod-like bacteria known for their spores that can persist for years. *B. anthracis*, the cause of anthrax in all species, may cause death in fox hounds and other animals that feed on infected carcass flesh.

bacillus, pl. bacilli Organism of the genus *Bacillus*; or it can be used to describe any rod-shaped bacterium.

bacitracin Antibiotic used mainly for skin infections, reputedly named after Mary Tracy, the patient who had a wound contaminated with the soil organism *B. subtilis*. The bacteria produced an antibiotic substance subsequently developed for clinical use.

backbone The name given to the spinal column; composed of individual vertebrae, it extends from the base of the skull to the tail tip.

back-cross Term used in breeding that implies the mating of an offspring to one or another of its parents. It is a test for breeding a heterzygote to a homozygote, so that the subsequent litter can be studied.

background radiation Additional radiation hazard experienced by all the population, caused by natural isotopes, radiation from outer space and previous earth-based nuclear accidents.

Backhaus towel clamp Clip used for fixing drapes to the patient during an operation. It should be applied with care as the needle-like blades can easily puncture the fingers of the person applying the clamp to the patient.

backscatter Radiation risk to attendants during radiographic procedures, as radiation can be deflected more than 90° from the main X-ray beam; the risk is increased with metallic objects or dense bone deflecting the ionising radiation.

bacteraemia The invasion of the blood stream by living bacteria: a sign of infection.

bacteriocidal Able to kill bacteria.

bacteriostatic Preventing the growth or increase in numbers of bacteria.

bacterium, pl. bacteria A group of micro-organisms that lack a distinct nucleus; most bacteria have a rigid cell wall or capsule. The capsule is associated with virulence and protects the organism against phagocytes; some antibiotics work by dissolving this capsular wall, e.g. penicillin and cephalosporins.

Bain system Anaesthetic circuit based on fresh gases passing up a central tube to the patient and exhaled gases passing down an outer sleeve. Allows for a degree of rebreathing and low respiratory resistance, *see also* COAXIAL.

balanced anaesthesia The use of several drugs to produce a satisfactory level of anaesthesia that allows the surgeon to operate and causes minimal damage to the patient.

balanitis Inflammation of the penis, the glans may become red and sore from repeated licking.

balanoposthitis Inflammation of the penis and the prepuce, often associated with a green or yellow discharge from a dog's prepuce.

baldness *see* ALOPECIA.

ball and socket joint *see* ENARTHROSIS.

ballottement Diagnostic test using the finger tips to palpate for an object floating in fluid; may be used with caution during examination late in pregnancy.

bandage A roll of material used for wrapping round the body either to support or to compress as in the case of haemorrhage and limb oedema. Bandages are also used to keep dressings applied closely to the skin surface, *see also* COTTON CONFORM, FIGURE-OF-EIGHT, PLASTER OF PARIS, ROBERT JONES.

barbiturates Group of drugs that induce sleep; may be used in anaesthesia and commonly used in overdose strength as a method of euthanasia. Thiopentone sodium is the most frequent barbiturate used for routine induction of anaesthesia.

Bard–Parker Surgical instrument name; known as a term for a scalpel handle but there are also forceps with this name as a description.

barium Radio-opaque material used in contrast radiography. A chemical element but is usually used as the sulphate; can be mixed with food or poured into the mouth as a suspension.

Barlow's disease Known as hypertrophic osteodystrophy, *see also* OSTEODYSTROPHY.

Barlow's sign A test for congenital hip luxation first used in new-born children. Heard as a click on flexing and abducting the joint; has been used to indicate hip dysplasia in puppies, *see also* HIP DYSPLASIA, ORTOLANI'S SIGN.

barrier cream A water-impervious cream used to protect the skin.

barrier nursing A term used in infectious-disease nursing to describe isolation of the patient, using separate utensils, ensuring scrupulous attention to hands and clothing disinfection, etc.

basal energy requirement (BER) The amount of energy used by an animal when it is resting completely in a cage kept at body heat.

basal metabolic rate (BMR) The amount of energy required for the maintenance of respiration, heart beat, peristalsis, body muscle tone, glandular secretions etc., *see also* BASAL ENERGY REQUIREMENT.

basal narcosis Term that was used in anaesthesia to indicate that a narcotic had been given before inducing general anaesthesia.

basophil Granular leukocyte with granules in the cytoplasm that stain with basic dyes; basophils are capable of ingesting foreign proteins and also produce heparin and histamine.

beak Structure formed of keratin that, together with the beak bone, makes the structure on the bird's head used for feeding and for attack. Beak trimming is necessary if there is any malformation, lack of wear or parasite infestation.

becquerel SI unit used to measure the radioactivity of a source, it has replaced the curie.

bed sore (decubitus ulcer, pressure sore) Found on the elbows of larger breeds of dog; any excessive or prolonged pressure on the skin when the dog lies on a hard surface is the commonest cause. Other sites of the body such as the hocks or the ischium may also be affected.

behaviour The way in which an animal performs; patterns of behaviour are the subject of much psychological study and the modification of behaviour has become a specialised science.

benign Indicates that it is not harmful, the opposite of malignant. The term, when applied to tumours, indicates that a full recovery is likely.

benzalkonium chloride Quarternary ammonium compound (Quat), used as a surface disinfectant with detergent properties.

benzathine penicillin *see* PENICILLIN.

benzimidazoles Group of anthelminthics more used in large animals than in small-animal practice.

benzodiazepines A group of sedative compounds used for sedation and behaviour modification.

benzoyl peroxide Preparation used on the skin for its keratolytic properties and for its antibacterial effect on *Staphylococcus*. May cause adverse reactions in some dogs so should be used with care.

beta-blocker Drug that blocks the action of adrenaline at the organ level with a beta-adrenergic receptor. This effect is used on the heart to increase the contractility and the rate, cause vasodilation of the arterioles and improve the airway by relaxing the bronchial muscles.

betamethasone A synthetic glucocorticoid with great potency if used on the skin surface; orally the duration of effect may not be to the animal's benefit.

bicarbonate A salt containing hydrogen, carbon and oxygen that can be easily broken down by the body to provide an alkali reserve. Bicarbonate is one of the extracellular buffers that can take up excess hydrogen ions and, with the help of the enzyme carbonic anhydrase, will produce waste products of water and carbon dioxide both of which can be excreted easily by the body.

biceps muscles The two-headed muscle; the dog and the cat have such a muscle in the foreleg as well as the back leg. Biceps brachii is a shoulder extensor and elbow flexor muscle on the cranial surface of the humerus. Biceps femoris is an extensor muscle lying caudo-lateral to the femur.

bicuspid The heart valve with only two cusps is found on the left side of the heart between the atrium and the ventricle; also known as the mitral valve, *see also* MITRAL.

b.i.d. Dispensing instruction for a medicine to be given twice a day. [L. bis in die, used by early physicians as a code.]

bile Clear orange fluid produced in the liver that is stored in the gall bladder. Strongly alkaline, it has an important role in the emulsification of fats as an aid to their digestion, *see also* BILIOUS VOMITING SYNDROME.

bile duct The tube that connects the gall bladder to the opening in the duodenum. Many small ducts unite to form the main bile duct; the cystic duct leads from the gall bladder to form the common bile duct.

bilious vomiting syndrome Condition in some dogs that vomit first thing in the morning; believed to be the result of an empty stomach collecting acid and perhaps bile reflux. Usually treated by dietary change, feeding carbohydrate in the late evening.

bilirubin One of the bile pigments produced by the breakdown of haem from the blood; it normally circulates in the plasma and is processed by the liver. Bilirubin which is yellow gives colour to the faeces.

biliverdin A green-coloured bile pigment, converted to bilirubin in the liver.

bioavailability The portion of a drug that is available at the site (tissue) where its action is required. Drugs given by mouth may have a low proportion of their content absorbed into the circulation.

biodegradable An important feature whereby a chemical product can be broken down by natural means such as enzymes or bacteria.

biological value (BV) A measure of the availability of proteins; it is the percentage of absorbed nutrient that is utilised and not lost immediately by excretion.

biopsy Taking living tissue from the body, usually for microscopic examination for the purpose of diagnosis or assessing cancer risks after tumour removal.

biotechnology The science of biology used for manufacturing and commercial purposes.

biotin One of the vitamin B group. Rich sources of the vitamin are egg yolk, yeast and liver and it is unlikely that deficiency would occur on normal feeding.

bistoury knife A surgical instrument of historic use, consisting of a long narrow blade used for lancing abscesses and opening up sinuses.

bladder The storage organ of the urinary tract; lined by transitional epithelium it has a smooth muscle wall that allows for great distension. The outer layer is the peritoneum, *see also* CYSTOCENTESIS.

bland Description used for a mild, non-irritant substance such as a 'bland ointment' e.g. K-Y jelly used when clipping up the eyelids to prevent hairs falling on the cornea.

blast cells Immature cells; usually applied to those of the bone marrow and those that would not normally appear in the peripheral circulation, *see also* MYELOBLAST.

bleeding *see* HAEMORRHAGE.

bleeding time A measure of the ability of the blood to clot; an incision is made in the gum or skin and the time taken for the blood to stop flowing is measured in minutes; often used as a quick test for thrombocytopenia and for haemophilia.

blepharitis Inflammation of the eyelids; the upper or lower eyelids may be affected at the edges; often seen as yellow dry crusts.

blepharospasm Spasm of the obicularis muscle of the eyelid, often the result of a foreign body or corneal injury.

blindness An inability to see but this may not be easily detected if a dog or cat has lost its vision slowly, *see also* NIGHT BLINDNESS.

bloat Condition of a distended abdomen either the result of gorging food or from an accumulation of gas in the stomach, *see also* GASTRIC DILATATION, TYMPANY.

block *see* HEART BLOCK.

blood Fluid tissue that circulates throughout the body in the arteries, capillaries and veins. Consists of a liquid component called plasma and a cellular component that gives the red colour.

blood–brain barrier The division between the body circulation and the brain substance; it is only slightly permeable to electrolytes and other ionic solutions. Many therapeutic substances with large molecules cannot readily reach the brain for this reason.

blood clot A solid mass formed from the elements of the blood either within the blood vessel or elsewhere, *see also* THROMBOSIS.

blood group The antigenic structure of the surface of the erythrocytes means that a first transfusion of blood can be given without risk but subsequent transfusions may result in haemolysis and even death. Cross-matching blood and recent information about the blood groups of dogs and cats reduces this hazard.

blood 'poisoning' The presence of bacteria or their toxins in the circulating blood is usually associated with severe illness.

blood pressure (BP) The pressure of the blood inside the walls of the main arteries. The highest BP is recorded during systole (systolic blood pressure) and corresponds to ventricular contraction. The lower diastole BP occurs as the heart relaxes and fills.

blood urea nitrogen (BUN) The urea content of serum or plasma, as measured by the nitrogen content.

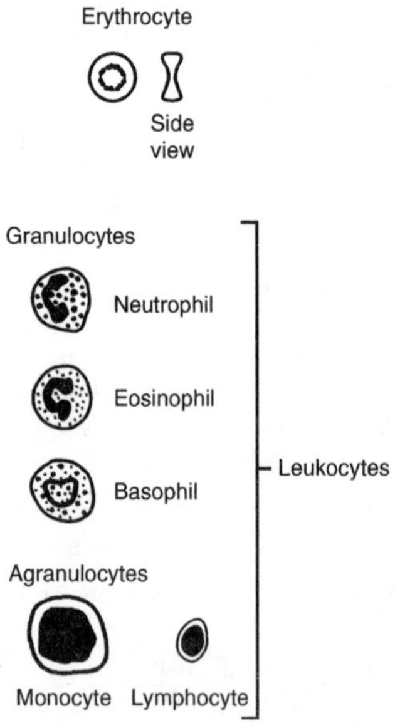

Blood cells. Erythrocytes and leukocytes

blue eye A popular description of a corneal opacity due to oedema of the interstitial cells. Particularly associated with the Afghan hound breed when live CAV 1 virus was first used for vaccination against hepatitis but blue eye may occur in the dog recovering from a hepatitis virus infection.

blue–green algae Cause of poisoning in dogs that have bathed or drunk from stagnant pools. Poisoning is most likely in warm weather after the sudden growth of the algae and the dog may show signs within 20 minutes of swallowing some of the water.

blunt dissection A method used by surgeons to separate fascial planes with minimal haemorrhage. Unless used with skill it could cause tissue damage and shock.

body bag Description of any container used for dead dogs or cats. Popular term derived from crime series, *see also* WASTE.

body cavity Refers to those areas within the body lined with serous membrane. The peritoneal cavity, the thoracic cavity and the pericardial cavity are all potential spaces but only contain a minute quantity of fluid between the viscera in the healthy animal.

bolus injection Method of giving intravenous medication in a concentrated mass. Used also in contrast radiography when giving an opaque substance.

bonding In psychology, developing a close but selective relationship. Important in puppy and kitten socialisation, *see also* IMPRINTING.

bone Hard rigid tissue that forms the internal skeleton of mammals, *see also* ENDOCHONDRAL OSSIFICATION.

bone marrow Vascular tissue mixed with fat, the soft contents of the long bones that has the important function of producing platelets, red and white cells for the blood.

booster vaccine Method of increasing immunity by administering vaccine after the initial vaccination course has been completed. Essential for vaccines using a killed antigen such as Leptospira and in general use for most dog and cat vaccines on a once-a-year basis although some animals have longer lasting immunity.

borborygmus Noises from the abdomen associated with gas or fluids passing into a larger hollow area of the intestinal tract, *see also* BOWEL NOISES.

Bordetella Bacteria associated with respiratory-tract infections of the dog and cat. *B. bronchiseptica* is considered to be one of the causes of kennel cough and infectious bronchitis.

botulism Poisoning, usually fatal, from ingestion of animal matter contaminated with *Clostridium botulinum*. An acute toxaemia.

Bovine spongiform encephalopathy (BSE) Affected many cattle in the late 1980s and early 1990s but it is now uncertain whether it caused a similar condition of spongiform encephalopathy in cats. Dogs were never known to be infected although many have consumed specified raw offal.

Bowie–Dick indicator tape Tape used to seal up plastic instrument packs; it has heat sensitive markings that change to dark brown at 121°C; it does not show if the inside of a pack has reached the required temperature for the required time to sterilise.

bowel clamps Surgical instruments with a fine long blade, used to isolate a length of intestine before incision. Various surgeons have given their to names to these – Doyens, Gillman, etc.

bowel noises Due to increased peristalsis and liquids squirting from the small intestine into the gas containing large intestine, *see also* BORBORYGMUS.

Bowman's capsule The envelope, two cell layers thick, that encloses the tuft of capillaries in the nephron that constitutes the glomerulus.

Box turtle An imported species from America, requires less water in its living space and is essentially carnivorous.

Boyle's law Quoted in anaesthesia, essentially it means that as the pressure of a gas is reduced the volume of the gas increases; assuming that the temperature does not alter.

brachial plexus The nerve centre for the foreleg, originates from the sensory branches of the last four cervical and first two thoracic nerves; it is located medial to the shoulder joint and can be damaged after some chest injuries.

brachycephalic Description of the short-faced, wide-head condition seen in normal boxer, King Charles spaniel and pug dogs etc. The condition of the skull bones may cause obstruction of the nasal passages and other airway obstructions; the lower lip folds may become moist and chronically infected.

brachycephalic airway obstruction syndrome (BAOS) A condition of short-nosed dog breeds where the airway is restricted by narrow nares and nasal cavity, a long soft palate, overlarge tongue base or a narrowed trachea.

bradycardia Slow heart rate often associated with hypokalaemia.

braided suture Multifilament plaited material used in suturing and said to hold a firmer knot. May be absorbable or non-absorbable. The wick-like effect can be a problem limiting its use as a skin suture.

brain The encephalon comprises all the nervous system within the cranium. It contains fluid ventricles and is divided into the fore-, mid- and hind brains.

brain death Sign of cessation of neurone function, loss of pupil response, slower breathing and other reflexes.

brainstem The base of the brain responsible for connecting the higher centres to the spinal cord; includes the pons, medulla oblongata and the thalamus.

brainstem auditory evoked response (BAER) Test used to assess hearing in dogs and people; assessing hearing acuity (in the sedated pet) by measuring electrical activity in the brain.

branchial The position in the neck where in the embryo the fish gills might have arisen; a cyst may develop at this site in dogs; filled with saliva it is thought to represent the branchial arches of the embryo.

breech birth Term used to describe posterior presentation of the puppy or kitten when the legs remain flexed and forward rather than the 'normal' hind toes first followed by tail then the rump.

breed standard A specification laid down by a Kennel Club committee to which a pedigree dog must conform.

breeding The animal's pedigree or the physical act of mating, *see also* CROSS BREEDING.

breeding season Those times in the year when an animal can be mated, *see also* SEASON.

brisket Part of the body at the base of the neck composed of fat and connective tissue that extends between the front legs.

broad ligament The suspensory ligament of the uterus, *see also* MESOMETRIUM.

broad-spectrum antibiotic One that has a wide range of activity against many bacteria.

broken down Breeder's terminology for the bleeding that indicates the onset of pro-oestrus. A greyhound with tendon injuries may also be referred to as 'broken down'.

bronchial Adjective relating to some conditions of the bronchi.

bronchiectasis Medical condition, the result of chronic dilation of the bronchial tubes frequently associated with a secondary infection.

bronchiole A smaller airway tube than a bronchus; each tube subdivides until the terminal bronchiole so that air reaches the alveoli by the alveolar ducts.

bronchitis Inflammation of one or both bronchi. May be caused by inhaled particulate irritants, dust, spores, pollen or smoke, but it is equally caused by virus or bacterial infections. The signs of repeated coughing and increased bronchial sounds on chest auscultation are characteristic.

bronchodilator Substance that increases the width of the airway in the lungs by increasing the lumen or preventing a spasm of the constricting smooth muscle.

bronchoscope Endoscope designed to examine the lining of the lower respiratory tract; it can also be used to obtain samples by aspiration or by washing, and to remove inhaled foreign bodies.

bronchospasm Disorder due to contraction of the muscles of the smaller bronchioles, possibly due to an inhaled irritant substance. Bronchospasm may occur in the anaesthetised animal, *see also* ASTHMA.

bronchus, pl. bronchi One of the larger airways entering the lung from the trachea; some smaller bronchi supply the lung lobes.

brown fat Fat deposited in connective tissue that is more easily mobilised; it is important in young and in hibernating animals as a rapid release form of energy store.

brown hypertrophy of the cere Overgrowth of the base of the budgerigar's upper beak; hyperplasia of the keratin may be caused by parasites and will lead to breathing difficulties and weight loss.

Browne's tubes Sealed glass tubes used during autoclaving to confirm that sterilisation in the centre of the pack is adequate; a colour change from orange–brown to dark green occurs with heat; tubes for temperatures of 121°C up to 134°C can be selected. Tubes for hot-air-oven monitoring can also be used.

Brucella canis Gram-negative bacteria often considered to be one of the causes of abortion in kennels of dogs.

bruising The effect of trauma with discolouration and haemorrhage; where there is a blood clotting disorder bruises may develop from very trivial injuries. Colour changes in bruises are the result of the breakdown of the haemoglobin.

bruit A sound similar to a murmur, usually less noticeable and the result of blood being forced past a small constricted area of the vascular system.

buccal Adjective used to describe the mouth cavity towards the cheek.

buccinator muscle One of the cheek muscles.

bucket muzzle Form of restraint in the dog used to prevent biting but one that is loose enough not to restrict breathing; the original patterns were made of steel with air holes punched in the base of the 'bucket' nearest the nares.

Bucky grid A moving grid used in radiography to control secondary scatter but avoiding the parallel lines on a plate where a stationary grid has been used. [Sometimes called POTTER-BUCKY.]

buffers Reagents used to combat acidity or alkalinity.

buffy coat Used in haematology as a rough measure of platelets and white cells; seen in a centrifuged blood sample as a layer above the red cells.

bulbar conjunctiva The portion of the outer layer of the eyeball that covers the white sclera.

bulbo-urethral gland Glands responsible for part of the ejaculate of the male. The glands lie between the prostate and the perineum.

bulbus glandis The swelling at the base of a dog's penis caused by vasodilation; its function is to retain the penis in the vagina as part of the 'tie'.

bulla Blister, usually can be seen to contain serous fluid.

bullous (adj.) Used to describe skin with many large blisters or in the lung condition of emphysema where there are air-filled cavities present, *see also* PEMPHIGUS.

bundle of His Specialised fibres that conduct the electrical impulse across the heart; also called the atrioventricular bundle.

bunny hopping A term used to describe a dog's movement when both hind legs are advanced together, often used to indicate abnormal gait with hip dysplasia or some spinal disorder.

buprenorphine An analgesic lasting 6 or 8 hours. Recognised by the trade name Temgesic.

bur (burr) A surgical instrument used to enlarge a cavity or to debride a bone.

burn A severe injury to tissue caused by dry heat, chemicals, radiation or electricity. Injuries are characterised by necrosis and pealing of skin, etc. Fluid losses may be anticipated, treatment for shock should be given and attempts made to prevent infection of the burn.

bursa, pl. bursae A small fluid-filled sac occurring in tissue, often the result of repeated injury or friction.

butorphanol A synthetic morphine-like substance used both as an analgesic and to suppress coughing.

butyrophenones A group of drugs used for pre-anaesthetic medication, not licensed for animal use at present.

C

cachexia Condition of weight loss, general bodily decline and weakness. Muscle loss is most noticeable on the skull's temporal muscles and can be a sign of progressive diseases such as neoplasia.

cadaver The body of a dead animal.

caecotrophy Process of extending the period for cellulose breakdown adopted by rabbits, where the soft faeces are removed from the rectum and ingested to pass through the alimentary tract a second time to produce hard dry pellets of faeces.

caecum The proximal part of the large intestine. Relatively narrow in the dog and cat but enormous in the rabbit for fermentation in the digestion processes.

Caesarean Birth of the fetus by an incision through the abdominal wall then the opening into the uterus.

calcaneus One of the bones of the tarsus; a square structure in the proximal row of the bones that forms the point of the hock.

calcification The process of depositing calcium salts in the tissue, *see also* HYPERPARATHYROIDISM.

calcinosis cutis Calcium deposited in the epidermis, characteristic of hyperadrenocorticism. The skin is usually thin and hairless and nodules can be felt with the finger tips.

calcitonin Hormone secreted by the parafollicular cells of the thyroid gland. It reduces blood calcium levels and limits the uptake from bone.

calcium Chemical element required in the food as it is an important constituent of bones, teeth and blood; nutritional diseases are more common in the young growing animal. Calcium is important physiologically for muscle contraction so calcium-channel blockers are used in treatment of heart arrhythmia.

calcium oxalate Crystalline salt found in the urine, associated with acid urines where there is an excessive excretion of oxalates. This may be a metabolic defect in some breeds, *see also* UROLITHIASIS.

calculus, pl. calculi Any unusual deposit of mineral salts as found in the bladder (urinary calculi), but may also occur in the kidney (renal calculi), the prostate or the teeth (dental calculus or tartar).

Calicivirus A virus of the cat commonly associated with 'cat flu' signs.

calling Popular term for the breeding season of the cat; oestrus is associated with a raucous cry in some cats.

callus (1) Tissue laid down during the repair of fractures, eventually becomes organised into harder dense bone. (2) Callus also refers to the hard leathery skin on the elbows of larger breeds of dogs, the result of pressure sores or of friction.

calorie Measure of food value defined as a unit of heat necessary to raise the temperature of 1 g of water through 1°C (strictly from 14.5 to 15.5°C). Now replaced in food value measurement by the joule. [1 calorie = 4.1855 joules.]

Calvé–Perthes disease Disease of the hip, *see also* LEGG–CALVÉ PERTHES DISEASE.

Campylobacter Gram-negative motile micro-organism which grows best in microaerophilic to anaerobic conditions. *C. jejuni* is a cause of infectious diarrhoea in dogs which has zoonotic implications.

canal Passageway; used anatomically: alimentary, auditory, nasolacrimal, semicircular, etc.

canaliculi A narrow passageway used as in bone canaliculi for the histological structure of bone or as in bile canaliculi from liver to bile ducts.

cancellous Description of open bone tissue of the medullary cavity as opposed to compact cortical bone. Cancellous bone has an open trabecular structure with large sinusoids containing bone marrow.

cancer Abnormal growth of tissue: implies neoplasia and usually means a malignant tumour.

Candida **(thrush)** Yeast-like fungal infection, not common in dogs and cats but the infection in humans is sometimes called *Monilia.*

canine tooth The corner tooth of the mouth with the longest point, used in carnivores for skin penetration and gripping prey. The four deciduous canines are replaced by permanent canines in the growing animal.

canker Term applied to ear disease in dogs; implies overgrowth of tissues; may be seen in advanced chronic otitis.

cannabis A Schedule 1 drug (S1) recognised as an addictive drug in the *Misuse of Drugs Act* 1971. Has some medicinal properties and may be the cause of small animal poisonings, either accidental or after deliberate experimental use on pets.

cannula A tube for insertion into a body opening – a lacrimal cannula for the tear ducts or an intravenous cannula that will then occupy the lumen of the vein.

canthotomy Incision of the canthus for greater exposure of eye structures during surgery.

canthus The angle at the corner of the eyelids, known as nasal (medial) and temporal (the lateral) canthi.

capacitation Part of the reproductive process where the sperm in the ovarian tubes finally mature to allow fertilisation of the ova to take place.

Capillaria Parasitic nematodes mainly found in birds. Species of *Capillaria* also affect small rodents and fish.

capillary refill time (CRT) Test used for quick assessment of shock or circulatory failure; pressure applied to the gum causes blanching and the time until the gum is pink again is measured in seconds.

capsule (1) The membrane like sheath that encloses some anatomical structure, a joint capsule being an example; also is used to describe the covering of some neoplasms. (2) Used in pharmacy for a small gelatine container for some unpleasant tasting medication. (3) The outer protective layer of bacteria that may be attacked by antibiotics.

capsulotomy (lens) Technique used in cataract surgery of the eye so that an intracapsular lens extraction can be performed by first incising the outermost layer which then remains to keep the vitreous in place.

captopril Medication used in cardiac disease, one of the ACE inhibitors.

caput The head of; used anatomically as in caput epididymis.

car sickness Motion sickness more common in dogs than cats; if medication may be required in cats it is best to use chlorpromazine.

carapace The dorsal shell of tortoises and turtles.

carbaryl An insecticide with less toxicity than other similar synthetic preparations.

carbohydrate Chemical compounds containing carbon, hydrogen and oxygen of great nutritional importance; they can be stored in the body as glycogen or, if excessive amounts are fed, fat will be laid down.

carbolic acid A phenol, formally used as a kennel disinfectant but due to its toxicity is now limited to laboratory use to disinfect glassware. Classified as a corrosive poison.

carbon dioxide Gas, the result of the oxidisation of carbon compounds, that is found in exhaled breath in higher concentration than in air, *see also* RESPIRATION.

carbon monoxide Gas with poisonous properties causing damage to the central nervous system and asphyxiation. Birds are particularly sensitive to such toxic fumes as produced by smouldering matter or gas fires where there is insufficient room ventilation.

carbonic anhydrase An enzyme, found in red blood cells and of importance in removing carbon dioxide from the tissues. Inhibitors of carbonic anhydrase are used in the treatment of glaucoma to reduce aqueous formation; the action on the eye is entirely separate from any diuretic effect.

carboxyhaemoglobin The product of carbon monoxide poisoning where the blood appears cherry red; usually fatal as tissues become starved of oxygen, *see also* CARBON MONOXIDE.

carcass (carcase) disposal Legal requirement in the UK is that bodies must be treated as clinical waste materials and handled as semi-hazardous substances. A dispensation allows the body to be treated as the legal property of the owner, so allowing burial of pets of all sizes in the owner's garden.

carcinogen Substance that causes neoplasia or cancer. Hazardous substances may be labelled carcinogenic and adequate precautions must be taken in their handling.

carcinoma A malignant neoplasm.

cardia The part near the opening of the stomach from the oesophagus, distal to the cardiac sphincter.

cardiac Relating to the heart.

cardiac arrest The cessation of the heart's action as a pump, a 3 minute emergency requiring well planned action, *see also* RESUSCITATION.

cardiac massage A method of resuscitation during cardiac arrest.

cardiac tamponade An effusion of blood or other fluid in the pericardial space surrounding the heart causing excessive pressure on the heart muscle. The heart shadow on X-ray is enlarged and the heart sounds are muffled.

cardinal signs Traditionally the most important clinical signs: pulse, temperature, respiration rate.

cardiomyopathy Degeneration of the heart muscle so that the heart fails progressively as a pumping organ, usually accompanied by dilation of the heart.

cardiopulmonary arrest (CPA) Cessation of both the heart beat and the respiration.

cardiopulmonary resuscitation (CPR) Nurses action is to follow the ABC routine of clearing the airway, ventilation of the lungs preferably with oxygen then chest compression and massage of the heart area, *see also* RESUSCITATION.

cardiovascular Adjective used to describe conditions of both the heart and the blood vessels.

caries Disease of the teeth with erosion of the enamel and pitting of the dentine.

carina (1) The pointed keel of the bird's breast. (2) A part of the bronchus dorsal to the heart; can often be identified on X-rays of the chest.

carminative Medical substances used to relieve flatulence and colic.

carnassial tooth Upper fourth premolar tooth (three rooted) and the lower jaw first molar tooth, used together as a shearing cutter. In the cat the upper third premolar and the lower molar are developed for the same purpose.

carotid Relates to anything near the carotid artery, the main blood vessel to the brain in the neck.

carotid body Chemoreceptor area at the bifurcation of the common carotid arteries that can influence the medullary respiratory centre.

carotid sinus A dilated area at the base of the internal carotid artery containing blood pressure receptors.

carotid sinus reflex A reflex induced by stimulating the upper neck area that will slow the heart.

carpal Adjective for the area of the foreleg known as the carpus; it is equivalent to the wrist.

carrier Implies an animal that has a low-grade infection but one that is still capable of infecting other animals. It may also be used for a heterozygous animal carrying recessive genes.

cartilage Dense connective tissue, found chiefly at joints and between bones.

cast In veterinary work, it is a method of external support using a mouldable material, e.g. plaster cast used in fracture repair, *see also* PLASTER OF PARIS.

castration Surgical (or chemical) removal of the testes, used to prevent breeding and undesirable social behaviour. The word can be used to describe the neutering of both sexes but in the UK it is restricted to the male animal. Sometimes it is considered that the operation involves entering a body cavity, although the scrotum is external in dogs and cats.

cat 'flu Upper respiratory tract infection caused by a variety of bacteria and viruses.

catabolism Process of breakdown of cells, a negative metabolic state.

catalyst Substance that promotes or alters the rate of a chemical reaction. The catalysts of biochemical processes are known as enzymes.

cataract An opacity of the lens. Described as congenital or acquired, also as central, cortical, post-polar, etc.

catarrh Discharge of mucoid material from a surface, often the result of inflammation.

catecholamine Substance released at nerve endings that helps to combat stress.

catgut Absorbable ligature or suture material produced from sheep intestine prepared in a sterile manner.

catheter A flexible tube introduced into the body for administering fluids or withdrawal of unwanted fluid or laboratory specimens. Intravenous catheters and urethral catheters are the two commonest veterinary types used.

cathode The negative electrode of the X-ray tube head from which electrons are emitted.

cauda equina syndrome A condition of the lumbo-sacral articulation characterised by incoordination of the hind limbs; it may be painful and there is often incontinence as the nerve control is damaged.

caudal Relates to the tail of the animal, so is most commonly used when describing the posterior or 'backwards' direction in anatomy.

cautery A method of controlling haemorrhage or removing excess tissue. Often an electric current, a hot instrument or a chemical agent such as silver nitrate is used.

Cavia (cavies) One group of the rodent family, commonly seen as guinea-pig pets for children. Noted for its inability to manufacture vitamin C and for a pregnancy time that is as long as a dog's.

canine Relating to the dog.

canine distemper (CD) A virus infection, *see also* DISTEMPER.

canine hip dysplasia (CHD) *see* HIP DYSPLASIA.

cell The basic structure of the living organism.

cell-mediated immunity Protection against infection involving cytotoxic T lymphocytes.

cellulitis Infection in the loose tissue below the skin, often seen in cats when bites have introduced bacteria into the subcutaneous space.

central nervous system (CNS) The portion of the nervous system that includes the brain and the spinal cord.

central progressive retinal atrophy (CPRA) Eye disease characterised by dark pigment accumulating in the retina. Genetic in origin, the disease was first identified in the briard but CPRA affects many large breeds and it is now thought that a dietary cause contributes to the appearance of the disorder, *see also* DYSPLASIA, RETINA.

central venous pressure (CVP) Pressure measured in the jugular vein; can be used to study the flow of blood back to the heart and is important in monitoring shock.

centrifuge A laboratory device to rotate liquids such as blood or urine at high speed, to separate out the more solid constituents from the liquid ones.

centriole Two cylindrical structures found in cell cytoplasm near the nucleus and the Golgi apparatus.

centrosome The part of the cytoplasm containing the centrioles.

centromere Temporary attachment of the chromatids during cell division.

centrum The body of the vertebra.

cephalic Relating to the head end of the body – the cephalic vein is located on the cranio-medial aspect of the forelimb.

cephalosporin A group of broad-spectrum antibiotics that are active mainly against Gram-positive bacteria.

cerclage Encircling a bone with a loop of wire, as in fracture stabilisation.

cere The firm bulge at the base of the bird's beak. Useful in sex discrimination of budgerigars as the female's has a light brown to pink colour and the male's is blue.

cerebellum Part of the hind brain, the cerebellum is responsible for involuntary control of balance, posture and coordination of movement.

cerebrocortical Relating to the cerebrum (fore brain).

cerebrospinal Relating to the brain and the spinal cord.

cerebrospinal fluid (CSF) A protective fluid layer that surrounds the spinal cord and brain, and circulates nutrients within the brain ventricles.

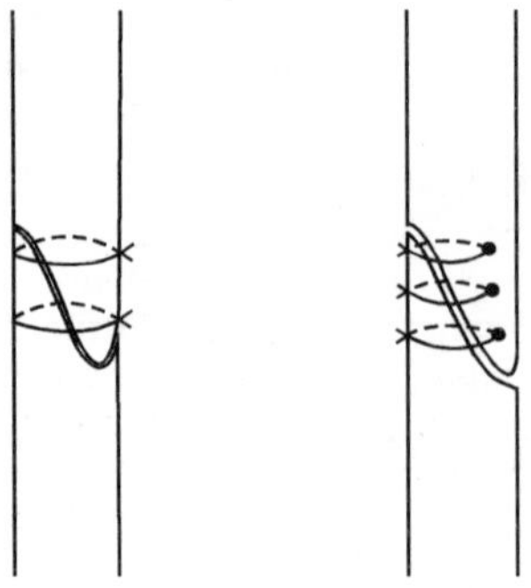

(a) (b)

Cerclage wiring. (a) Cerclage wiring; (b) hemicerclage wiring

cerebrum The largest part of the brain, often called the 'cerebral hemispheres'.

cerumen Waxy secretion of the glands of the outer ear.

cerumenolytic A substance used in ear cleaning to dissolve wax.

cervical Relating to the animal's neck or the neck of the uterus.

cervix Narrow portion of the uterus where it joins the vagina.

cestode Parasitic worm that is flat and has no alimentary tract – tapeworms.

cetaceans Group of sea mammals that includes harbour porpoise and bottlenose dolphins, both are found off the UK coast.

chalasia Relaxation of a body opening such as the cardiac sphincter, *see also* MEGAOESOPHAGUS.

chalazion (meibomium cyst) Swollen sebaceous gland in the eyelid.

chameleon Small reptile kept as a pet; has the ability to alter its body colour.

charting (records) The keeping of clinical records; in veterinary nursing helps the veterinary surgeon to know of the patient's progress.

Cheatle's forceps *see* FORCEPS.

cheilitis Inflammation of the lips.

cheilorrhaphy Surgical repair of the congenital defect of a hare lip.

Chelonia Members of the reptile family of chelonians.

chemoreceptor A cell or group of cells that responds to a specific chemical compound, e.g. the taste buds and receptors in the mucous membrane of the nose.

chemoreceptor trigger zone (CRTZ) Found on the floor of the fourth ventricle, it connects to the vomiting centre and relates to the vestibular apparatus. The zone is susceptible to a variety of stimuli including blood-borne substances such as toxins, usually results in reflex vomiting.

chemosis Oedema of the conjunctiva often causing the eyelid to bulge outwards.

chemotherapy The treatment of illness by chemical means particularly relevant to cancer therapy.

cherry eye Prolapse of the nictitans gland of the third eyelid, *see also* NICTITANS GLAND.

Cheyletiella Group of surface-feeding mites, noted for excess skin scaling in dogs (walking dandruff), also found on cats and rabbits and a cause of pruritic vesicles in humans.

Cheyne–Stokes respiration Type of automatic breathing seen in respiratory failure where the patient deeply inhales air followed by a period of shallow or invisible chest movement. The breathing pattern is repeated periodically at short intervals. It occurs particularly in states of coma and just before death.

Chick Martin test A traditional test for the efficiency of antiseptics and disinfectants.

chigger Name for larva mites of the genus *Trombicula,* also known a harvest mites.

chipmunk Squirrel-like creature sometimes kept as an attractive domestic pet.

chitonaside Product from sea shells that has a moisturising effect when incorporated in skin dressings and makes the active principle effective for longer.

Chlamydia A genus of bacteria that are extremely small and can live within the cell. *C. psittacci* is an important cause of animal and bird disease, *see also* CHLAMYDIOSIS, PSITTACOSIS.

chlamydiosis Disease caused by specific organism: in birds known as PSITTACOSIS or ORNITHOSIS. Also causes chronic conjunctivitis in cats, and in sheep is a cause of abortion. The human eye disease trachoma has *C. trachomatis* as its causal agent and there is also a sexually transmitted human infection of importance but it is not related to the feline disease, *see also* PSITTACOSIS.

chloramphenicol Antibiotic effective against a wide range of organisms, now most widely used as a topical application such as eye ointment.

chlorhexidine An antiseptic used in solution as an effective skin disinfectant before surgery.

chlorine An extremely pungent and toxic gas but used in the form of liquid 'bleach' can be a very effective kennel disinfectant.

chlorpromazine One of the phenothiazine antipsychotic drugs; has been used as a mild 'tranquiliser' in dogs and cats as an alternative to acepromazine. It is an effective anti-emetic for cats especially when travelling.

chlortetracycline Antibiotic effective against many bacteria but used mainly for oral medication or in the form of eye ointment.

choanae A funnel-shaped structure; used to describe the area at the back of the pharynx where the paired openings lead from the nasopharynx.

chocolate agar Heated blood agar used in bacteriology to culture fastidious pathogens such as *Neisseria.* The heat treatment breaks down haemoglobin and gives the agar the brown colour.

chocolate poisoning Accidental poisoning of pets from overeating. Sickness and diarrhoea are usual with elevated liver enzyme levels but rarely there are more severe affects on the heart, *see also* THEOBROMINE.

cholangitis Inflammation of the bile duct.

cholemesis Vomiting of bile.

cholesterol Steroid found in animal fat, present in the blood and frequently measured during biochemical screening tests. Elevated blood levels (hypercholesterolaemia) are associated with thyroid disease but diet influences the sample collected.

choline Basic compound involved in the transport of fat in the body; phospholipids and acetylcholine are two products for which it is needed. At one time was listed as part of the vitamin B group but no longer as it can be synthesised by all animals from serine. It may be given as an oral supplement in the treatment of liver disease.

cholinergic Describes those autonomic nerves that release acetylcholine as the neurotransmitter. Also used to describe drugs that mimic the actions of acetylcholine, *see also* PARASYMPATHOMIMETIC.

cholinesterase An enzyme that splits acetylcholine into acetic acid and choline. With any organophosphorous poisoning the enzyme is inhibited and the effect may be shown on muscle fibre contraction with tremors; often sickness and diarrhoea follows initial salivation.

chondrocyte A mature cartilage cell.

chondrodystrophy A disorder of cartilage formation.

chondroma Benign tumour of cartilage.

chordae tendineae The 'strings' in the ventricles that stop the A–V heart valves everting.

chorea Rapid involuntary muscle movements often most noticeable in the muscles; usually considered to be a sequel to canine distemper infection, *see also* FITS.

chorioallantois The fetal membranes that lie outermost, and therefore may be described as the first 'water bag' as it is the amnion that lies closest to the fetus.

chorionic gonadotrophin Hormone produced by the placenta during pregnancy and may be collected from urine. After refinement it may be injected as a source of luteinising hormone.

choroid The middle coat in the eyeball, richly supplied with blood vessels, contains the sensory receptor cells and associated pigment cells.

choroid hypoplasia A congenital disease of collie breeds where defects in the development may cause loss of vision, *see also* COLLIE EYE ANOMALY.

Christmas disease (haemophilia B) Hereditary disease of specific dog breeds and short-haired cats with a blood-clotting defect. Carrier females exist that can be identified by blood testing.

chromatid Found in the nucleus of the cell during division; each chromosome forms two identical chromatids.

chromic catgut Natural product used in suturing; prepared from sheep intestine and hardened by immersing in chromic acid to delay its breakdown (and loss of strength) when in the animal's body.

chromosome One of the thread-like strands in the nucleus that carry genetic information. Composed of two coils of DNA.

Chronic degenerative radiculomyelopathy (CDRM) Progressive wasting disease of the hind limbs, usually affecting the German shepherd breed; of unknown cause, *see also* RADICULOMYELOPATHY.

chronic disease One that has been present for some time and does not immediately progress to cause the death of an animal.

chronic pulmonary osteoarthopathy Seen as hard swellings above the toes of all four legs. A disease state of boney enlargement due to reduced oxygen supply after certain chronic lung diseases. Known also as hypertrophic pulmonary osteopathy.

CHV1 Canine herpes virus 1, *see also* HERPES VIRUS.

chyle Milky fluid, the product of digestion in the intestines which is carried in the lacteals to the thoracic duct.

chylothorax The presence of chyle in the pleural space, often the result of traumatic damage to the thoracic duct or neoplasia of the mediastinum.

chyme The semi-liquid product of digestion in the stomach, a mixture of food, saliva and gastric secretions that passes through the pylorus into the duodenum; normally will have a low pH.

cicatrix Contracted area as seen when a wound heals leaving a scar.

cilia Fine hair-like processes that cells can use to waft away mucous material. Cilia are also used to describe the eye lashes, *see also* ECTOPIC CILIA.

ciliary body An important part of the eye that supports the lens and contains muscles that by squeezing the contents help the lens to focus. The ciliary body connects the choroid with the iris, and produces the aqueous humour for the anterior chamber of the eye.

cimetidine An H_2 receptor antagonist, used in tablet form to reduce the acidity of the stomach. Allows certain drugs to reach the small intestine that would be damaged by a low pH.

ciprofloxacin Antibacterial agent, effective mainly against Gram-negative aerobes. Used in gastro-intestinal and urinogenital infections; the ability to penetrate intracellularly makes it suitable for treating *Chlamydia* and *Pseudomonas*.

circle system An anaesthetic system in which oxygen as the carrier and anaesthetic gases are delivered to the patient and carbon dioxide is removed.

circulation Refers to the passage of blood around the body.

circulatory shock Develops from circulatory insufficiency as the result of a fall in cardiac output; dilated capillaries with pervious walls lead to inadequate perfusion of the peripheral tissues.

circum-anal glands Sebaceous glands situated just outside the anus in a ring, *see also* ANAL ADENOMA.

cirrhosis A liver disease characterised by loss of normal hepatic cells and fibrosis causing scarring of the liver lobes.

clavicle The collar bone; only of importance in the domestic cat. The dog has a tendon band but no bone.

clean-contaminated (wound) Description of a surgical wound that was sterile but has become contaminated. One example is the accidental leakage of the intestinal contents during an enterotomy.

clearing time During the development of an X-ray plate, the milky appearance of the plate after it is put in the fixer should become 'clear' after 30 seconds but the plate should be left longer to fix.

cleft palate A fusion failure seen in the new-born animal. New-born kittens and puppies should always have their mouths examined for congenital defects; the defect in the palate may allow milk to reflux down the nose while feeding, *see also* HARE LIP.

clindamycin Synthetic antibiotic used for treating contaminated wounds and for oral infections.

clinical audit Assessment of the progress of a case.

Clinical Waste Regulations Legislation to regulate the disposal of undesirable materials. The *Control of Pollution Act*, *Collection and Disposal of Clinical Waste Regulations* and the *Environmental Protection Act* should all be consulted.

cloaca The external orifice of birds and reptiles; fulfils a dual function of excretion and of reproduction.

clone Replica produced by artificial division of the DNA as a form of asexual reproduction; all clones contain the same genetic material.

Clostridium Group of bacteria characterised by their ability to survive for long periods away from the animal by forming resistant spores. They can cause serious illnesses such as tetanus, botulism poisoning and bacterial endotoxaemia.

closed angle glaucoma The type of raised intra-ocular pressure due to a shallow anterior chamber of the eye and a narrowed junction between the cornea and the iris causing an obstruction to the normal fluid outflow.

closed wounds Those where the skin surface is unbroken, *see also* CONTUSION, HAEMATOMA, RUPTURED SPLEEN.

clot A solid mass of blood (or lymph).

cloxacillin Broad-spectrum antibiotic, one of the semi-synthetic penicillins.

Cnemidocoptes Parasite of birds. One type *C. pilae* causes scaly beak in budgerigars.

coagulase Enzyme produced by staphylococci; an antigenic substance often found in more pathogenic strains and related to thrombus formation in infected tissues.

coagulation Process of stopping bleeding by the clotting of blood.

coagulation disorders A general term for any condition of prolonged bleeding due to an impaired clotting mechanism, includes von Willebrand disease, DIC and haemophilia.

coagulopathy A disorder of blood coagulation, *see also* DISSEMINATED INTRAVASCULAR COAGULATION, HAEMOPHILIA.

coaption The bringing together of tissue surfaces to aid healing.

coaxial Used to describe one tube running inside another; utilised in anaesthetic circuits with low resistance to expiration, *see also* LACK, BAIN SYSTEM.

cobalamin The vitamin B_{12} compound notable for containing the metal cobalt. Its measurement is used to assess absorption from the small intestine, *see also* MALABSORPTION.

Coccidia Single-cell organisms characterised as Sporozoa; they can live parasitically inside gut epithelial cells. Other species affect the liver cells. As a cause of diarrhoea signs are seen in rabbits and in poultry, and sometimes also in puppies and kittens. Infection is through ingesting faeces as resistant oocysts can remain viable in the soil for months.

coccidiosis Disease due to multiplication within the body of minute protozoal parasites. *Eimeria* are a common cause of diarrhoea in the domestic rabbit. Treatment is by medicating the drinking water and improving hygiene. *Isospora* (or *Levineia*): two species that infect dogs and another two species affect cats, uncommon except in puppies, kittens and immunosuppressed adults.

coccygeal Referring to the tail area.

cochlear Relating to the spiral tube in the inner ear known as the cochlea.

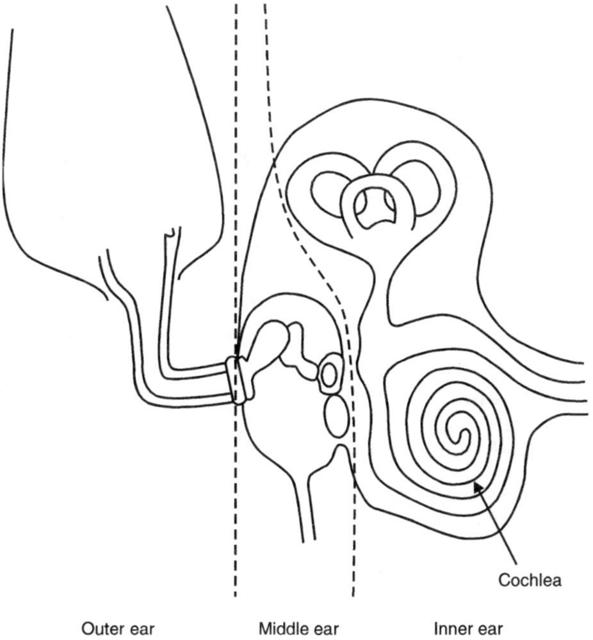

The cochlea

coeliotomy Incision into the abdomen, *see also* LAPAROTOMY.

cognition Mental facility to recognise and reason; an animal's first reaction is to investigate; subsequent processing of the information depends on the individual.

coitus Sexual union through the penis being inserted into the vagina to promote the release of semen for the intra-abdominal fertilisation of eggs by the sperm, *see also* REPRODUCTION.

colectomy Excision of the colon is rare but subtotal colectomy is sometimes a preferred treatment in chronic constipation of the cat when the ileo-caecal junction is preserved.

colic Pain in the abdomen due to stretching of the viscera from gas or from calculi, foreign bodies, etc., *see also* PAIN.

colitis Inflammation of the colon, a medical condition often associated with excessive mucoid faeces, sometimes alternating with periods of normal faecal output. Severe cases show tenesmus and blood, *see also* COLONIC INFLAMMATORY DISEASE.

collagen Protein substance that supplies strength to fibres in the body.

collateral A side branch to an anatomical structure.

collateral ligament *see* LIGAMENTS.

collie eye anomaly (CEA) A group of signs in the dog's eye that may result in blindness from a retinal haemorrhage. A hereditary disease most frequently found in the Shetland collie, *see also* RETINAL DYSPLASIA.

colloid solution A solution in which small particles are permanently suspended. Colloidal particles will not pass through a semipermeable membrane, *see also* SEMIPERMEABLE MEMBRANE.

coloboma Defect of structure, often a pit; when applied to the eye it means a developmental defect in the sclera wall so that the choroid bulges through it. Eyelids lacking shape may be described as having a palpebral coloboma.

colon Part of the large intestine stretching from the caecum to the rectum. Plays an important role in the absorption of water and salt. Particularly well developed in herbivores such as the rabbit.

colonic inflammatory disease Disease of the colon may be of a chronic inflammatory nature and there are many possible causes; neoplasia and motility disturbances are separate diseases.

colorimeter Laboratory instrument for measuring fine colour differences.

colostrum The first fluid available to the new-born animal. Rich in proteins it carries maternal antibodies and is replaced by the milk from the lactating animal's mammary glands.

coma State of deep unconsciousness from which the patient refuses to be aroused.

comedo, pl. comedones Blocked sebaceous glands often contaminated by skin bacteria, *see also* ACNE, HYPOTHYROIDISM.

comminuted fracture Injury where the bone is broken into many small pieces as after impact with high-speed vehicles or crushing injuries.

communicable disease A disease that may pass from one animal to another, either by direct contact, by an object such as a brush or by a vector such as an insect bite. All communicable diseases are transmissible unlike metabolic diseases.

compensatory hyperdynamic shock In shock there is an immediate rise in the heart rate, with both arterial and venous constriction, that helps to increase the circulating blood volume and raises the blood pressure. Unfortunately this response may not last and treatment for shock with fluid therapy and other measures is needed and would be more suitable.

complete blood cell count (CBC) An abbreviation frequently used when haematology is requested for a blood sample.

compress Pressure pad applied to a bleeding wound or after a sprain or strain a cold application would be used.

compulsive behaviour Described as a ritualistic behaviour pattern such as tail chasing, flank sucking (particularly in the Dobermann), wool sucking (Siamese cats) and fly biting.

computed scan (CAT) Axial tomography, a method of studying deep structures by looking at 'slices' of the body with scanning X-rays.

conception The start of pregnancy, following fertilisation of the ovum.

concussion Trauma to the central nervous system causing a limited period of unconsciousness. Usually a head injury following a road traffic accident is the cause.

condyle A rounded prominence on a bone, forming part of an articular surface.

cones, retinal Receptor cells in the retina more associated with colour vision but this does not necessarily apply to animals.

congenital Condition present at birth; it may be hereditary or develop after some injury during pregnancy.

congestive heart failure A serious condition where the pumping action of the heart is no longer adequate to maintain the circulation; signs are dilated veins and enlarged heart chambers, *see also* MYOCARDIUM.

conjunctiva The surface lining the eyelids and covering the sclera up to its junction with the cornea.

consensual light reflex The constriction or dilation of the pupil of the eye opposite to the eye that is being stimulated (by light changes).

constipation Faeces retained in the rectum and large intestine; hard lumps may be difficult to pass and straining may alert an owner to the problem. May be diet related or due to a painful prostate or pelvic injury.

consultant A fully trained specialist who accepts responsibility for the diagnosis and advises on the treatment, *see also* SPECIALIST.

contagious disease Originally only a disease spread by direct animal-to-animal contact, today the term is often used for any communicable disease.

continuing education The ongoing process that involves attending courses, reading books and journals, etc. to stop the qualified person 'stagnating', *see also* CONTINUAL PROFESSIONAL DEVELOPMENT.

contrast media In radiography, any substance that highlights a hollow organ. Positive contrast is provided by barium- and iodine-type compounds, negative contrast is provided by air.

Control of Substances Hazardous to Health (COSHH) A set of regulations in the UK for safe and healthy working conditions.

controlled drug Specified category of POM drugs, consists of five groups or schedules, but only four have veterinary application. Stringent regulations relate to their purchase, storage and recording of their use. In the UK, the *Misuse of Drugs Act 1971* and the *Misuse of Drugs Regulations 1985* must be strictly adhered to.

contusion Injury to tissue by a blunt object – similar to a bruise; the skin usually remains unbroken.

coprophagia Undesirable habit of eating faeces, often acquired kennel behaviour due to attractive food residues. The rabbit has a similar process to digest cellulose in the food but then the soft faecal pellets are taken directly from the rectum into the mouth, *see also* CAECOTROPHY.

copulation The act of sexual union; the word usually is only applied to animals, *see also* COITUS.

corium Part of the skin equivalent to the dermis.

cornea Surface of the eye that is transparent to light as it totally lacks blood vessels and it is composed of layers of parallel tissue: epithelium, stroma and Descemet's membrane.

corneal lens A protective plastic cap placed over the cornea at the front of the eye; previously reused human contact lenses were put into use in dogs with corneal erosion.

corneal sutures Must be very fine and with low irritancy; Ethilon 4/10 to 10/0 may be favoured.

coronavirus Single-strand RNA viruses, associated with feline infectious peritonitis and with diarrhoea in dogs.

coronoid process There are two such bony prominences of importance in animals: one is found on the mandible that lies near the temporomandibular joint. The other site is the medial coronoid process of the ulna where the heads of the radius and ulna articulate with the humerus, *see also* OSTEOCHONDROSIS.

corpus luteum Literally 'yellow body', a structure found in the ovary after ovulation, responsible for hormone production (progesterone).

corpus spongiosum Part of the penis characterised by its vascular beds that allow the penis to stiffen prior to mating. Forms the bulb proximally and the glans distally.

cortex Refers to the outer part; variously applied to the forebrain, the filtering part of the kidney and the hardest part of the bone.

cortical bone Compact bone covered by periosteum.

cortical cataract Lens opacity that is first seen at the edge of the lens but then spreads across the capsule causing loss of vision.

corticosteroid Steroid hormone produced by the adrenal cortex or synthesised in the laboratory.

coryza Profuse discharge from the mucous membrane of the nose applies especially to birds.

cotton conform bandage Type of open mesh flexible bandage that makes applying dressings to limbs of the dog easier than using white open wove (WOW) bandages.

cough Expulsive effort originating in the thorax, usually a reflex action to expel mucus or foreign matter but it may be caused by unusual pressure on airways, e.g. cardiac cough from a dilated atrium.

coupage A physiotherapy manoeuvre used to assist the removal of fluids from the thorax; a chopping action of percussion over the ribs; from the French word *couper*, to cut.

coxa plana Flattening of the head of the femur is one of the radiographic signs of damage to the epiphysis.

coxa vara Deformity of the hip joint with a change in the angle of articulation.

coxitis Inflammation of the hip joint.

continual professional development (CPD) A system of further training often associated with credits for hours attended that may lead to the issue of certificates of competency in specialised areas.

cramp A general term applied to painful muscle spasms.

cranial Closest to the head or the cranium.

craniocaudal Means in simple terms from the front to the rear. Used as the direction of entry of the X-ray beam as when examining the elbow joint.

craniomandibular osteopathy A specific disease of the West Highland white terrier breed as an autosomal recessive but also seen in Scotties, other terriers and rarely in large breeds such as the Pyrenean and boxers. Known also as 'lion jaw' it is a non-neoplastic proliferation of bone that may affect the joint, causing difficulty in opening the mouth due to a symmetrical enlargement of the bones of the mandible; other skull bones may also be affected.

cranium The dome of the skull, and the other bones that surround the brain.

creatine A non-protein substance synthesised by the body from amino acids.

creatinine A product of creatine metabolism and constantly formed in muscle; it can be measured in the blood as a reliable indicator of renal function; normally there is a constant excretion of creatinine in the urine.

cremaster Muscle found in the spermatic cord, responsible in the male rabbit for retracting the testes into the abdomen outside the breeding season. Most other domestic animals have very restricted voluntary control of this muscle.

cremation Disposing of a body by burning; considered environmentally sound, *see also* CLINICAL WASTE REGULATIONS.

crenation Appearance of erythrocytes often due to slow air drying of films or from shrinkage when blood is placed in a hypertonic solution.

crepitus Grating feel or noise when broken bone fragments move across each other or roughened cartilage. Similarly a sound is heard with the stethoscope when there is a dry lung inflammation; also known as crepitations.

Creutzfeld–Jakob disease (CJD) Human disease of spongiform encephalopathy; the 'new form' variant has been related to the ingestion of beef products. Characterised by a very long incubation period of 10 years or more. The main effect of control regulations for pets is that hard beef bones are no longer freely available for dogs to chew, as a result of perceived disease risks.

cricoid A ring structure but usually means one of the cartilage structures that makes up the larynx.

crop Digestive organ of the bird found proximal to the gizzard.

cross breeding Indicates an out cross of two different strains of the same species; this will help to reduce the effect of recessive genes that may be harmful in close breeding.

cruciate Shaped like a cross, usually applied to the ligaments between the femur and tibia – the anterior and posterior cruciate ligaments.

crura (of diaphragm) Bands of fibromuscular tissue that arise in the lumbar veterbrae and attach to the central tendon of the diaphragm.

cryosurgery Method of surgical treatment using an intense cold source to freeze tissue.

crypt A blind pit used anatomically as in the crypts of Lieberkuhn of the intestine.

crypto- Meaning hidden, usually combined with another word.

cryptorchid Usually indicates that at least one testis has not descended into the scrotum but strict definition would mean that both testes are hidden in the abdominal cavity.

Cryptosporidium Coccidia-like parasites that may enter the drinking water supplies affecting humans and house pets; another species *C. meleagridis* causes disease in birds.

crystalloid Substances of inorganic origin dissolved in water, commonly used to describe the 'salts' group of intravenous fluids. The other group of replacement fluids are known as colloids.

Ctenocephalides The commonest genus of fleas of the dog and cat.

curette Surgical instrument shaped like a long handled spoon used for cleaning out diseased tissue in a wound, obtaining cancellous bone graft, etc.

Cushing's disease Hyperadrenocorticism; may be due to an adrenal cortex tumour or overstimulation by the pituitary gland, *see also* PDH.

cushingoid Describes any disorder with signs of increased thirst, muscle weakness, pendulous abdomen and hair loss that is not due to hyperadrenocorticism.

cusp A small flange as seen in a tooth or the tricuspid heart valve's structure.

cutaneous Relates to the skin surface.

cutdown, venous Method of introducing a cannula into a vein by making a small skin incision immediately above the vein; a hypodermic needle or a scalpel blade may be used.

cuticle The outermost covering sometimes used to describe the skin, the outermost part of the hair shaft, part of the nail or in birds the eggshell covering.

cutis Alternative skin name, *see also* DERMIS.

cyanosis Bluish appearance of the skin, tongue or mucous membranes due to insufficient oxygen reaching the tissues. An alternative term used is 'dusky' and remedial action is urgent, *see also* RESUSCITATION.

cyclophosphamide Cytotoxic agent effective in neoplasia treatments especially proliferative lymphoid tumours.

cyclopegia Term used in eye disease where the pupils do not constrict with light; the paralysis may be the result of medication or nerve injury when there is fixed dilation of the pupils, *see also* MYDRIASIS.

cyesis Pregnancy, *see* PSEUDOCYESIS.

cyst Defined as a fluid-filled cavity, some are called retention cysts. The prostate cyst is one example of a cause of prostate enlargement but may only account for 5% of prostate disease in the dog.

cystic endometrial hyperplasia Condition of the lining of the uterus that may develop in metoestrus, *see also* PYOMETRA.

Cysticercus tenuicollis Larval stage of the tapeworm of the dog *Taenia hydatigena* found in offal of sheep, pigs and wild ruminants on which dogs may feed.

cystine calculi One of the more common types of calculi in dogs as they form in acid urine; may cause obstructions; they are 'stones' produced by errors of the metabolism of cystine and lysine.

cystitis Inflammation of the bladder, may be due to bacterial infection or irritation from calculi.

cystocentesis Surgical procedure to puncture the bladder via the abdominal wall in order to obtain a urine sample.

cystogram An X-ray picture of the bladder, usually involves a positive or a negative contrast agent, *see also* PNEUMOCYSTOGRAM.

cystopexy Procedure to fix the bladder wall to the abdominal wall; may help to draw the vagina out of the pelvic canal and contribute to the control of urinary incontinence.

cystoscopy Endoscopic examination of the urinary bladder.

cystotomy Surgical procedure to open up the bladder; first involves a laparotomy incision.

cytokines Substances that are involved in the inflammatory response and are part of cell-mediated immunity.

cytology The study of the cell structure.

cytopathic Toxic substances that work at individual cell level causing disease and cell death.

cytoplasm The substance of the cell other than the nuclear material, *see also* PROTOPLASM.

cytotoxic An agent that destroys the cells; may be used in neoplasia treatments.

Czerny–Lambert An inverting suture at one time much in favour for repair of intestinal incisions as the suture material passed through the mucosa only.

D

dacroadenitis Inflammation of the lacrimal gland of the eye.

dacrocystitis Inflammation of the lacrimal sac, usually occurring when the duct draining the tears to the nose is blocked, *see also* LACRIMAL GLAND.

dactyl- Relates to a digit or toe.

Dangerous Dog Act Act of Parliament introduced in 1991, which was designed to stop people from keeping those specific breeds of dogs traditionally used for fighting.

Dangerous Wild Animals Act Act of Parliament from 1976 prohibiting the keeping of any dangerous animal unless a licence has been issued by the Local Government Authority; the premises and the animal will be inspected prior to licensing by a veterinary surgeon accompanied by an environmental health officer and there is an annual relicensing inspection; a list of animals considered dangerous is available.

darkroom Area set aside for developing radiographs and reloading X-ray cassettes, usually a light-proof room.

dartos The muscle under the skin of the scrotum that causes it to wrinkle and helps contract the size of the scrotal sac.

deadly nightshade Garden and hedgerow weed that has berries containing atropine that could cause death if eaten in any quantity.

dead space (1) Surgical term used to describe a poorly apposed gap in the tissues that is likely to fill with serum or blood and then become infected. (2) In the respiratory system it represents the part that contains air but does not exchange oxygen and carbon dioxide at alveolar level.

deafness Total or partial loss of hearing in one or both ears. Obstruction in the external canal and loss of sensory nerve routes (sensoneural deafness) are the two most frequent causes, *see also* BRAIN STEM AUDITORY EVOKED RESPONSE.

deamination A process of metabolism in the liver when protein from the diet is used to produce new amino acids or to provide energy and ammonia is released. Normally the liver converts the ammonia to urea for excretion by the kidneys.

death, signs of Traditionally the six signs must be tested before a pronouncement is made: absence of heart beat, no respiratory movement, dilation of pupils with loss of eye reflexes, loss of corneal reflex, glazing of the cornea, body cooling and eventual rigor mortis in 12 hours.

debility Weakness, loss of body strength; multiple causes of this condition, *see also* ANAEMIA.

debridement Cleaning up a wound by removal of contaminating foreign matter and devitalised tissue, healing then takes place by granulation if coaption is impossible, *see also* WOUNDS.

debulking procedure Technique used in tumour surgery to remove the majority of the neoplastic mass to make the remainder more suitable for chemotherapy or radiotherapy.

decompression Applied to acute neurological situations, raised pressure of fluid on the brain being an example of a need for urgent surgical or medical attention.

decubital ulcers A skin ulcer produced by prolonged lying down, usually affects the point of the elbow where there is little soft tissue between the bony prominences and the skin.

decussate Cross, especially in a Y-shape.

decussation The point at which two or more objects in the body cross over, applies especially to nerve tracts, *see also* OPTIC CHIASMA.

deep pain sensation Pain measured by the animal's attitude and behaviour. Not always easy to assess but is an important prognostic indicator in spinal injuries.

defecation (defaecation) Act of passing faeces through the anus from the rectum, involves both conscious expulsion and involuntary peristaltic movement to fill the rectum.

deferent (1) Vessel or nerve that conducts away from the centre. (2) Relating to the vas deferens.

defibrillator Electrical equipment used in ventricular fibrillation to give a controlled electric shock to restore normal heart rhythm in cases of cardiac arrest.

deficiency Anything caused by a lack of a substance; deficiency diseases result from insufficiency of some essential nutrient in the diet, *see also* RICKETS, TAURINE.

definitive host Point in the life cycle of a parasite where the sexual stage of the infecting organism occurs.

degenerative joint disease (DJD) Progressive condition leading to erosion of cartilage and new bone deposits around the joint, *see also* ARTHRITIS.

degloving injury Major injury after accidents when the skin is peeled back from the subcutaneous tissue with loss of associated blood supply. Skin flaps may be non-viable and have to be removed before surgery involving skin transplantation techniques, *see also* AVULSION.

deglutition Swallowing. Birds have a special swallowing mechanism that allows the crop to fill even when the head is down for floor feeding.

degranulation Mast cells release histamine and other cells can similarly lose granules as a part of the secretory process.

dehiscence Splitting open, often after trauma; a surgical wound that opens.

dehydration A reduction in the total body water content and the signs associated with deficiency of water in the tissues and circulation due to diseases, shock or inadequate fluid intake.

delayed suture Method for dealing with contaminated wounds, where after debridement and coaption of tissues, the skin is left open to granulate before being closed by suturing once the tissues have cleaned.

delayed union Term used for a bone fracture that heals more slowly than expected.

delivery Term to denote activity in parturition.

demi- Prefix denoting half of.

***Demodex* spp.** Ectoparasitic mites that inhabit hair follicles and may cause little irritation. Each species is specific to the host. In immunosuppressed and growing animals the parasites cause a pruritic response with hair loss and sometimes secondary bacterial infection, *see also* PUSTULE.

demulcent Substance used to protect and soothe mucous membranes, relieves irritation by coating the surface, milk and honey are used in first aid.

demyelination Degenerative process of nerve tissue where the myelin sheath is destroyed or removed.

denature Remove a principle or alter a protein structure.

dendrite Tree-like arrangement of branches from a nerve cell, involved in nerve conduction.

denervation Interruption of the nerve supply to the muscles or section of a nerve that conducts sensation to the central nervous system.

dens Tooth or tooth-like structure. The second cervical vertebra has a cranially projecting process known as the dens.

dental Relating to the teeth; may be used to describe a nurse or a hygienist. The dental formula is a table of teeth numbers, different in each species.

dentigerous cyst A cyst of dental origin, causing a local swelling on the jaw.

dentine Sensitive calcified tissue forming the bulk of the tooth, it is covered by the outer enamel and there is a central pulp cavity, *see also* TOOTH.

dentistry The profession of caring for, repairing and repositioning teeth.

dentition Normal teeth in the dental arches of the mouth, may be deciduous or permanent.

deoxyribonucleic acid (DNA) The basic structure of all genes, consisting of a double helix of deoxyribose sugars, linked by the purines adenine and guanine, and the pyrimidines cytosine and thymine.

dermal Relating to the skin.

Dermanyssus gallinae Poultry mite which occurs in many aviary-reared birds, known also as red mite; it can cause severe anaemia in the host.

dermatology The scientific study of skin disease.

dermatome (1) Instrument for taking split-thickness skin grafts. (2) Area of skin innervated by a single spinal nerve.

Dermatophagoides Very small mites that feed on household dust and are now considered one of the most important causes of skin allergies in dogs.

Dermatophilus congolensis Gram-positive parasitic bacteria that causes dermatitis; infection often arises acutely in horses after heavy rain – hence the colloquial names of rain scald and mud fever.

dermatitis Any inflammatory condition of the skin, especially from some outside influence such as bacteria, parasites, fungi and mechanical damage.

dermatomycosis Fungal infection of the skin, *see also* RINGWORM.

dermatomyositis Disease syndrome characterised by muscle weakness and dermatitis.

dermatophytosis Fungal infection of the skin, *see also* RINGWORM.

dermatosis Any non-specific disorder of the skin.

dermis The true skin layer, lying immediately beneath the epidermis; it contains blood vessels, lymphatics, nerve endings, glands and hair follicles, *see also* CORIUM.

dermoid cyst A cyst containing curled round hair, sebum and skin debris; often found along the back or on the head representing the fusion sites of the embryo's ectoderm.

Descemet's membrane The innermost lining of the cornea; this structure is important in the healing of corneal wounds.

descemetocoele A bulging of Descemet's membrane that may appear when the overlying corneal layers are eroded, as in a deep corneal ulcer; requires urgent attention.

descenting Surgical procedure performed more commonly in the USA; it involves the removal of the anal sacs in an effort to reduce the odour associated with skunks and ferrets.

desensitisation Medical procedure to reduce an allergic response by giving small but progressively increasing doses of antigen by injection, *see also* HYPOSENSITISATION.

desquamation Sloughing of epidermal cells.

detrusor Smooth muscle of the bladder that contracts to expel urine.

develop Chemical process that converts grains of silver halide on an X-ray film that has been exposed to X-radiation to black silver particles.

developer Solution used as a reducing agent as the first stage of X-ray film processing; consists of either phenidone-hydroquinone or metol-hydroquinone.

devitalisation Loss of blood supply to tissue; seen especially after trauma and makes the tissue non-viable.

dewclaw Vestigial first digits that still have a function in racing dogs when cornering at speed; hind dewclaws are better removed when the dog is young, although the tendency now is to leave the front claws, unless, as in some terrier breeds, the claw grows in a half circle penetrating the flesh.

dewlap The loose fold of skin hanging below the neck of rabbits, etc.

dexamethasone A synthetic analogue of cortisol with a potent anti-inflammatory action; available as oral, injectable and topical preparations; may produce polyuria/polydipsia, and sudden withdrawal of the drug after long-term use may predispose to Addison's disease.

dextran Used in fluid therapy, it consists of a polymer of glucose with side chains to prolong the osmotic action. A large molecule, it remains in the circulation and is not lost via the kidneys. Used as a plasma expander and useful if plasma is not available.

dextrose saline Crystalloid solution used in fluid therapy mainly to replace water and chloride deficits as the strength of the isotonic solution does not allow sufficient glucose to be provided as an energy source.

diabetes insipidus A condition characterised by polyuria and polydipsia, and the production of urine with a low specific gravity and without glucosuria; most commonly caused by defective ADH secretion by the pituitary gland; also a less common nephrogenic form where the kidney is insensitive to ADH; diagnosis is based on a water deprivation test and response to ADH.

diabetes mellitus Metabolic disease where carbohydrate, fat and protein metabolism is defective due to a failure to produce or respond to insulin. Diagnosis is based on elevated fasting plasma glucose levels, and if these exceed the renal threshold, glucose will be present in the urine. The most common form in animals is type I diabetes mellitus, where B cells in the islets of Langerhans of the pancreas fail to produce sufficient insulin; treatment for this form of the disease includes regular administration of insulin and other hypoglycaemic agents, and diet. Type II (non-insulin dependent) arises when the body fails to respond to secreted insulin, *see also* INSULIN.

diagnosis The art and science of determining the cause of illness by considering the patient's signs and symptoms, the history provided by the owner, together with such laboratory tests and imaging techniques as needed.

dialysis Form of filtration where mineral salt molecules diffuse through a semi-permeable membrane. **Peritoneal dialysis** Use of the peritoneum as a semi-permeable membrane; isotonic fluid is injected into the abdomen and then withdrawn – solutes may pass from the blood stream into the fluid, and hence be removed from the body.

diapedesis The outward passage of blood cells through the capillary walls into tissue spaces.

diaphragm Muscular structure that divides the thoracic cavity from the abdominal cavity; there are tendinous parts nearer the abdominal floor and important entry points for major conducting structures that need to pass from one cavity to the other, such as the aorta and oesophagus.

diaphragm, ruptured An abnormal tear in the diaphragm, usually after abdominal trauma; the tear may allow abdominal viscera to enter the thoracic cavity, causing rapid breathing, collapse and death if untreated, *see also* HERNIA.

diaphysis The shaft of a long bone; consists of a tube of hard cortical bone with a marrow cavity.

diarrhoea Rapid passage of soft faecal matter from the intestines to the exterior; the passage of abnormally soft or liquid faeces is accompanied by fluid and electrolyte losses (particularly bicarbonate and potassium).

diarthrosis Joint articulation where there is free movement between the bone ends through the joint capsule and supporting structures, *see also* SYNOVIA.

diastole The part of the contraction cycle of the heart that represents the relaxation of the atria and ventricles and the time when they are filling again with blood.

diastolic blood pressure The lowest blood pressure, measured when the heart is in the relaxed phase of the cardiac cycle.

diathermy Method of using high-frequency electric currents to elevate the temperature of a small area of tissue so that blood coagulates; at a higher frequency it can be used to cut tissue; a type of diathermy is also used to deliver moderate heat for physiotherapy purposes in the treatment of deep-seated pain.

diazepam A sedative and anxiolytic; may be used as a premedicant prior to general anaesthesia and is also used to control epileptiform seizures; when given intravenously it can be used to stimulate the appetite in cats, *see also* EPILEPSY.

diencephalon The thalamus and hypothalamus; a relay station between the forebrain and the brainstem, controls autonomic and endocrine functions.

diet Mixture of foods that the animal eats; the diet should meet the minimum nutritional requirements for that animal and specific diets may be advisable for certain disease states.

dietary hypersensitivity Allergy to a component of the diet, where certain foods precipitate responses varying from severe gastroenteritis to skin rashes; the basis of treatment is to feed an elimination diet which is bland and contains a 'novel' protein source that the animal is unlikely to have come into contact with before; other elements can then be added one at a time, to identify the allergen.

differential white cell count Laboratory technique where the white blood cells are counted manually on a thin blood smear or using an automatic processor; the relative numbers of neutrophils, eosinophils, basophils, lymphocytes and monocytes are obtained to assist in diagnosis.

diffusion The random movement of particles in a solution or gas so that they eventually become evenly distributed.

digestible energy (DE) Measure of the proportion of the food consumed that is available as energy as opposed to the amount lost in faeces, etc.

digestibility Amount of the food in the diet that can be absorbed and not lost in the faeces.

digestion Process of breaking down complex dietary substances into smaller particles and constituents that can be absorbed through the intestinal wall.

digital extensor muscles Group of muscles running on the cranial aspect of the fore- or hind limb that will extend the toes during locomotion.

digital flexor muscles Group of muscles running on the caudal aspect of the fore- or hind limb that act to flex the toes and push the animal forwards.

digoxin Traditional medicine derived from the foxglove leaf; as a glycoside it slows and strengthens contraction of the cardiac muscle, *see also* INOTROPIC.

dilatation Stretching or enlargement, usually applied to a hollow organ or opening. **Gastric dilation** Distension of the stomach with gas; a disorder usually affecting the larger breeds of dog; arises mainly soon after feeding and can rapidly become life-threatening as it impairs respiration, *see also* AEROPHAGIA, TYMPANY.

diluent Substance that makes a solution more dilute; in the case of a freeze-dried vaccine it is the fluid that is added to dissolve the pellet prior to injection.

Dioctophyma renale Type of worm occasionally found in the kidneys of dogs and wild carnivores.

dioestrus The luteal phase of the reproductive cycle, between metoestrus and the next oestrus, *see also* METOESTRUS.

Dipetalonema reconditum A filarial worm of the dog, transmitted by fleas and lice; microfilariae may be found in the blood stream and adult forms in connective tissue and viscera.

Diphyllobothrium latum Known as the fish tapeworm, may inhabit the intestine of cats or dogs fed on raw fish.

Dipylidium caninum The most common tapeworm of pet dogs and cats in the UK; fleas and lice are the usual intermediate hosts.

diploid Having the normal number of chromosomes; all cells of the body are diploid, apart from ova and sperm, which are haploid and have only half the number of chromosomes; the diploid number is restored when an ovum is fertilised.

Dirofilaria immitis Heartworm of the dog, living in the heart and large blood vessels; microfilariae may be demonstrated in blood smear; transmission is by mosquito bites and the condition occurs in tropical and subtropical regions, or in imported animals.

dirty Unclean or contaminated, *see also* WOUNDS.

disbud Term used for the removal of the growing horn buds in young animals such as goats.

disc Round, flattened structure such as the optic disc, where the optic nerve enters the eye, or an intervertebral disc between adjacent vertebrae.

discharge Fluid flowing from a wound or body cavity.

discharge procedures Routine that the nurse should follow whenever a patient leaves the hospital accommodation.

discoid lupus erythematosus Rare auto-immune condition, seen as small skin plaques often on feet or around the nose; the plaques may ulcerate and the condition is often exacerbated by sunlight; biopsy confirmation is advised, *see also* LUPUS, SLE.

discospondylitis Bacterial infection of an intervertebral disc and the adjacent end plates of the vertebrae.

disease Any morbid disorder with a specific cause; signs and symptoms can be recognised; injuries and accidents are excluded from this definition.

disinfect The process of eliminating micro-organisms from contaminated instruments, surfaces, skin, etc. by the use of physical or chemical means, does not include killing spores.

disinfectant Agent that destroys or removes all bacteria, viruses and fungi, includes environmental and skin disinfectants; the major types of disinfectants are alcohol, bleaches (hypochlorite), aldehydes, chlorhexidine, iodophors and quaternary ammonia compounds, *see also* ANTISEPTIC.

dislocate Disruption of a joint so that there is loss of contact between the articular surfaces, *see also* LUXATED.

dispensing Method of controlling the issue of effective medication; some products, e.g. flea collars, are on a general sales list and can be sold 'over the counter' under the exclusions of the *Marketing Authorisation for Veterinary Medical Products Regulations 1994*. Pharmacy and merchant list (PML) drugs can only be sold from pharmacies and licensed premises. Prescription Only Medicine (POM) can be supplied directly by veterinary surgeons to 'animals under their care', and also by pharmacists on production of a valid prescription.

disseminated intravascular coagulation (DIC) A serious disorder where activation of the coagulation and fibrinolytic pathways lead to the formation of thrombi in small vessels, and an increased tendency to haemorrhage; associated with some viral infections, neoplasia, heat stroke and liver disease; the prognosis is very poor.

dissociative anaesthesia Type of general anaesthesia produced by agents such as ketamine; the agent produces good analgesia, with only superficial sleep – the patient is dissociated from their surroundings; muscle relaxation may not be sufficient for some procedures; respiratory depression is mild, and blood pressure may rise with these agents.

distad Distally, towards the periphery.

distal Furthest away, distad, *see also* PROXIMAL.

distal denervating disease A syndrome in the dog characterised by progressive, severe, flaccid paralysis of all four limbs; reflexes are depressed or absent, although sensation remains intact; the aetiology remains obscure; prognosis is good, with most animals making a full recovery, although this may take several months.

distemper Specific morbillivirus infection principally affecting the dog and ferret, but largely controlled by the use of effective vaccines; contagious and produces severe-to-fatal disease primarily in puppies; clinical signs include pyrexia, oculonasal discharge, cough and neurological signs; post-recovery dogs may develop hard pad, distemper teeth and old dog encephalitis, *see also* CHOREA, HARD PAD.

distemper teeth Adult teeth with pitted, discoloured enamel, resulting from distemper infection in puppyhood.

distichiasis Presence of a double row of eye lashes at the lid margin that may rub against the cornea.

disuse atrophy Wasting of a limb muscle as a result of reduced use of the limb; causes include pain, fracture, soft tissue injury, etc.

diuretic Drug that increases urine output.

diverticulum Sac or pouch opening from a hollow structure such as the alimentary tract.

docking Deliberately removing all or part of an animal's tail; defined as an act of veterinary surgery. There are advisory rules on who shall carry out docking and in what circumstances it should be done.

dog Member of the Caniidae, with very many varieties (breeds) of domesticated dogs; wild dogs, foxes, jackals and wolves make up the rest of the group.

dog catcher Piece of equipment consisting of a pole with a distendable rope loop for securing free-running dogs.

dog warden Person appointed by a local authority with a statutory function to control the stray dog population and educate the public on the need for dog controls.

dolichocephalic Dogs with long pointed skulls, such as the saluki; the shape of the skull will be in the breed standard.

dolor Latin for pain; one of the four classic signs of inflammation.

dominant (1) Term used to denote a gene or trait that will always show its effect in the next generation. (2) Behavioural characteristic where one animal ranks higher than others in its social group.

domitor Commonly used, reversible sedative and premedicant, *see also* MEDETOMIDINE.

dorsal Towards the spine or back surface, *see also* VENTRAL.

dorsum The back or often the upper (top) exposed body surface, e.g. the upper surface of the paw.

dose Measured amount of drug required to obtain a therapeutic effect.

dosimeter Instrument used to measure radiation, *see also* FILM BADGE.

doxapram A CNS stimulant often used sublingually to stimulate respiration in the new-born.

drain (1) Method of removing fluid from a cavity. (2) Channels in buildings to remove waste water. **Penrose drain** Soft rubber tubing that can be inserted into the region requiring drainage, with the lowest end protruding; works by capillary action, drawing fluids down the inner and outer surfaces of the tube – should not be fenestrated as this reduces the surface area of the tube. **Chest drain** Tubing inserted into the thoracic cavity in the lower third (to remove fluid) or the upper third (to remove free air). The external end must be carefully connected to a vacuum pump (for continuous drainage) or sealed with a tap or spigot (for intermittent drainage); a gate clamp or second seal should also be used for security; the internal end may be fenestrated to increase the number of openings that fluid can move through, *see also* HEIMLICH VALVE. **Sump drain** Consisting of outer and inner tubes; suction is applied to the inner tube, while the outer is perforated to allow fluid to be drawn in.

drape Cloth or paper, presterilised and used to cover the patient before and during surgery.

dressing Wound protection or material applied to the surface with or without medication to provide cover and assist in healing.

drill Apparatus used in orthopaedic surgery to make the screw holes.

drip set Apparatus for continuous injection (infusion) of fluids into a vein; consists of an attachment that links to the drip bag, a measuring chamber, a length of tubing and a luer connection; giving sets specifically for blood also contain a filter to remove any small clots.

dropsy Oedema fluid in the abdomen, *see also* ASCITES.

drowning Death by asphyxiation if water is inhaled into the lungs; the liquid prevents the exchange of oxygen and carbon dioxide, resuscitation should always be attempted unless there has been a prolonged period of immersion.

drug Any therapeutic agent other than food used to prevent, diagnose or treat a disease, *see also* CONTROLLED DRUG.

drug eruption Hypersensitivity to a drug, characterised by acute pruritus, erythema and red wheals, *see also* ANAPHYLAXIS.

dry eye Disorder due to inadequate tear secretion, *see also* KERATO CONJUNCTIVITIS SICCA.

duct Channel or passageway used for excretion and secretion.

ductus arteriosus A fetal blood vessel connecting the pulmonary artery and the aorta, so that blood is diverted from the lungs; after birth the vessel closes and becomes a fibrous remnant, *see also* PATENT DUCTUS ARTERIOSUS.

duodenum First part of the small intestine running from the pylorus to the jejunum; produces many digestive juices and receives secretions from the pancreas and liver.

dura mater The outermost of the three membranes that protect the CNS (meninges); the dura is tough and blends with periosteum in the cranium, *see also* EPIDURAL.

durotomy Surgical incision of the dura mater, necessary for intracranial procedures and to get access to the nervous tissue of the spinal cord.

dynamic compression plate (DCP) Metal plate used for internal fracture fixation; the plates are available in a variety of lengths and thicknesses; the screw holes are oval in shape, so that screws inserted eccentrically will provide compression across fracture gaps, *see also* ASIF.

dys- Prefix for difficult, abnormal or impaired.

dysautonomia Disease affecting the autonomic nervous system, *see also* KEY–GASKELL SYNDROME.

dyschezia Difficult or painful passage of faeces from the rectum, usually the result of a long period of voluntary suppression.

dyschondroplasia Abnormal skeletal development, *see also* OSTEOCHONDROSIS.

dyscoria Unequal size of the pupils or an abnormal shape of the opening.

dyscrasia Presence of abnormal cells and particles in the blood.

dysecdysis Skin moulting in reptiles; may be incomplete especially when due to malnutrition or an unsuitable environment.

dysentry Term used for severe diarrhoea with blood and mucus, *see also* PARVOVIRUS.

dysmetria Unequal movements of the limbs due to damage to the cerebellum.

dysphagia Difficulty in swallowing.

dysphonia Difficulty in voice production; may be due to a disorder of the larynx, pharynx, tongue or mouth, sometimes psychogenic.

dysplasia Abnormal development leading to disease, *see also* HIP DYSPLASIA, RETINAL DYSPLASIA.

dyspnoea Laboured or difficult breathing; may be due to obstruction of the airway, various diseases of the bronchial tree and lung tissue or from heart disease.

dysrhythmia Abnormal heart rhythm, *see also* CARDIAC.

dystocia Difficulty giving birth; it is traditionally divided into fetal and maternal categories, *see also* PRESENTATION, POSITION.

dysuria Painful passage of urine or difficult flow from the bladder.

E

ear The organ of hearing and balance. **Inner ear** The deepest chamber of the ear, located within the petrous part of the temporal bone of the skull; consists of the semicircular canals (vestibular apparatus), the coiled cochlea and the vestibule (composed of utricle and saccule); the vestibular apparatus provides positional information concerning head movements and balance, while the cochlea provides hearing, *see also* DEAFNESS, OTITIS INTERNA, SEMICIRCULAR CANAL. **Middle ear** The chamber of the ear, within the tympanic part of the temporal bone, housing the auditory ossicles – the malleus, incus and stapes; it transmits sound from the external ear canal (across the tympanic membrane) to the oval and round windows of the cochlea, *see also* COCHLEA, OTITIS MEDIA. **Outer ear** The pinna (ear flap) and external auditory canal, *see also* OTITIS EXTERNA.

ear canal The funnel-shaped, cartilaginous canal of the outer ear, running from the ear flap to the tympanic membrane; composed of vertical and horizontal parts; external auditory canal.

ear canal ablation *see* TOTAL EAR CANAL ABLATION.

ear drum Tympanic membrane; the thin membrane dividing the external and middle ear; transmits sound waves from the external ear to the malleus, incus and stapes of the middle ear.

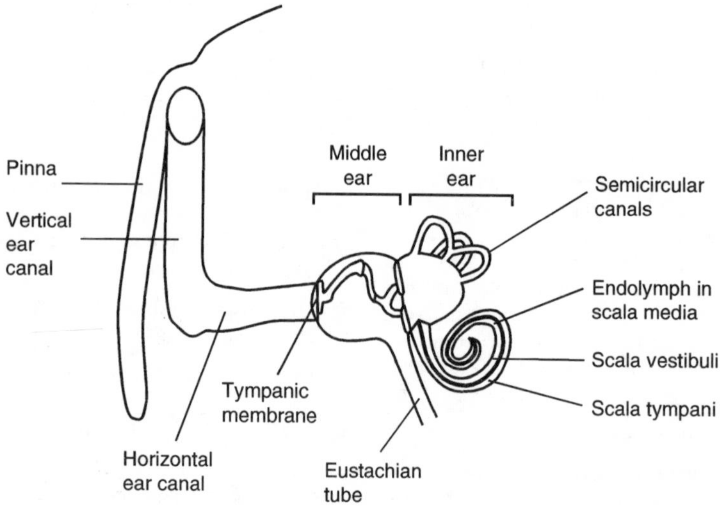

Ear

ear mites *Otodectes cynotis*; surface-living, visible to the naked eye and can be seen on auroscopic examination; a common cause of otitis externa, all animals within the household will require treatment, as the mites are not host specific; cats in particular can tolerate a large ear mite burden with few clinical signs; repeated treatment may be necessary to break the life cycle of the mites.

eburnation Sclerosis of bone; usually a response to chronic injury, such as degenerative joint disease; the subchondral bone plate thickens and hardens, becoming less able to absorb concussive forces during locomotion.

ecbolic A drug that stimulates smooth muscle contraction, *see also* OXYTOCIN.

ecchymosis Leakage of blood into the tissues to cause a bruise, *see also* PETECHIA.

Echinococcus granulosus Small tapeworm of the dog; the larvae infect ruminants, pigs and horses, and can infect humans, where they cause hydatid cysts (hydatidosis) in the liver and lungs; control measures include effective, regular worming of dogs, good hygiene and not feeding uncooked offal to dogs.

echocardiography Ultrasound scanning of the heart and major vessels.

eclampsia Nervous signs resulting from low blood calcium levels; occurs shortly before parturition or 4–6 weeks after, when milk demand is at its peak and large calcium reserves have to be mobilised by the mother; signs vary but can include fits; treatment includes slow intravenous infusions of calcium borogluconate and calcium tablets; offspring should be removed and hand-reared.

-ectasis Distension of any tubular structure.

ectoderm The outer layer of cells in the embryo, giving rise to the skin and its associated structures.

-ectomy Surgical removal of a part, e.g. splenectomy.

ectoparasite A parasite that lives on the outer surface of the body e.g. mites, lice, ticks, fleas.

ectopic Aberrant, occurring in the wrong place, e.g. ectopic ureters enter the bladder at a site other than the trigone, and may even enter the vagina or urethra, ectopic ureters are often a cause of urinary incontinence.

ectopic beats Contractions of the heart which are initiated by a region other than the sinoatrial node.

ectopic cilia Single hairs or small hair clusters that arise from the conjunctiva and irritate the cornea; usually require surgical removal, *see also* DISTICHIASIS.

ectropion Outward drooping of the lower eyelid, usually an inherited defect; treatment is surgical.

eczema General term for any patch of inflamed skin.

efferent Conducting away from, e.g. an efferent nerve carries an impulse away from the spinal cord to a gland or muscle; efferent blood vessels take blood away from an organ.

effusion Fluid that leaks out from blood vessels or lymphatics, e.g. joint effusion collects within a traumatised joint, pericardial effusion collects within the pericardial cavity.

eggbound Lodging of an egg within the oviduct of birds and reptiles; calcium borogluconate may be given, but manual manipulation or surgical removal may be required.

Ehlers–Danlos syndrome Rare disorder characterised by hyperelasticity of the skin and increased joint laxity.

Ehmer sling Hind leg sling used to maintain the limb in flexion and prevent weight bearing; may be used after replacement of luxated hips; requires careful padding and application to ensure that it does not rub, slip or impair circulation.

ehrlichiosis Disease caused by *Erhlichia canis*; the Gram-negative bacterium gives rise to neurological signs and is spread by ticks; rare in the UK, but more common in the USA.

***Eimeria* spp.** Coccidia; many species of protozoal parasites that cause enteritis in their host animals.

ejaculation The expulsion of semen from the penis.

elbow The ginglymus (hinge) articulation between the distal humerus, radial head and proximal ulna.

elbow dysplasia Developmental disease with a high genetic component; affects mainly large and giant breeds; primary lesions include ununited or fragmented coronoid process and osteochondritis dissecans; leads to irreversible DJD.

electric burn Tissue damage due to the passage of a large electric current through an area.

electric shock Passage of a large electrical current through the body, resulting in muscle spasm (which may affect the heart muscle leading to cardiac arrest); can occur in puppies that chew electric flex, etc. Care must be taken to ensure that the causal electrical equipment is switched off and unplugged before approaching an animal that has just had an electric shock. Use rubber gloves or a broom handle to first make contact.

electrocardiograph (ECG) Electrical tracing of activity in the heart; usually obtained by attaching three recording leads to the animal placed in right lateral recumbency.

electrocoagulation Haemostasis using a small metal blade that is electrically heated, or by passing an electric current through the localised blood vessel.

electrodiagnostic testing (EDT) Use of fine needle electrodes and nerve stimulators to record nerve conduction velocities and the response of muscles to nervous stimulation.

electroencephalograph (EEG) Trace of the electrical activity in the brain; as little is known about EEG patterns in animals the test may provide limited information.

electrolyte A salt that can conduct electricity in solution as it breaks down into positive and negative ions, e.g. NaCl, $NaHCO_3$.

electromagnetic radiation (EMR) Waves of radiation including radio waves, infra-red, light, ultraviolet radiation, X-rays and gamma radiation.

electromyograph (EMG) The recording of electrical activity in muscles, by introducing fine needle electrodes into the tissue; part of electrodiagnostic testing.

electron Elementary particle that carries a negative charge and circles around the nucleus of an atom;

electricity results from a flow of electrons.

electrophoresis Movement of particles when an electric field is applied; negative particles will move towards the positive anode, while positive charges will move towards the negative cathode.

electroretinograph (ERG) Trace of the electrical activity of the retina in response to light; may be used to test retinal function prior to cataract surgery, when the lens opacity prevents ophthalmoscopic examination of the retina.

enzyme-linked immunosorbant assay (ELISA) Rapid laboratory test where a colour change is linked to enzyme activity; used to detect FELV for example.

Elizabethan collar 'Buster' collar; plastic cone that fits around the neck but extends up to or beyond the end of the nose; prevents the animal scratching or rubbing the head, or chewing at the body, widely used post-operatively, e.g. after ocular surgery, to prevent wound interference, etc.

emaciation Extreme thinness; may be due to starvation, chronic disease, etc.

embolism Obstruction of a blood vessel by an embolus.

embolus, pl. emboli Plug of fibrin and platelets that blocks a blood vessel.

embrocation Liniment or ointment.

embryo The developing fertilised egg before becoming the fetus.

emesis Vomiting.

emetic An agent that induces vomiting, e.g. a side-effect of xylazine in the dog which may be used if the animal has eaten recently but requires emergency surgery, or if the dog has ingested a non-corrosive poison, *see also* WASHING SODA.

emollient An agent that softens the skin.

emphysema Dilation of the alveoli; if alveolar membranes rupture air can also enter the connective tissue between alveoli; the condition leads to expiratory dyspnoea and cyanosis.

empyema Pyothorax.

emulsion Mixture of two liquids, one suspended as fine particles within the other.

enamel Hard substance forming the outer covering of teeth.

enarthrosis Ball and socket joint, such as the hip.

encapsulated Enclosed within a limiting membrane.

encephalitis Inflammation of the brain tissue.

encephalomeningitis Inflammation of the brain and its meninges (meningoencephalitis).

encephalomyelitis Inflammation of the brain and spinal cord.

encephalopathy Any disease or disorder of the brain.

encephalon The brain.

endarteritis Inflammation of the endothelial lining of an artery.

end artery An artery that is the sole supply to a region and has no collateral vessels; thus, should the artery be occluded the area of tissue it supplied will become devitalised, e.g. retinal vessels, coronary vessels.

endemic Disease that is always present within a given population.

endocarditis Vegetative lesions on the atrioventricular valves due to seeding of bacterial infection from a remote location via the blood stream; common septic foci include teeth and gums, bite wounds and infective arthritis; organisms involved include *Staphylococcus*, *Streptococcus* and *E. coli*.

endocardiosis Progressive degeneration of the cardiac atrioventricular valves; a common occurrence in ageing dogs, and younger animals in breeds such as the Cavalier King Charles spaniel; may also be accompanied by degenerative changes within the chordae tendinae; leads to valvular incompetence and congestive heart failure (predominantly left-sided).

endocardium The inner membrane lining the chambers of the heart and covering the valves.

endochondral ossification Type of ossification occurring at growth plate regions in long bones (epiphyseal plates) and beneath the articular cartilage, brings about limb lengthening and enlargement of the articular surfaces; cartilage cells proliferate and form long columns of hypertrophied cells; the cartilage matrix mineralises and the chondrocytes are replaced by osteocytes which remodel the matrix to form bone.

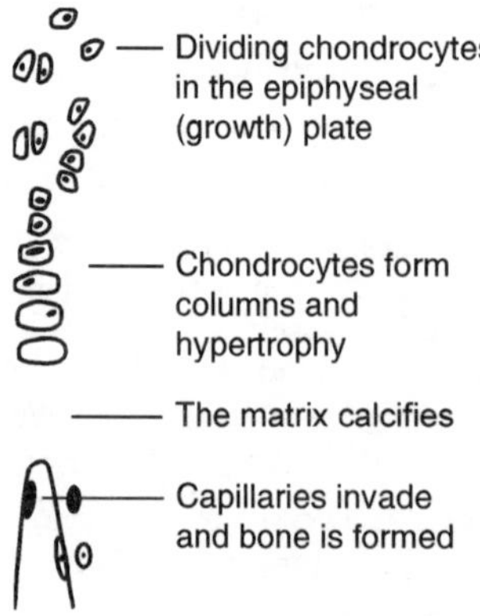

Dividing chondrocytes in the epiphyseal (growth) plate
Chondrocytes form columns and hypertrophy
The matrix calcifies
Capillaries invade and bone is formed

Endochondral ossification

endocrine Internally secreted.

endocrine glands Ductless structures that secrete hormones directly into the blood stream, e.g. adrenal gland, thyroid.

endocrinology The study of endocrine glands and the hormones they produce.

endolymph The fluid contained within the scala media of the inner ear.

endometrium The lining of the uterus.

endometritis Inflammation of the lining of the uterus, usually due to infection; may occur after parturition.

endomysium The connective tissue layer surrounding a muscle fibre.

endoneurium The innermost connective tissue layer surrounding a nerve fibre.

endoparasite Parasite living within the body of the host; including roundworms, tapeworms, protozoa, lung worm, etc.

endoplasmic reticulum Folded membranous structures within a cell, close to the nucleus; rough endoplasmic reticulum is encrusted with ribosomes and synthesises proteins; smooth endoplasmic reticulum lacks ribosomes and produces lipid secretions.

endoscope Instrument with a light source and viewing channel; the first endoscopes were rigid structures, but the use of fibre-optics has allowed them to become flexible.

endoscopy Examination of body cavities using an endoscope.

endosteal Relating to the endosteum or lying adjacent to it, e.g. endosteal blood vessels.

endosteum Membrane lining the medullary cavity of the long bones.

endotendinium Connective tissue sheath surrounding a strand of tendon.

endothelium Thin lining membrane of body cavities and blood vessels; derived from the embryonic endodermal layer.

endothermic Chemical reaction that takes in, or requires, heat.

endotoxic shock Caused by the release of endotoxins from bacterial infection.

endotoxin Harmful substance released by some bacteria when their cell wall ruptures; most commonly ingested in rancid food, causing abdominal discomfort, vomiting and diarrhoea. *E. coli* produces an endotoxin causing necrosis.

endotracheal tube (ET tube) Rubber or polymer tube placed into the trachea of anaesthetised animals to maintain a patent upper airway and allow the administration of anaesthetic gases. Available in a wide range of sizes, with and without inflatable cuffs; the cuffs should be inflated to limit the escape of anaesthetic gases into the environment and prevent aspiration of water, saliva, blood, etc.

end plate potential The electrical potential developed at the motor end plate, where a nerve axon contacts a muscle fibre.

end-to-end anastomosis Surgical technique for the repair of resected intestine, blood vessels, etc. where the open ends of two hollow structures are sutured together to make one continuous tube.

enema, pl. enemata A liquid introduced into the rectum; may be used to encourage defaecation and evacuate the bowel, administer a drug or as part of a radiographic contrast study of the terminal digestive tract.

enfloxin Derivative of quinalones developed in the early 1990s with very little antibiotic resistance, largely effective in treatment of skin, respiratory and urinary infections. Well tolerated by exotic pets, *see also* FLUOROQUINALONES.

enflurane (Ethrane) Volatile anaesthetic agent; sweet-smelling; provides rapid anaesthesia and recovery but is relatively expensive.

enophthalmos Retraction of the eyeball into the socket, e.g. after debilitating illness where the retrobulbar fat pad reduces in size, *see also* HORNER'S SYNDROME.

enteral Via the gut; enteral nutrition is the supply of nutrient into the gastrointestinal tract by routes other than the mouth, e.g. nasogastric tube, PEG tube.

enterectomy Surgical removal of a portion of small intestine.

enteric Relating to the small intestine.

enteritis Inflammation of the small intestine.

enterolith Concretion of hardened material, usually faeces, that may cause intestinal obstruction.

enteropathy Any disease of the intestines, e.g. protein-losing enteropathy, mucoid enteropathy of rabbits.

enterotomy Surgical incision into the small intestine to remove a foreign body for example; care must be taken to ensure that the rest of the abdomen is not contaminated with intestinal contents.

enterotoxin A toxin that has its effect on the gastrointestinal tract, *see also* ENDOTOXIN, EXOTOXIN.

entropion Curling inward of the eyelid margin, so that hairs may contact the cornea and cause irritation; hereditary in many breeds, such as the sharpei and cocker spaniel; requires surgical correction.

enucleation Total removal of the eyeball.

enzootic Describes a disease occurring within a particular region or area, e.g. rabies is enzootic in much of Asia.

enzyme Protein produced by a cell and that catalyses a specific chemical reaction; routinely used as biochemical markers to locate damage to specific organs, e.g. raised alkaline phosphatase levels may indicate increased bone turnover.

eosin Red stain used routinely for histological examination of tissues, *see also* HAEMATOXYLIN.

eosinopenia Reduced number of circulating eosinophils, most commonly a result of corticosteroid therapy.

eosinophil Granular type of white blood cell; have striking red granules within the cytoplasm; they contribute to the allergic response and are important in the inactivation of histamine; produced by the bone marrow.

eosinophilia Raised number of circulating eosinophils; causes include tissue injury (with the release of histamine), parasite burden, allergic responses or oestrus.

eosinophilic The adjective is used to describe diseases such as a type of chronic enteritis where there are collections of eosinophils in the intestine wall. The non-healing eosinophilic ulcer of the cat's nose and upper lip, also known as rodent ulcer, is sometimes neoplastic.

eosinophilic myositis Inflammatory myopathy affecting the masticatory muscles, especially in German shepherd dogs; occurs in acute, recurring bouts and may lead to marked atrophy and fibrosis of affected muscles; often responds to steroids; the exact aetiology remains unclear.

epaxial Muscles around the vertebral column along the dorsum, lying above the level of the transverse processes; comprises the iliocostalis, longissimus and transversospinalis muscle systems; act to extend the spine and produce lateral movements.

ependyma Thin membrane lining the ventricles of the brain and the central canal of the spinal cord.

epicondyle Bony prominence on a condyle; usually a site of soft tissue attachments.

epidemic Outbreak of disease above the normal expected levels.

epidemiology The study of the patterns of disease within populations.

epidermis Superficial layer of the skin.

epididymis Convoluted duct attached to the ventrocaudal aspect of the testis; conveys sperm from the testis to the vas deferens.

epidural Outside the dura mater; epidural anaesthesia is achieved by injecting local anaesthetic into the fat-containing epidural space outside the spinal cord.

epigastric Region around the stomach.

epiglottis Cartilage at the base of the tongue; acts as a stopper to close off the airway during swallowing.

epilepsy Abnormal patterns of activity within the brain, resulting in collapse, loss of consciousness and convulsions, *see also* GRAND MAL.

epimysium Fibrous outer connective tissue sheath surrounding a muscle.

epineurium Fibrous outermost connective tissue surrounding a nerve.

epiphora Overflow of tears; chronic epiphora leads to tear-staining of the facial hair coat; commonly due to blockage of the nasolacrimal duct.

epiphyseal Relating to the epiphysis.

epiphysis Proximal and distal extremities of a long bone; form from separate centres of ossification from the shaft of the bone and are separated from the shaft by growth plate regions in skeletally immature animals, *see also* ENDOCHONDRAL OSSIFICATION.

epiploic foramen Connecting opening between the abdominal cavity and the omental bursa, also known as the foramen of Winslow.

episcleral Around the margins of the sclera of the eye.

episiotomy Surgical incision into the vulva to help the delivery of offspring.

episodic weakness Periods of muscle weakness and collapse; associated with conditions such as alkylosis, hypoglycaemia and myaesthenia gravis.

epispadias Congenital abnormality where the urethra opens out onto the dorsal surface of the penis.

epistaxis Nosebleed.

epithelioma Neoplasm arising from any of the elements of the epithelium.

epithelium The surface of the body, including skin, mucous membranes, cornea, serous surfaces and associated glands; types include ciliated, columnar, cuboidal, pseudostratified, stratified and squamous.

epizootic Epidemic.

epulis A hard, neoplastic proliferation of the gums.

equator of the lens Peripheral region of the lens, where the supporting zonules attach.

equine Relating to the horse, e.g. equine veterinary nursing.

erection Filling of the corpus cavernosus with blood so that the penis becomes erect.

eructation Belching, regurgitation of free gas from the stomach, *see also* AEROPHAGY.

erysipelas Skin disease caused by *Erysipelothrix rhusiopathiae*; characterised by the acute appearance of inflamed, reddened patches; can also cause bacterial endocarditis.

erythema Reddening of the skin due to dilation of capillaries.

erythroblast Immature forms of erythrocyte, e.g. normoblast, reticulocyte.

erythrocyte Mature red blood cell; the most numerous cell in the blood stream; lack a nucleus (except in birds) and are packed with haemoglobin, which carries oxygen to the tissues; discoid in shape and deformable, so they can pass easily through capillaries.

erythrocytopenia Abnormally low number of circulating red blood cells; causes include haemorrhage, haemolysis, reduced production by the bone marrow and heavy parasite burdens, *see also* ANAEMIA.

erythrogenesis The formation of red blood cells, erythropoiesis is a similar word.

erythrolysis Haemolysis, the breakdown of red blood cells.

erythron Erythrocytes and all the tissues that produce red blood cells.

erythropoiesis The process of red blood cell formation; occurs within the red bone marrow; maturation time is approximately 4–7 days.

Escherichia coli Gram-negative, rod-shaped bacteria; widely distributed and part of the normal gut flora; pathogenic strains produce enterotoxins that cause diarrhoea. A cause of death of young puppies, *see also* FADING PUPPY/KITTEN SYNDROME.

Esmarch bandage Rubber bandage that can be used to exsanguinate a limb prior to surgery, to control haemorrhage; the bandage is applied from distal to proximal, squeezing blood out of the limb; the distal end is then unwrapped to expose the required surgical site, but a loop is left proximally to act as a tourniquet; operating time is limited as tissue hypoxia can occur; the bandage may also mask haemorrhage, blood loss only becoming apparent when the bandage is removed.

ethanol An alcohol, each molecule containing two carbon atoms.

ether One of the earliest volatile anaesthetic agents; highly inflammable and explosive; decomposes readily so has to be stored in dark glass; irritant to mucous membranes, commonly causes post-operative nausea; superseded by agents such as halothane and isoflurane; may be applied to ticks to facilitate removal.

ethics Code of practice for correct conduct of all veterinary staff.

ethmoid Like a sieve; the ethmoid bone of the cranium is perforated with many fine holes that allow the passage of fibres of the olfactory nerve as they run cranially to innervate the nasal membranes and organs of smell.

ethmoturbinates Scrolls of bone arising from the ethmoid bone and dividing the nose into nasal chambers.

ethylenediaminetetraacetic acid (EDTA) An anticoagulant used in blood collection tubes if the sample requires haematological tests.

ethylene glycol Antifreeze; has a sweet taste and is a common form of poisoning in dogs, signs include vomiting, weakness, collapse, haematuria and convulsions.

ethylene oxide Vapour used to sterilise equipment; the gas is highly effective against micro-organisms and spores; the process can also be carried out at room temperature, so heat-sensitive items can be sterilised; however, the procedure takes at least 24 hours (items have to be left to air) and specialist fume cabinets are required.

eukaryote Cell possessing a membrane-bound nucleus.

Eustachian tube Running from the middle ear to the nasopharynx; a route for ascending middle ear infections.

euthanasia Humane destruction of an animal; means 'good death'.

euthyroid Having normal thyroid function, *see also* THYROID.

euthyroid sick syndrome Syndrome where the thyroid secretes a normal level of T_3 and T_4, but circulating levels are low due to starvation, surgery, hepatic or renal disease, diabetes mellitus or other chronic illness.

evacuant A laxative enema.

evolution The process of genetic change and development.

exacerbate Make worse or more severe.

excision Surgical removal of a part.

excision arthroplasty Surgical removal of an articular surface, e.g. femoral head excision for Legg–Calvé–Perthes disease.

excitement, involuntary The second stage of general anaesthesia; the animal is unconscious, but there may be struggling and paddling; breath-holding is common.

excitement, voluntary The first stage of anaesthesia; the animal is conscious and may struggle to prevent induction.

excoriation A scratch.

excretion The elimination of waste materials from the body.

exercise Physical activity; a minimum level of regular activity is required to ensure the animal maintains healthy locomotor and cardiovascular systems; activity also helps to relieve boredom.

exhale Breathe out.

exhaustion Severe tiredness and collapse after strenuous, sustained effort.

exocrine Secretion via a duct, e.g. the secretion of saliva from the parotid salivary gland is via the parotid duct.

exocrine pancreatic insufficiency (EPI) Reduced function of the exocrine pancreas, due to atrophy of the acinar cells or a sequel to chronic pancreatitis; the lack of lipase, amylase and trypsin normally produced by the exocrine pancreas gives rise to the symptoms of weight loss, poor condition and fatty, odorous faeces; diagnosis may be confirmed by measuring trypsin-like immunoreactivity in a serum sample. Treatment includes supplementation with pancreatic extracts, vitamins, and feeding a low-fibre, low fat diet, *see also* TRIPSIN-LIKE IMMUNOREACTIVITY.

exophthalmos Protrusion of the eyeball; considered normal in some breeds, such as the Pekinese; exposed cornea may be prone to ulceration.

exostosis Proliferation of hard tissue; may be a benign neoplastic change; cartilaginous exostoses are found predominantly affecting the digits and metacarpal/tarsal regions.

exothermic Chemical reaction that gives out heat to the surroundings.

expectorant An agent that increases the elimination of secretions from the respiratory tract by increasing the activity of cilia, stimulating cough reflexes, etc.

expiration Breathing out; a passive process brought about mainly by elastic recoil of thoracic structures.

expiratory reserve volume The difference between the amount of gas exhaled for a given level of activity, and the maximum amount that could be exhaled.

expiratory valve The valve in a semi-closed, non-rebreathing anaesthetic circuit that allows exhaled gases to be removed.

exploratory laparotomy Surgical opening of the abdomen to visually examine the enclosed organs and reach a diagnosis.

exposure Use of X-rays to image an area of the body.

express (1) Press or squeeze out. (2) Show physical outward signs that reflect genetic make-up, e.g. a dog with certain coat-colour genes will have a black coat.

exsanguinate Remove the blood from.

extensor Muscle whose action is to extend a joint.

external fixation Techniques of fracture fixation where the support is applied externally, for example using an external fixator or a cast.

external fixator A frame of metal pins, connecting bars and clamps that are used externally to support bone fractures; the pins are driven through the skin and into the bone fragments, the pins are then clamped onto the connecting bar which is placed close to (but not touching) the skin surface.

external verifier Person appointed by the RCVS to assist in veterinary nurse training at ATACs and assess the portfolios.

extinction Death of the last remaining members of a species, so that the species no longer exists.

exotoxin Toxic substance produced by growing bacteria and released into the tissues.

extra-articular Outside a joint.

extracapsular Outside a capsule.

extracellular Outside the cell; often used to describe the spaces between cells within the tissues.

extracellular fluid (ECF) Tissue fluid that bathes all the cells of the body; filters out of capillaries and is collected up into the lymphatic system, returning to the circulation via the thoracic duct.

extraction Surgical removal, e.g. extraction of teeth, lens, etc.

extradural Outside the dura mater.

extravasation Escape of fluid (usually from a damaged blood vessel) into the tissues.

extremity The distal part of a limb.

extubation Removal of the endotracheal tube during recovery from anaesthesia; this should be done as soon as the protective laryngeal reflexes are regained.

exudate The fluid that oozes slowly out of damaged capillaries and dries to form a scab.

eye The organ of sight; generally forward-pointing in species that hunt and more laterally located in herbivores.

eyeball The globe of the eye, sitting within the bony orbit; comprises the cornea, aqueous (anterior chamber), lens and ciliary body, vitreous (posterior chamber) and sclera.

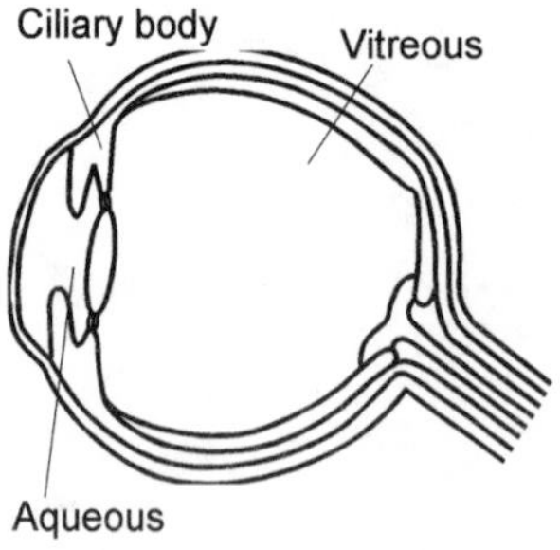

Eye. Cross-section

eyelid The upper and lower folds of skin that move over the eye during the blink reaction; act to protect the eye and spread the tear film over the cornea, *see* ECTROPION, ENTROPION.

eyepiece Lens on a microscope nearest to the user's eyes; contributes to the overall magnification of the object; microscopes may have one or two (binocular) eyepieces.

F

fabella, pl. fabellae Small, paired sesamoid bones that lie just caudal to the stifle joint; they are located in the origins of the gastrocnemius muscle, within the medial and lateral heads where they arise from the respective femoral condyles.

face mask Conical rubber mask that fits over the muzzle of an animal to allow the administration of anaesthetic gases; although available in a variety of sizes, they may not fit all animals and thus, there is increased likelihood of environmental pollution with anaesthetic agents.

facet Small, flat surface on a bone; often a region for muscle attachment or articulation with another bone.

facetectomy Surgical removal of an articular facet; removal of the articular facets of adjacent vertebrae may form part of the dorsal or lateral approach to the spine.

facial nerve Seventh cranial nerve, running from the ventral aspect of the brain, through the facial canal in the petrous temporal bone, and exiting the skull via the stylomastoid foramen. The facial nerve innervates the muscles of facial expression, the lacrimal glands, part of the tongue (carrying taste sensation) and some salivary glands.

facial nerve paralysis Syndrome caused by any lesion along the length of the facial nerve, resulting in paralysis of the facial muscles; more commonly unilateral, but bilateral if the lesion is central within the brain; the face and ear appears to droop on the affected side, saliva may dribble from the mouth, eyelids droop and the blink (menace) response is poor or absent.

facultative Adjective describing bacteria that are able to adapt and live under various conditions.

fading puppy/kitten syndrome A perinatal condition where offspring initially feed well and appear to thrive, but then lose condition, become weak and moribund, and may die. It affects puppies and kittens within the first few weeks of life; generally caused by bacterial or viral infections, particularly herpes virus; non-infectious causes include hypothermia and cardiopulmonary failure; treatment is symptomatic and supportive; the incidence of the condition can be minimised by maintaining good hygiene and ensuring neonates receive adequate colostrum. *E. coli* toxins may cause necrotising pneumonia and renal damage.

faecalith Hard concretion of faeces; may cause tenesmus and pain on defecation, and obstruction of the rectum; faecaliths may also become tangled in the coat around the anus.

faeces Waste material excreted from the gastrointestinal tract; consists of unabsorbed food (mainly fibrous matter), digestive secretions and water.

Fahrenheit Temperature scale; converted to centigrade by applying the formula: degrees centigrade = $^5/_9 \times$ (degrees Fahrenheit – 32).

fainting Syncope; transient loss of consciousness due to insufficient oxygen reaching the brain; boxers are particularly prone to fainting attacks, possibly as a result of high vagal tone slowing the heart rate; also associated with a number of cardiac diseases.

falciform Sickle-shaped, curved.

Fallopian tube Oviduct; tube arising near each ovary and running to the body of the uterus; Fallopian tubes have a fimbriated end at the ovary; they collect the ova released at ovulation and convey them to the uterus, *see also* ECTOPIC.

false pregnancy Pseudopregnancy, phantom pregnancy, pseudocyesis; a condition occurring to some degree in all non-pregnant bitches 6–8 weeks after a season (during metoestrus); the intensity of the signs is variable, it may be unnoticed in some bitches, while others show marked signs; behavioural changes such as nest-building, excitability and protective aggression over toys, etc. are common; the mammary glands enlarge and milk may also be produced; false pregnancy had survival value for ancestral dogs living in packs as it allowed a non-pregnant bitch to provide milk for other puppies whose mother may have had an inadequate supply or a large litter; the condition arises because the corpora lutea that develop in the ovaries after ovulation remain for a similar length of time irrespective of whether the bitch is pregnant or not. With increasing age, false pregnancy is more likely to be complicated by pyometra; treatment options include oestrogens and diuretics and, in the long-term, neutering during anoestrus is advisable.

familial Occurring within close relatives or within a certain line.

Fanconi syndrome A renal disease characterised by multiple defects in absorption from the proximal tubules of the kidney; inherited in the Basenji but may also be secondary to renal injury such as heavy-metal poisoning; protein and glucose appear in the urine, and there may be other electrolyte imbalances; affected animals are polyuric/polydipsic and renal failure may occur acutely.

faradism Physiotherapy technique where specific superficial muscles are stimulated electrically, using pads placed over them; some animals may resent the skin sensation associated with the treatment.

fascia Fibrous connective tissue, also containing fat, which surrounds the body beneath the skin and ensheaths muscles and muscle groups.

Fasciola hepatica Liver fluke; a parasitic trematode worm using a specific snail as an intermediate host and affecting ruminants, horses, man, rats, mice and rabbits; ingested immature flukes migrate to the liver where they develop into the adult form, causing damage to hepatic and biliary tissues; can be controlled by using flukicidal wormers, by draining marshy areas where the snails live or preventing livestock having access to such areas.

fat A large molecule consisting of a glycerol core linked to three fatty acid side chains; in the diet it is a source of fat-soluble vitamins, essential fatty acids and energy; it also enhances the palatability of the food; fat has a higher calorific density than either carbohydrate or protein; surplus dietary calorie intake

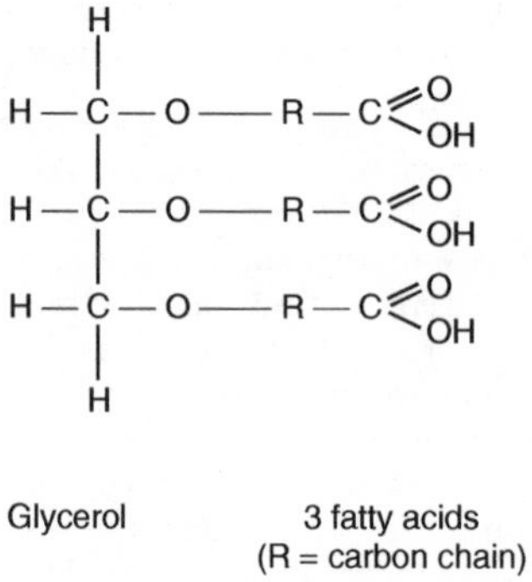

Fat molecule

is stored by the body as fat; most body fat is white fat, but the 1–5% brown fat, deposited mainly around the shoulders and chest, is important for heat production. Radiographically fat is less dense than other soft tissues and thus is useful to outline organs such as the kidneys.

fat pad Triangular area of fatty tissue within the stifle joint, just caudal to the patellar ligament; because the fat pad is less radiodense than the surrounding soft tissue, it appears radiolucent on lateral stifle radiographs and can be useful for assessing joint effusion.

fat soluble Having an affinity for fatty substances and able to be concentrated and stored within them; a number of vitamins are fat soluble, e.g. vitamins A and D.

fatigue Tiredness; may be associated with over-exertion or disease; muscle fatigue describes the physiological response of a single muscle fibre to repetitive stimulation, such that the strength of the contraction reduces as the muscle exhausts its energy supply.

fatty acid A component of fat; some fatty acids cannot be synthesised by the body and must be acquired from the diet. The essential fatty acids include linoleic acid and arachadonic acid (cats only); such fatty acids form part of cell membranes and are used in the synthesis of prostaglandins; deficiency leads to reproductive failure, poor coat and skin, delayed wound healing and emaciation.

feather The plumage of birds, consisting of primary (flight and tail) and secondary feathers and underlying down; each feather has a central shaft that supports many barbs; these in turn give rise to the smaller barbules which interlock with those on adjacent feathers to form a vane, a surface that will produce lift when swept through the air.

feather plucking Common condition of caged birds, possibly due to boredom; may be difficult to correct as it rapidly becomes a habit; changing the environment or providing another bird nearby for company may help; birds may also peck at each others feathers if they are kept in overcrowded conditions.

febrile Pyrexic; having an elevated body temperature; usually a response to infection or pain.

fecundity Fertility.

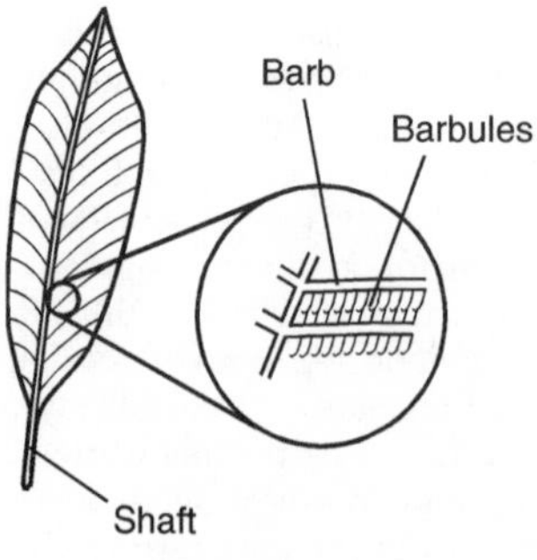

Feather

feedback Part of physiological regulatory responses, where the levels of a particular substance are detected and either increase (positive feedback) or reduce (negative feedback) the production of that substance.

feeding Intake of food; feeding patterns for pets generally fall into one of three categories – free access (*ad libitum*, food always available), time-restricted (food is available for 5–30 minutes at intervals during the day) and meal-restricted (a set amount of food is fed); anorexic patients may be encouraged to feed by feeding a highly palatable diet, adding oil to the diet, warming the food, hand feeding or smearing small amounts on the paws; other feeding techniques include force-feeding, intravenous alimentation, gastrotomy or PEG tube, pharyngostomy or nasogastric tube feeding; intravenous diazepam can also be used to stimulate feeding in cats; calorie and nutrient requirements in the diet should match the metabolic needs of the animal, and it must be remembered that these are increased in disease states.

Felicola subrostratus The cat louse; a macroscopic ectoparasite with six legs and sucking mouth parts; host specific, causing pruritis and alopecia.

feline acquired immunodeficiency syndrome (FAIDS) Syndrome in cats who are immunocompromised, usually secondary to FeLV infection, and thus become susceptible to other pathogens; common conditions associated with FAIDS include gingivitis, enteritis, rhinitis, pyoderma and FIP; secondary bacterial infections may respond to antibiotics, but the prognosis is poor.

feline calici virus (FCV) Small, RNA virus causing oculonasal discharge and oral ulceration after an incubation period of 2–5 days; recovery is usually uneventful, but virulent strains may cause life-threatening pneumonia; treatment is supportive.

feline dysautonomia *see* KEY-GASKELL SYNDROME.

feline herpes virus (FHV) *see* FELINE VIRAL RHINOTRACHEITIS.

feline immunodeficiency virus (FIV) *see* FELINE LEUKAEMIA VIRUS.

feline infectious anaemia (FIA) *see* HAEMOBARTONELLOSIS.

feline infectious enteritis (FIE) *see* PANLEUKOPENIA.

feline infectious peritonitis (FIP) Two disease syndromes caused by a corona virus. The 'wet' form is characterised by a chronic peritonitis, with fluid collecting in the abdomen and chest; this fluid is typically straw-coloured and a sample will foam slightly if shaken. The 'dry' form is more variable in its presentation, but tends to affect the kidney, eye and CNS; serology confirms exposure to the virus; disease often becomes apparent if the cat also acquires FeLV infection.

feline leukaemia virus (FeLV) The virus associated with lymphosarcoma (affecting lymph nodes, thymus, spleen and gut wall); non-regenerative anaemia is common, but only about 10% of cases are actually leukaemic; as the virus damages lymphoid tissue, affected cats become immunosuppressed and more likely to develop other secondary diseases; diagnosis can be confirmed by rapid ELISA testing; vaccines are available.

feline miliary eczema Flea-allergy dermatitis, feline hormonal alopecia; small crusting skin lesions develop predominantly on the dorsum, but may be generalised; these can often best be detected by running a hand through the coat; affected cats spend considerable time licking at pruritic areas and may inflict serious self-trauma, with marked alopecia over the thighs and abdomen; the cause of this common condition is an allergic response to flea bites and thus, rigorous flea control of all animals and the environment is required; corticosteroids may be used in the short term to break the itch–scratch cycle and antibiotics may also be required if the lesions are infected.

feline urological syndrome (FUS) Sandy deposits of struvite (triple phosphate) crystals that commonly block the penile urethra in male, neutered cats; possibly associated with high magnesium dry food diets; if the urethra blocks totally the situation is an emergency; in the short term the obstruction is cleared and the bladder catheterised; in the long term prescription diets can be fed, or urinary acidifiers used to help dissolve crystals.

feline viral rhinotracheitis (FVR) Severe upper respiratory tract disease caused by a herpes virus, with profuse ocular and nasal discharges, pyrexia, buccal ulceration and cough; contagious and may be more severe in young kittens or immunocompromised animals; treatment is supportive; vaccines are available; many recovered cases will become carriers and may shed virus continuously or when stressed, *see also* CAT FLU.

female Individuals having an XX genotype and female reproductive organs.

feminisation Development of external female characteristics by a male; associated with some tumours and hormone treatments.

femoral Relating to the femur and the thigh region.

femur The thigh bone, running from hip to stifle.

fenbendazole A worming preparation.

fenestrated drape Surgical drape with an opening or window cut out of it.

fenestration Cutting out a window or opening.

fentanyl A short-acting opioid analgesic, often combined with a neuroleptic for neuroleptanalgesia.

feral Wild, used to describe colonies of free-living cats.

ferritin A protein found in the liver that acts as a reserve of iron for the body.

fertile Able to reproduce.

fertilisation The penetration of an ovum by a sperm, with fusion of the gametes.

fetal Relating to the fetus.

fetal membranes The two layers surrounding the unborn puppy or kitten are known as the allanto-amnion and the chorioallantois. Usually only recognised when the 'water bag' appears at the vulva during the birth process.

fetid Foul-smelling.

fetus Unborn offspring. The embryo after the fetal membranes develop until birth.

fever Pyrexia; having an elevated body temperature.

fibre Thread-like structure.

fibreglass Mixture of resin and fibres that hardens on contact with air; bandages impregnated with fibreglass can be used for external fracture fixation; the resulting cast is light, waterproof, but more expensive than plaster of Paris.

fibril Filamentous structure; often a fibre will be made up of several fibrils.

fibrillation Rapid, small contractions of muscle fibres, rather than coordinated contraction of the whole muscle.

fibrin An important clotting protein in the blood; formed by the action of thrombin on fibrinogen.

fibrinogen Precursor of fibrin; a globulin protein found in the blood.

fibrinolysis The dissolution and removal of fibrin clots.

fibrinous Made of fibrin.

fibroblast Immature fibrous connective tissue cell that can produce collagen fibres.

fibrocartilage Cartilage rich in type I collagen fibres; found where tendons and ligaments blend into bone.

fibrocyte Mature fibrous connective tissue cell, often dormant and relatively inactive.

fibroma Benign tumour of fibrous connective tissue.

fibrosarcoma Malignant tumour of fibrous connective tissue.

fibrosis Fibrous reaction to an injury.

fibrous Made of fibrous tissue.

fibula Thin bone on the lateral aspect of the hind leg; runs alongside the tibia from the stifle to the hock; distally the fibula forms the lateral malleolus which contributes to the stability of the tibiotarsal joint.

fight wounds Various wounds that result from fights between animals; may be inflicted by teeth or claws; the potential for infection must always be considered; teeth puncture wounds may appear less serious, but damage to deeper structures must always be borne in mind.

field (of microscope) Area within which objects are visible at any particular magnification.

field of vision Area that can be seen by one eye at any one time.

figure-of-eight bandage Method of applying white open-wove (non-conforming) bandage to ensure even pressure is obtained; may also be used when conforming bandage is applied to a tapering region, e.g. tail.

filamentous Made of thin threads.

Filaroides osleri The most common nematode lungworm of the dog; ingested larvae travel in the lymphatics and circulation to the lungs, where they migrate to the tracheal bifurcation; causes a chronic tracheobronchitis and cough, and is usually associated with kennelled animals; diagnosis is best confirmed by bronchoscopy, where characteristic nodules at the tracheal bifurcation or within the bronchi are seen; treatment with suitable anthelminthics is usually effective, *see also* *OSLERUS OSLERI*.

filariasis The presence of filariae in the body tissues or circulation.

film badge Personal radiation monitoring badge, worn on the trunk by staff undertaking radiographic procedures; consists of various thicknesses of metal overlying sensitive film; badges are sent to the National Radiological Protection Board at statutory intervals to ensure that body radiation is below legal limits.

film focal distance (FFD) The distance between the radiographic film and the focal spot in the X-ray tube head; the distance affects the exposure, according to the inverse square law – that is, if the FFD is doubled, the exposure will have to be quadrupled; the greater the FFD, the sharper the image as there is less penumbral blurring, *see also* PENUMBRA.

filter Sheet of aluminium or copper in the X-ray tube head that absorbs radiation of a low energy that would not contribute to a diagnostic image.

filum Thread-like structure.

filum terminale Thin, fibrous continuation of the pia mater (the innermost meningeal layer) from the end of the spinal cord to the coccygeal vertebrae.

fimbrium, pl. fimbria Fringe, e.g. at the end of the oviduct.

fin Webbing of skin stretched across supporting bones and used for locomotion by fish.

fin rot Term used to describe various conditions of the fin; may be caused by bites from other fish, *Oodinium* spp. and infections; treatment depends on the specific cause.

firearms certificate Licence granted by the police that must be held by all veterinary surgeons who have humane killers such as captive bolt pistols.

first aid Immediate life-saving aid that may be given without the need for any drugs, medication or specialist equipment.

first intention healing How sutured surgical wounds heal – the epithelial layers are held in apposition, fibroblasts migrate across the wound and there is minimal scarring.

fissure Deep furrow.

fistula Abnormal tube connecting two epithelial surfaces, e.g. vaginorectal fistulae linking the vagina to the rectum may occur after whelping; if material regularly passes through the fistula the connection develops its own epithelial lining and becomes permanently patent, e.g. teat fistulae will not heal while the animal continues to produce milk which passes through the opening.

fit Lay term for a convulsion or seizure, *see also* EPILEPSY.

fixation, external Any method of fracture fixation using apparatus applied to the outside of the limb, e.g. splinting, casting, external fixator frames.

fixation, internal Any method of fracture fixation involving the use of implants within the bone or on the bone surface, e.g. intramedullary pinning, plating, tension band wiring, rush pinning, etc.

fixative (1) A chemical that denatures protein, hardening and preserving tissue samples, e.g. formalin. (2) In radiography, the chemical solution that dissolves and removes unexposed silver bromide crystals from the radiographic film, and hardens the film.

flaccid Limp, relaxed, lacking tone.

flagellum Whip-like tail attached to many protozoa, some bacteria and cells such as sperm; used for locomotion.

flail chest Segment of the thoracic wall which becomes free-moving as a result of multiple rib fractures; the free segment is sucked inwards by the negative pressure produced during inspiration, and compromises respiratory function; treatment consists of stabilising the fragment to an external frame.

flank Lateral body wall between the last rib and the hind leg.

flare, aqueous Bright reflection of light from particles within the anterior chamber of the eye.

flatulence Gas in the digestive tract.

flea Common ectoparasitic insect, living mainly in the environment, but moving onto warm-blooded animals to feed on their blood; intermediate host for part of the lifecycle of *Dipylidium caninum*, the common tapeworm of the dog; life cycle can be as short as 3 weeks under suitable conditions, or eggs can remain dormant for many months if necessary.

flea allergy dermatitis *see* FELINE MILIARY ECZEMA.

flexion Movement of a joint such that the angle between the articulating bones reduces.

flexor Muscle whose action is to bring about flexion of a joint.

flexure A bend.

floaters Small bodies within the vitreous of the eye.

flocculent Tending to precipitate and form irregular fluffy masses.

flotatation Laboratory technique where faecal samples are mixed with sugar or salt solutions of a high specific gravity; worm eggs will float in this solution and stick to a cover slip floated on the surface.

flowmeter Part of an anaesthetic circuit used to regulate the flow of gases to the patient; scale is marked in l/min, and a float in the chamber is used to take the reading, most floats have a dot on them which shows that the float is rotating and gas is flowing (rotameter).

fluid therapy The use of blood, plasma or synthetic fluids to replace deficits; may be administered intravenously, subcutaneously, intraperitoneally and intraosseously; fluid therapy supports the cardiovascular system, maintains renal perfusion and urine output; an important component of the treatment for many disorders, including shock.

fluothane *see* HALOTHANE.

fluorescein Fluorescent dye that can be used to demonstrate corneal ulcers, check the patency of the nasolacrimal duct, etc.

fluorescent Able to absorb light of one wavelength and emit light of a longer wavelength.

fluoroquinolones Important group of antibacterial agents effective against Gram-negative organisms. Used in the treatment of otitis media due to *Pseudomonas* and for enteric infections such as *Salmonella*, *see also* ENFLOXIN, CIPROFLOXACIN

fluoroscopy Radiographic technique where X-rays are generated and passed continuously through the area of interest; the image is formed on a fluorescent screen, providing a moving image; useful for guided catheterisation of vessels, evaluating gut peristalsis/swallowing, etc.

focal Restricted to one defined area.

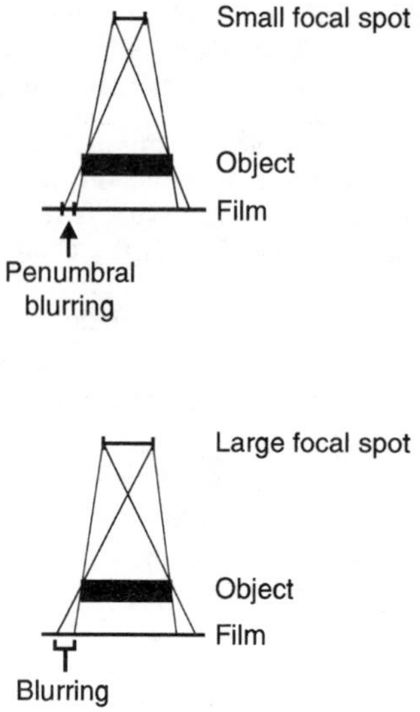

Focal spot

focal spot The area on the target in an X-ray tube head where the electrons strike; the region where the radiation is produced; the smaller the focal spot the sharper the resulting radiographic image as there is less blurring.

fogging Radiographic term describing lack of definition in the finished radiograph; causes are overdevelopment or inadequate rinsing after fixation.

folate One of the vitamin B complex.

Foley catheter Indwelling urinary catheter with a soft bulb at one end that can be inflated with air or water to hold the catheter tip in the bladder.

follicle Collection of cells with a central hollow or cavity, e.g. ovarian follicles surrounding developing ova.

follicle stimulating hormone (FSH) Hormone released from the anterior pituitary; stimulates the formation and maturation of Graafian follicles within the ovary; in the male it increases spermatogenesis.

folliculitis Inflammation of hair follicles, with the formation of papules and pustules.

fomentation Application of heat to an area, e.g. use of a poultice.

fomite An inanimate object, such as a grooming brush or feed bowl, that may transmit disease-causing organisms.

fontanelle The junction between two cranial bones in the immature animal.

food Dietary material that is consumed to meet nutritional needs.

food hypersensitivity Allergic reaction to a component of the diet, *see* WHEAT-SENSITIVE ENTEROPATHY.

foot and mouth disease Highly contagious, viral, notifiable disease of cloven-hoofed animals; characterised by the appearance of vesicles around the mouth, between the digits, etc; the MAFF must be informed if the disease is suspected, and a slaughter policy operates in the UK.

foramen Hole or aperture.

foramen magnum The opening in the occipital bone of the skull that allows the exit of the spinal cord and its enveloping meningeal membranes.

foramen ovale The hole in the septum between the atria in the fetal heart; this allows blood to bypass the lungs in the fetus, and it normally closes at birth.

foramenotomy Surgical enlargement of a foramen; may be used as part of the lateral surgical approach to the spinal cord, where enlargement of a spinal foramen between two adjacent vertebrae allows decompression of the exiting spinal nerve.

force feeding Providing food for a patient who refuses to eat voluntarily.

forceps Instrument for gripping and holding tissues; common types include Allis tissue forceps, bone holding forceps, dressing forceps and rat-toothed forceps.

forearm Region from the elbow to the carpus.

forebrain Cerebral hemispheres and thalamus.

foregut The cranial portion of the gut in the developing embryo, becoming the pharynx, oesophagus, stomach and duodenum.

foreign body Any object within the body that is not self, e.g. piece of grit, shard of glass, barley awn, swallowed golf ball, etc.

formaldehyde Formic acid; a pungent disinfectant and tissue fixative; the vapour is toxic.

formalin A 37% aqueous solution of formaldehyde, used as a standard tissue fixative.

formulation The chemical preparations of a drug, e.g. ointment, tablet, powder, liquid.

formulary A collection of drug formulae and dosing information, e.g. *British National Formulary*.

fornix Arch-shaped structure.

fossa Dent or depression, usually in the surface of a bone.

fovea Cup-shaped depression or small pit.

fractionate Separate out the components of a mixture.

fracture Complete break in the integrity of a bone; usually a result of trauma, but can occur with little force if the bone is diseased, e.g. fracture at the site of an osteosarcoma.

fracture disease Less than optimal return to function after bony union at a fracture site; may be caused by malunion, nerve damage, muscle contracture, fibrosis, etc.

fracture healing The physiological method by which a fracture heals; if there is a gap of more than a few millimetres between the bone ends, the initial haematoma organises into a fibrous callus which calcifies and finally ossifies; if the fracture is rigidly immobilised and there are no gaps or only small gaps between the fragments, direct bony union can occur; direct bony union is the more rapid process, but the repair is not as strong initially as callus.

fracture-separation Type of fracture occurring in skeletally immature animals, where the fracture line is at the level of a growth plate; commonly divided into the Salter–Harris types I–V.

fragmented coronoid process The most common lesion of elbow dysplasia; the medial coronoid process of the ulna fails to develop correctly, and forms one or more loose fragments which irritate the joint and cause secondary arthrosis, *see also* ELBOW DYSPLASIA.

French moult Rapid shedding of flight and tail feathers, making affected birds unable to fly; exact cause is unknown.

frenulum Band of connective tissue on the ventral aspect of the tongue.

friable Brittle, crumbling.

frontal bone Bone of the skull forming the forehead and dorso-medial aspect of the orbit.

frontal sinus Air spaces within the frontal bone which communicate with the nasal passages.

frostbite Damage to tissue due to extreme cold; ear tips, toes and tail are most commonly affected; affected areas become erythematous initially but then slough.

fructose Fruit sugar.

frusemide Commonly used diuretic, promoting the excretion of potassium and loss of water via the kidneys. A loop diuretic.

full-pin splintage Type of external fixator frame where the pins enter the limb, penetrate both cortices of the bone and exit through the skin on the far side, thus allowing connecting bars to be placed on two sides of the limb.

fulminating Occurring suddenly and rapidly worsening.

fumigation Use of a gas or vapour to disinfect the environment.

fundus The lowest part of a hollow organ, or the part furthest away from the opening. Used to describe the posterior surface of the eyeball as seen by the ophthalmoscope.

fungal Relating to a fungal infection.

fungus, pl. fungi Yeasts and moulds; some are commensals, some are opportunistic pathogens while others always cause disease, *see also* *CANDIDA*, *MALASSEZIA*, *MICROSPORUM CANIS*, MYCOSIS, RINGWORM, *TRYCHOPHYTON* SPP.

funicular Cord-like.

fur The hair coat of animals, characteristic of mammals.

furunculosis Deep pyoderma, *see also* ANAL FURUNCULOSIS.

fusiform Spindle-shaped.

G

gags Metal objects used in veterinary dentistry; sometimes a roll of bandage between the molar teeth or a wooden block with a drilled hole is utilised to help pass a stomach tube.

gagging Description of a choking/retching mechanism often associated with vomiting as a reflex.

gait Movement.

galactic Relating to milk.

galactose Monosaccharide derived from lactose, important in kitten and puppy nutrition and it is converted to glucose in the liver.

gall bladder Structure in the liver for bile storage, connects by the bile ducts to the duodenum.

gallipot Small container used in pharmacy for ointments and lotions.

gallop rhythm Heart disorder where the beat is very rapid and similar to the beat of a horse's fastest gait.

gamete Mature sex cell – the sperm of the male or the ovum of the female.

Gamgee Dressing composed of a thick layer of absorbent cotton between two layers of gauze.

gamma (γ) Third letter of the Greek alphabet; was often used to describe newer words for globulins and in radiation studies, *see also* GAMMA RAYS, GLOBULIN, RADIATION.

gamma globulin Any of a class of protein present in the blood stream, as almost all are immunoglobulins; often used as a measure of immunity.

gamma linoleic acid (GLA) One of the lipids responsible for mediating the anti-inflammatory reaction.

gamma rays Rays emitted by radioactive substances that have severe cytotoxic effects.

ganglion A group of nerve cells important in the interchange of signals, some distance away from the central nervous system, *see also* PARASYMPATHETIC NERVOUS SYSTEM, SYMPATHETIC.

gangrene Death and decay of part of the body, due to a failure of the blood supply, toxins, burns, etc., *see also* NECROSIS.

gangrenous mastitis Toxins from infections such as *Staphylococcus* may cause necrosis of part of the mammary gland.

gas Usually invisible vapour in which the particles are diffusely suspended, e.g. anaesthetic gas. **Alveolar gas** The gas used in respiration that remains in the alveoli, *see also* ANATOMIC DEAD SPACE.

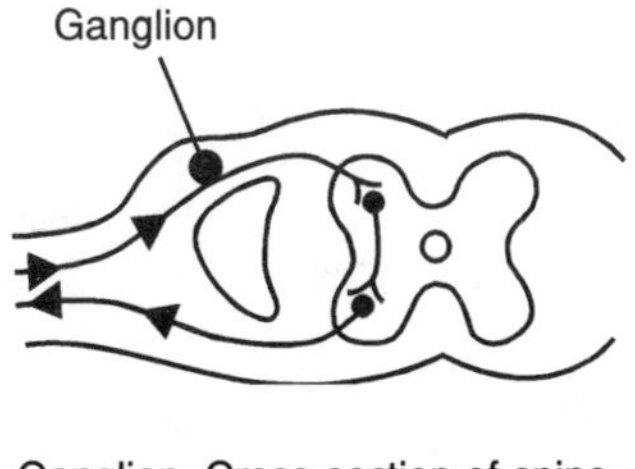

Ganglion. Cross-section of spine showing dorsal root ganglion

gaseous products of digestion (GPD) Gases that escape from the body as part of the digestive process.

gaskin Portion of the hind leg muscles proximal to the hock. This term is rarely used in dogs.

gastric Relates to the stomach.

gastric dilation Distension of the stomach with gas, a disorder usually affecting the larger breeds of dog; arises mainly soon after feeding and can rapidly become life-threatening as it impairs respiration. May be due to pyloric dysfunction or a foreign body, torsion, atonic muscles, *see also* AEROPHAGY, TYMPANY.

gastric dilation/volvulus (GDV) Acute illness seen in deep-chested dogs where the stomach inflates and then rotates, often involving a rotation of the spleen and then a profound vascular change affecting venous return; this is an emergency.

gastric emptying time Physiologically important, can be demonstrated with contrast radiography; may be used diagnostically.

gastric haemorrhage Blood appears in the vomit; indicates a bleeding ulcer or a foreign body.

gastric lavage Used to remove toxic or excess stomach contents; a technique using two tubes: one to pump in and a wider bore one to drain out gastric contents; can be improvised.

gastric torsion The disease state where the stomach has rotated through 180° or 360° so that gas can no longer escape up the oesophagus.

gastric tympany A condition when the stomach is gas filled and there has been some inability to release it.

gastric ulcer Occurs in the mucosal layer, of significance when medication has been used, *see also* NON-STEROIDAL ANTI-INFLAMMATORY DRUG.

gastrin Hormone produced by the 'G' cells of the fundus; stimulates the production of acid secretions.

gastritis Inflammation of the lining of the stomach. Bacteria such as *Helicobacter*, or food toxins in the stomach or some disease elsewhere in the body, may be involved.

gastro- Relating to the stomach.

gastrocentesis Puncture of the stomach to relieve gas distension, usually an emergency procedure.

gastrocnemius Muscle of the hind limb connecting the distal femur to the os calcis of the tibia, extends the hock on contraction.

gastroenteritis Inflammation of the lining of the stomach and the intestine – usually seen as sickness and diarrhoea or 'd and v'.

gastroscope Endoscope designed to examine the interior of the stomach; it is necessary that it should be flexible to curve to see all the surfaces of the organ.

gastrotomy Incision into the stomach.

gauze, absorbent Wound dressing with open mesh weave.

gecko Small reptile, sometimes kept as an exotic pet.

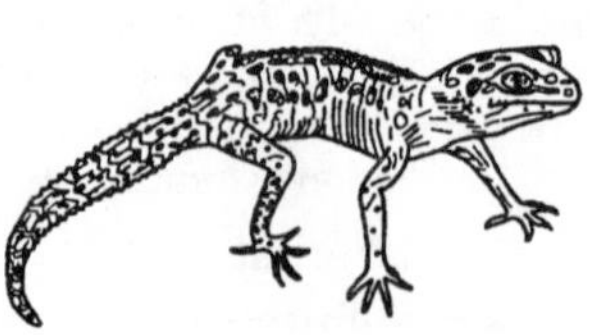

Gecko

gel Suspension of colloid with a firm consistency. Used in laboratory tests for diffusion techniques.

gelatin Pliable substance produced by digesting collagen; is used for medicinal capsules and in a modified form as a surgical dressing often as a foam.

geld Traditional word for neutering farm animals. The sow gelders had basic surgical skill but no anaesthetics. Castrated horses are still known as geldings.

gene The basic unit of genetic material found on the chromosome in the cell nucleus, a sequence of base pairs on the DNA strand. **Dominant gene** One that produces its effect in the offspring regardless of the other allele. **Lethal gene** One that brings about the death of the organism. **Mutant gene** The 'rogue' that has mutated to produce a different characteristic. **Recessive gene** One that produces its effect in the offspring only when both alleles are the same, *see also* HOMOZYGOUS.

gene alleles Different forms of the same gene occupying the same locus on the chromosome.

gene mapping Modern technology used to study the gene locus.

gene selection Breeding strategies; eventually will eliminate hereditary disorders.

general anaesthesia Method of muscle relaxation with pain removal by rendering the central nervous system inert, produced by inhalation or injection of an anaesthetic or analgesic drug.

general anaesthetic (GA) Loss of consciousness brought about by administering anaesthetic agents.

General Sales List (GSL) Pharmaceutical category of medicines that may be sold to the pet owner without restriction.

genetics The science of studying inheritance.

genial Relating to the chin.

genicular Relating to the knee.

genital Relating to the organs of reproduction, especially the visible external organs. As an adjective, the word 'genitals' is incorrect, *see also* GENITALIA.

genitalia Popular term for the external parts of the reproductive organs, *see also* PENIS, VULVA.

genome The complete set of hereditary factors comprising all the genes in the chromosomes.

genotype The genetic make up that leads to a particular configuration, *see also* PHENOTYPE.

gentamicin Antibiotic effective against mainly Gram-negative bacteria but because of toxicity is often used as a topical application only.

Genu valgum Angulation of the femur and the tibia to produce a condition of the knee joint equivalent to 'knock knees'.

genus Group classification of organisms, higher than 'species'.

gerbil Small mammal and popular child's pet.

geriatric Refers to the state of ageing and to disease of old animals.

gestation The time of pregnancy from fertilisation to birth.

glomerular filtration rate (GFR) A measure of renal blood flow.

Giardia Parasitic organism, motile when examined in fresh faeces due to presence of flagellae. Species cause disease in cats and dogs, often an intractable diarrhoea with the presence of mucus and blood.

Giemsa Stain used in the microscopic examination of differential blood films, protozoal parasites, bacteria, etc.

Gigli saw Fine wire chain that is used to saw through bone as in the amputation of the forelimb through the humerus.

gill The external apparatus of the fish to obtain oxygen from the surrounding water, equivalent in function to the mammal's lung.

Gillies needle holder Needle holder with a short blade to cut the suture material included near the points of the forceps.

gingiva The gum.

gingivitis Inflammation of the gums, often seen as a red rim at the margin with the teeth, *see also* PERIODONTITIS.

ginglymus Joint in which movement occurs in one plane; the knee and the elbow joints are the commonest examples.

girdle An encircling structure, e.g. the pelvic girdle.

gizzard Muscular digestive organ in birds, often contains grit or small stones. It may be the site of parasitic worms.

gland A group of cells organised to produce a secretion or an excretion, traditionally divided into the two groups endocrine and exocrine.

gland of Harder Term once used for the nictitans gland on the inner surface of the third eyelid.

gland of Moll Modified sweat glands at the edge of the eyelid.

glans The tip of the penis, enlarges with altered blood flow.

glaucoma Increased intra-ocular pressure; pressure on the retina may result in loss of vision; a series of pathological conditions develop varying with the pressure increase and its consequences, *see also* AQUEOUS, CLOSED ANGLE GLAUCOMA, OPEN ANGLE GLAUCOMA, UVEITIS.

glenoid cavity Hollow depression in the ventral part of the scapula, for articulation with the head of the humerus.

glia (neuroglia) Special connective tissue of the central nervous system, glial cells make up about 40% of the brain.

gliosis The loss of neural elements, especially in the retina of the eye following some form of injury.

globe (eye) The optic globe is the equivalent of the eyeball.

globulin Protein substance with large molecules, imunoglobulins are produced by the plasma cells and have an important role in immunity. Serum protein electrophoresis divides the globulins into five groups ranging through α, β and γ. The gamma (γ) globulins have the most important function in 'humoral' immunity.

glomerular filtrate The product in the kidney of diffusion from the blood stream of low protein ultrafiltrate of plasma into the low pressure of Bowman's capsule ready to pass into the tubules.

glomerulonephritis Inflammation of the filtering glomeruli of the kidney, characterised by urine samples that are very rich in protein.

glomerulus The tuft of capillaries contained in the cup-like Bowman's capsule of a nephron. Fed by afferent arterioles and drained by efferent arterioles.

glossal Relating to the tongue.

glossotrichia Condition seen in cocker spaniels and other breeds, where hairs emerge from the tongue dorsum.

glottis The vocal apparatus, consists of a space between the vocal cords, and is that part of the larynx that produces sounds such as barking, mewing, purring.

glove, radiography Fine layers of lead within the gloves give some protection to the hands. The gloved hands should not be placed in the primary beam.

glove, surgical Latex rubber capable of being sterilised or already packed sterile. Closed and open gloving methods may be used in applying them to the hands.

gloving The procedure of donning sterile gloves so that there is no contamination from the hands or clothing, preserving the asepsis of the procedure.

glucagon Hormone produced by the pancreas, that causes an increase in the blood sugar level.

glucocorticoid Any one of a group of corticosteroids that are essential for the utilisation of carbohydrate, fat and protein by the body. Both natural production and synthetic hormones have powerful anti-inflammatory effects.

gluconeogenesis Biochemical process where glucose is synthesised from non-carbohydrate sources in the body.

glucose A simple sugar used by the body as an important energy source. Any glucose not needed for energy is stored as glycogen.

glucosuria The presence of glucose in the urine, *see also* DIABETES MELLITUS.

glutamic–oxaloacetic transaminase (GOT) *see* SGOT.

glutamic–pyruvic transaminase (GPT) *see* SGPT.

gluteal Muscle mass of the hip, used to extend, abduct and rotate the thigh.

gluten The protein found in wheat and in other cereal grains, *see also* DIETARY HYPERSENSITIVITY, MALABSORPTION, WHEAT-SENSITIVE ENTEROPATHY.

gluteraldehyde Compound used for the cold sterilisation of instruments such as endoscopes, produces irritant vapours and must be handled carefully. Also used as a tissue fixative for electron microscopy.

glycaemia Implies the presence of glucose in the blood, *see also* HYPOGLYCAEMIA, HYPERGLYCAEMIA.

glycerol Clear viscous solution with a sweetish taste, used as an enema in cats and topically to moisten the skin. Also known as glycerine when used pharmaceutically.

glycine A non-essential amino acid, functions as an inhibitory neurotransmitter in the CNS.

glycogen Storage form of carbohydrate, formed and stored in the liver and muscles.

gnatho- Relates to something involved with the jaws.

gnotiobiotic animal An animal reared in a way to exclude normal bacteria – born 'germ free' it may be infected with one organism to study the response.

goblet cell Simple glands whose function is to secrete mucus; may be found in the lining of epithelial surfaces.

goitre Condition seen as a swelling of the neck from enlargement of the thyroid gland.

Golgi Name given to the organelle complex in the cell, consists of a series of tubes that store lysosomal enzymes.

gonad Male or female reproductive gland that produces the gametes, *see also* OVARY, TESTIS.

gonadotropin Any of those hormones synthesised by the pituitary gland that have an effect on the gonads, *see also* FOLLICLE STIMULATING HORMONE, LUTEINISING HORMONE.

goniometer Special lens instrument for measuring intra-ocular pressure by measuring iridio-corneal angles, *see also* OPEN ANGLE GLAUCOMA, CLOSED ANGLE GLAUCOMA.

gonioscopy The junction between the iris and the cornea is viewed directly using the special lens.

gonitis Inflammation of the stifle (femoro-tibial) joint.

gouge A curved chisel used in orthopaedic operations to cut and remove bone.

gracilis muscle A fine 'slender' muscle that connects the pelvic symphysis to the tibial crest; adducts.

Graffian follicle Small follicles containing oocytes that develop in the ovary, they mature to release ova and become converted into corpora lutea.

Graefe's knife A knife with fine point used in cataract surgery.

graft operation Any tissue or organ that is removed from one site and located elsewhere.

gram Unit of mass equivalent to one thousandth of a kilogram.

Gram's stain Staining of bacteria by application of dyestuffs, iodine and ethanol: those that retain the crystal violet colour are Gram-positive and those that can be decolourised and retain carbol fuschin, a red dye, are Gram-negative organisms.

grand mal (fit) Major convulsive attack, as occurs in epileptic fits, *see also* EPILEPSY, SEIZURES.

granulation, healing by Process of wound healing where fibroblasts and vascular elements progressively fill up a wound defect so that eventually epithelium can grow across.

granulocytes White cells of the blood that have granules in the cytoplasm and a multilobed nucleus – neutrophils, eosinophils, basophils. Also known as polymorph leukocytes.

granuloma Description of a tissue mass that has an appearance similar to granulation tissue. May appear like a tumour but is usually due to a chronic inflammatory process.

grass seeds Spiky grass awns may penetrate the skin or cause severe irritation on entering orifices such as the ears, mouth, eye lids and prepuce, *see also* OTITIS EXTERNA, INTERDIGITAL ABSCESS.

gravid Pregnant, *see also* PRIMIGRAVIDA, MULTIGRAVIDA.

grazed wounds Abrasions, open wounds; often the result of friction in road accidents, etc.

grid Structure like a grating, used in radiography as a series of vertical lead strips that reduce or eliminate scatter from the primary beam.

griseofulvin An antibiotic administered by mouth to treat fungal infections of the skin such as ringworm; should be handled with care: teratogenic.

grit Part of a bird's diet, required by the gizzard to help process hard foods such as seeds.

growth hormone Anterior pituitary hormone that regulates the rate of growth of the long bone.

growth plate Known as the epiphyseal plate, is found as cartilage at the ends of most bones in young animals, *see also* PHYSIS, ENDOCHONDRAL OSSIFICATION.

gubernaculum Fibrous band that connects the testis to the scrotum aiding the descent of the gonad from the abdomen to the adult male's position.

guinea-pig Small mammal and a popular pet, of South American origin. Reputedly domesticated 3000 years ago, prefer a dry cold winter due to their original habitat.

guppy Small warm water fish, grows to 4 cm or more.

gut (1) Popular word for any part of the intestinal tract. (2) Name of soluble suture material, *see also* CATGUT.

guttate Resembling a drop of water.

gutter splint External splint shaped to support a fractured limb.

gynaecomastia The mammary glands of a male resembling those of a female about to lactate. A disease sign of some hormonal imbalance.

gyrus Convolution of the brain surface, in the cerebral cortex, between the sulci (clefts).

H

habit Behaviour pattern acquired by frequent repetition of some act.

hachement Used in physiotherapy as a hacking action to massage muscles.

hackles Hairs at the crest of the neck, raised during anger or fright situations to protect and to threaten. Most obvious in terriers and other dog breeds.

haem- Stem word to denote blood (hem- in USA).

haemagglutination Ability of an antibody or virus, etc., to cause agglutination clumping of erythrocytes.

haemagglutination inhibition (HI) test Method of testing for viral antibodies in serum.

haemangiectesis Blood under the skin surface associated with dilated blood vessels.

haemangioma Benign tumour of blood vessels, found especially in the spleen and sometimes under the skin.

haemangiopericytoma A vascular tumour containing spindle cells.

haemangiosarcoma Malignant tumour most commonly found in the spleen but occurs at other vascular sites of the body.

Haemaphysalis leporispalustria One of the common rabbit ticks, also lives on other small mammals and birds.

haematemesis The vomiting of blood. May appear bright red if fresh or a 'coffee grounds' appearance suggests contact of the blood with the gastric juices' acidity.

haematidrosis Appearance of blood in the sweat.

haematin Chemical derived from the breakdown of blood that still contains iron.

haematinuria The presence of blood in the urine.

haemato- Stem word for blood (hemeto- in USA).

haematocele An accumulation of blood in a cavity.

haematochezia Blood in the faeces that is obviously fresh and red, *see also* OCCULT BLOOD.

haematocrit The measurement of the percentage of erythrocytes in the whole of the blood. The term is also used for the tubes used to centrifuge heparinised blood, *see also* PACKED CELL VOLUME.

haematogenous Carried in the blood stream.

haematological tests Relating to the examination of blood cells; does not include blood biochemistry.

haematoma Swelling caused by extravasated blood; result of an injury to the blood vessels or a clotting disorder.

haematopoiesis Formation of blood cells.

haematosalpinx An accumulation of blood in the uterine tube.

haematoscheole Accumulation of blood in the scrotum after a castration.

haematoxylin Natural blue dyestuff used as a microscope stain, often combined with eosin to study tissues histologically. Haematoxylin and eosin stain is used in histology, known as H&E.

haematuria The presence of blood in the urine; the urine may be bright red or smoky brown in colour depending on how recently the blood was lost.

haemobartonellosis Haemolytic anaemia disease produced by a group of intracellular organisms that parasitise blood cells. *Haemobartonella felis* is the cause of feline infectious anaemia and may be associated with lowered immunity as with feline leukaemia.

haemoconcentration Loss of the fluid components of plasma leads to an increased concentration of blood cells, used to measure conditions such as shock and dehydration.

haemocytometer Counting chamber instrument (Improved Neubauer) for counting blood cells, used under the microscope – the kit includes pipettes and cover glasses.

haemodialysis Technique used to remove toxic products from the blood during renal failure, across a semi-permeable membrane.

haemoglobin Protein/iron compound found within the red blood cells, transports oxygen from the lungs to the body tissues.

haemoglobinuria Colouration of the urine due to the presence of haemoglobin; indicates severe blood haemolysis.

haemolysis Breakdown of red blood cells so that haemoglobin is released into the plasma. Occurs in samples of blood incorrectly handled and makes testing more difficult. Haemolysis will occur in the living animal in some types of anaemia, in toxic conditions and immune reactions.

haemolytic anaemia A reduction in the number of erythrocytes caused by an agent damaging the cells.

haemopericardium Accumulation of blood in the pericardial space; may result from chest injury, tumours or rupture of a blood vessel.

haemoperitoneum Blood loss into the peritoneal cavity; may be tested for by paracentesis.

haemophilia Disorder where blood clots slowly, hereditary disorder and may be a cause of neonatal death, *see also* VON WILLEBRAND DISEASE, VON WILLEBRAND FACTOR.

haemopneumothorax Life-threatening condition, often the result of a road accident, when there is an accumulation of both blood and air in the pleural space.

haemopoiesis The formation of blood cells including platelets.

haemoptysis Coughing up blood; rare in domestic animals but indicates lung trauma.

haemorrhage The loss of blood from arteries, veins or capillaries. Haemorrhage may be classified as internal or external, other descriptions describe the location or the time it occurred, *see also* EPISTAXIS, REACTIONARY, HAEMORRHAGE.

haemorrhagic gastroenteritis (HGE) An acute disease often associated with allergy or *E. coli* toxin.

haemosiderin Form of iron stored by the cells, usually derived from diet or excess haemolysis.

haemostasis The arrest of haemorrhage; involves pressure applied to blood vessels, natural retraction and clot formation.

haemostat (1) Method of stopping blood loss. (2) The name given to instruments such as artery forceps.

hair Keratinised thread-like structure arising from the hair bulb of the epidermis. Characteristic of mammals, pigmentation and hair length differs in the species and the individual strains, e.g. dog and cat breeds. **Guard hair** Stiffer hairs that form the outer protective coat. **Lanugo hair** Fine hairs formed during fetal development. **Wool hair** Hairs that form the undercoat, make up the soft 'puppy' coat and are the insulating layer closest to the skin of adults.

hairball Characteristic of cats that lick guard hairs which then accumulate in the stomach; most cats vomit these as sausage shaped pellets. If not removed can cause an obstruction.

half-life (1) The time taken for 50% of a drug to be excreted by the body. (2) Similarly, the time of radioactive isotope decay.

halide salts Chemical group of halogen elements, includes iodine, chlorine and fluorine. Silver halide is used in X-ray film.

halitosis Breath odour which is unduly offensive, *see also* LABIAL ECZEMA.

hallucogenic An agent that affects the brain and produces a false perception. Controlled drugs listed as Schedule 1 (S1) are not substances that veterinary surgeons may purchase in the UK.

halogen An element of the group bromine, chlorine, fluorine, iodine.

halothane Volatile liquid anaesthetic substance, administered by inhalation. It is made from a halogenated hydrocarbon which decomposes in ultra-violet light.

Halsted sutures Pattern of interrupted suture used in organ closure, of special value for friable tissue repair.

Halti Pattern of head collar used in dog training.

Hammondia Species of protozoa found in the intestine of cats. Oocysts appear similar to *Toxoplasma*; the intermediate host is the rat.

hamster Small brown mammal frequently kept as a child's pet. Includes the golden hamster *Mesocricetus auratus* and the common (brown) hamster *Cricetus cricetus*.

hangers Metal structures used in radiographic processing to stretch and dry film. Channel and clip varieties are used.

haploid Condition in the gamete cells where only half the normal number of chromosomes are present, *see also* DIPLOID.

hard palate Structure that forms the roof of the mouth, made up of the three bones maxilla, premaxilla and palatine covered with tough mucous membrane.

Harderian gland Name formerly used for the nictitans gland that occupies the inner surface of the third eyelid, *see also* NICTITANS GLAND.

hardpad Traditional name for the form of canine distemper where hyperkeratosis of nose and foot pads was seen. The word was associated in dog breeders' minds with severe or fatal virus infections.

hare lip Failure of the upper lips to fuse during embryonic development; a congenital disease, may be inherited as a recessive gene, *see also* CLEFT PALATE.

Hartmann's solution Solution used for fluid therapy, isotonic containing balanced sodium, potassium and calcium chlorides, phosphates and lactates. Known also as Ringer-lactate.

harvest mites Surface mites that cause intense pruritus of dog's feet, scabs and crusts may be present; most often seen in the autumn after walking in fields, etc.; caused by larval forms of *Trombicula* or *Neotrombicula autumnalis.*

Haversian system Bone structure of microscopic concentric lamellae with a central canal for nutrition of compact bone; carries blood vessels, nerves and lymphatics.

haws Protrusion of the third eyelid, a term used by cat owners for the third eyelid syndrome. Dog owners use the term to refer to exposure of the lower lid also.

hay Fed to rabbits or if used as bedding, it forms a diet supplement. Good quality hay has 8–12% protein, 30–35% fibre and is a good source of carotene.

Hayem's solution Laboratory solution used for diluting blood for red cell counts.

head The anterior part of a bone or more specifically the front of the animal that contains the brain and the organs of special sense.

'head-gland' disease Disorder of puppies characterised by oedematous nose and the face below the eyes; may become pus filled and local lymph nodes then discharge purulent material.

heart Hollow organ responsible for the blood circulation by the muscular contraction of the four chambers. Divided by a septum, the left and right chambers contract synchronously controlled by the electrical impulses from the sino-atrial (S–A) node.

heart block Term used to describe an interruption in the rhythm as the conduction of the electrical impulses from the S–A node is impaired.

heart failure Condition in which the pumping action of the ventricles is inadequate, *see also* MYOCARDIAL DEGENERATION.

heart valve One of four devices inside the heart that allow for the forward propulsion of blood when the heart muscles contract, squeezing the blood inside the heart. Variously known as aortic, mitral, pulmonary and tricuspid valves.

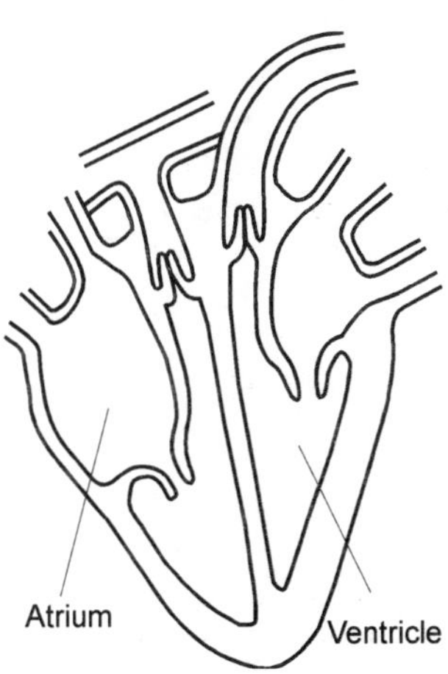

Heart. Cross-section

heartworm Parasitic condition in dogs, with blocking of the pulmonary artery by numerous *Dirofilaria immitis* worms. Confined mainly to southern areas of UK but widespread in USA.

heat In addition to the usual meaning of a raise in temperature, it is popularly used to describe the onset of oestrus in dogs and cats.

heat stroke Condition of collapse associated with an elevated body temperature, haemoconcentration and failure of body enzyme systems, *see also* HYPERTHERMIA.

heat of nutritient metabolism (HNM) Produced by the intermediary metabolism of absorbed nutrients.

hedgehog Small mammal with spiny exterior, species *Erinaceus*.

Heimlich manoeuvre Technique to dislodge a foreign body stuck in the trachea or the back of the throat. May be attempted in dogs with care.

Heimlich valve One-way valve put into a chest drainage system to prevent influx of air.

Heinz bodies Found on examining blood smears, as dark stains in the erythrocytes, in cases of haemolytic regenerating anaemia.

Helicobacter Bacteria found in the intestinal tract of domestic species, specially adapted to resist the acid of the stomach wall. Have been associated with gastritis, especially in cats which have their own subspecies *H. felis*.

helminth Description for parasitic worms that include cestodes, nematodes and trematodes.

hemeralopia Defective vision in bright light, also known as day blindness, *see also* CENTRAL PROGRESSIVE RETINAL ATROPHY.

hemi- Used to denote words where 'half' is the important feature.

hemianopia Blindness of one half of the visual field as in unilateral injury to the optic nerve tracts.

hemilaminectomy Operation to remove the vertebral lamina on one side of spine only.

hemimelia Congenital absence of all or the distal part of the limb, seen rarely in new-born puppies and kittens.

hemiplegia Paralysis of one side of the body only; indicates a brain lesion or high cervical injury, *see also* PARAPLEGIA.

hemisphere, cerebral Half of the forebrain, includes cortex, lateral ventricle and basal ganglia.

hemithyroidectomy Operation to remove one of the two thyroid glands.

Henle's loop Part of the kidney drainage system, the first U-loop after the nephron.

heparin Anticoagulant of natural origin from animal tissue. May be used to obtain plasma.

hepatic Relating to the liver.

hepatitis Inflammation of the liver but more specifically a virus infection or sometimes the result of toxicity.

hepatobiliary Refers to the liver substance and the bile duct system.

hepatoid cells Cells with microscopic appearance of liver cells, typically reported when anal adenoma tissue is biopsied.

hepatoma Tumour of the liver, may be confused with a benign enlargement of the liver.

hepatomegaly Enlargement of the liver, to the extent it can be felt beyond the rib cage (on the right). More common in the cat as in the dog the liver tends to reduce in size if diseased.

hepatoportal Involving the conduction system of fluids, the hepatic portal system; when bypassed as a congenital disorder it is known as a shunt, *see also* PORTOCAVAL

hepatosis Non-specific term for some dysfunction of the liver.

herbage One of the most common constituents of commercial feeds for smaller pets such as hamsters and guinea-pigs is alfalfa (lucerne). It can be supplied as pellets or in dried chopped form. It has a modest protein content, and is rich in fibre and minerals such as calcium but low in phosphorus.

hereditary Something that can be transmitted by one or more parent to the offspring.

Herring–Breuer reflex Regulates the filling and emptying of the lungs. Stretch receptors on the walls of the bronchi and bronchioles transmit impulses to the respiratory centre of the brain allowing for rhythmic breathing movements.

Herman's tortoise One of three species of tortoise found in the UK.

hermaphrodite Animal that contains both female and male reproductive organs.

hernia Defect or weakness of the body wall allowing the protrusion of viscera to occur through one of the body's normal openings.

herniorrhaphy Operation to incise the hernial sac and repair the defect.

herpes virus An important group of viruses for animals, causing diseases such as cat 'flu, abortion and fading puppies.

hetero- Word used to describe the opposite or dissimilar.

heterochromia Difference in colour, usually used to describe the iris of cats that have two different colours.

heterograft Tissue or organ grafting where material from one species is donated to another species, *see also* XENOGRAFT.

hiatus Opening or aperture; used anatomically for the apertures in the diaphragm for the passage of the oesophagus, blood vessels, etc.

hibernation The winter period of dormancy used by many cold-blooded animals to conserve energy. Nursing of hedgehogs and tortoises in the post-hibernation period is critical for anorexic animals.

hilus Anatomical term for a sunken pit – the hilus of the kidney, etc.

hind brain That portion of the brain that includes the pons, the medulla oblongata and the cerebellum.

hip The part of the body around the articulation of the femur with the pelvis or more specifically the hip joint itself (coxo-femoral articulation).

hip dysplasia Hereditary disease characterised by loose fitting joints; has an environmental component in the development of the disorder; usually diagnosed on X-ray and a control scheme exists administered in the UK by the BVA and the Kennel Club.

hippocampus Part of the brain that forms the floor of the ventricles of the cerebral hemispheres. The area is important to identify when diagnosing death from rabies.

histamine Enzyme found in all body tissues but particularly associated with allergic responses, *see also* ANTIHISTAMINE.

histiocyte Cell with phagocytic ability found in organs and in tissues, a fixed macrophage.

histogram Method of showing information as vertical blocks or similar portrayal of statistical information.

histology The study of tissue structure, usually by the microscopic examination of stained cells.

hive A raised skin plaque, *see also* URTICARIA.

hob Male ferret.

hock The hind leg joint also known as the tarsus that has the greatest flexion angulation, *see also* OSTEOCHONDROSIS.

Hodgkin's disease Name of a human disease of malignant lymphoma; does not occur in dogs but often the name pseudo-Hodgkin's disease is given to enlarged lymph node neoplasia in dogs.

holistic Total care involving physiological, psychological and sociological factors in nursing.

holistic dog training Method of bringing up dogs from puppyhood where there is continual training using sympathetic methods.

homatropine Medication used to dilate the pupil for a shorter time than obtained with atropine; a synthetic compound that acts by blocking the parasympathetic nervous system.

homeo- Word used to denote the same or like.

homeopathy Method of treatment involving the use of minute doses of substance that could produce similar symptoms to the illness if overdosed. Based on the theory that 'like cures like'.

homeostasis The ability to maintain the body to as close to the 'normal' state as possible. Internal control of the body symptoms in an attempt to overcome outside influences.

homo- Word used to indicate it is the same, e.g. homosexual behaviour.

homozygous The same genetic make up – identical alleles.

hookworm Nematode worms that were thought to attach themselves to the intestine wall by their 'hooks'; the dog species are *Ancylostoma canininum* and *Uncinaria stenocephala.*

hordoleum Localised purulent infection of the eyelid, commonly known as a 'sty'.

horizontal transmission Spread of infection or disease from one living in a group to another, *see also* VERTICAL TRANSMISSION.

hormonal Caused by some imbalance of hormone output by endocrine glands.

hormones Chemical transmitters secreted into the blood stream by endocrine glands, used to stimulate processes or sometimes to slow them down.

Horner's syndrome Group of signs affecting the eye due to a dysfunction of the sympathetic nerve supply; classic signs are of ptosis, miotic pupil, sunken eyeball and prominent third eyelid.

host Name for an animal that carries a parasite and may serve as a source of infection to others.

hot spots Popular term used in dermatology to describe acute weeping areas of skin; may start as an allergic response but the animal biting or licking the area makes the skin look worse.

house dust mite Important in veterinary dermatology as the most frequent cause of allergic responses; belong to *Dermatophagoides* species. *D. pharinae* and *D. pteronyssinus* are common house dust mites, faeces of these are allergenic.

Howell–Jolly bodies Remains of nuclei seen microscopically as opaque bodies in erythrocytes, found in some anaemias or conditions of the spleen.

human–animal bond Term used to denote a close relationship of an animal with its owner or keeper.

human immunodeficiency virus (HIV) Responsible for AIDS but not known to have any veterinary significance.

humane destruction Euthanasia performed in an acceptable manner.

humerus Bone of the foreleg loosely connected to the scapula and closely connected in the elbow joint to the radius and ulna, *see also* TROCHLEA, TUBERCLE.

humoral Relates to the body fluids, e.g. humoral immunity.

humour A body fluid. **Aqueous humour** The fluid of the anterior chamber of the eye. **Vitreous humour** Jelly-like fluid that keeps the retina in place through its 'filling' of the posterior chamber.

hyaline cartilage Description of the type of cartilage found in articular surfaces of the joints and the rings of the tracheal cartilage.

hyaline membrane Deposit found in the alveoli of the lungs composed of cell debris and fibrin, *see also* PNEUMONIA.

hyalitis asteroid Partial opacity of the vitreous humour due to minute calcified bodies fixed to the collagen framework, *see also* SYNCHESIS SCINTILLANS (distinguishable by wobbling of the small particles when the head moves).

hyaluronidase Enzyme that dissolves hyaluronic acid in connective tissue. An important virulence factor for pathogenic organisms such as *Streptococci* and *Staphylococci.*

hybrid Name for a cross-bred animal; increases vigour when the parents come from different strains or species.

hydatid A bladder-like cyst found in tissues, usually associated with *Echinococcus granulosus.*

hydration Relates to the fluid electrolyte balance of the body and its water content.

hydrocele Fluid-filled swelling sometimes found in the enlarged scrotum when fluid accumulates around the testes.

hydrocephalus Accumulation of fluid in the brain ventricles when drainage of the cerebrospinal fluid fails.

hydrocortisone Glucocorticoid; pharmaceutical name used for cortisol the hormone secreted by the adrenal cortex.

hydrogen Gaseous element with the atomic number 1, used as a measurement in a breath test for some intestinal absorption investigations.

hydrogen ion concentration Known by the symbol pH, it is a measure of hydrogen ions denoting acidity or alkalinity.

hydrogen peroxide Solution used in first-aid treatment that releases free oxygen when it comes in contact with organic matter. Mechanical cleansing effect is of especial value in contaminated wounds.

hydrolysis Any chemical reaction when a compound reacts with water to produce another end product.

hydrometer Instrument to measure specific gravity of fluids.

hydronephrosis The abnormal filling of the kidney with urine; may be the result of reduced drainage through the ureter.

hydrophobia The fear of water; popular term for rabies when one of the symptoms is of painful spasms of the throat muscles that are induced by swallowing.

hydrops Watery accumulation in body tissue, when in the fetus it is called hydrops amnii.

hydrotherapy Use of warm or cold water often combined with massage for treatment of disease – puppies and adults can be made to swim to strengthen legs. In labradors, their swimming in very cold water may lead to tail injury or temporary paralysis.

hydrothorax Fluid in the pleural space, usually serous in nature and not the result of infection, *see also* PYOTHORAX.

17-hydroxycorticosteroids Adrenocorticosteroid hormones with a C-17 hydroxyl group: includes cortisol, cortisone and others.

hygienist (dental) Person trained to practice certain preventive and curative treatments. For animals, the treatment must be prescribed by the veterinary surgeon and carried out under his/her supervision.

hygroma Fluid-filled cavity usually over a joint such as the elbow, the point of the hock or the carpus.

hyoid U-shaped structure, usually refers to the apparatus that suspends the larynx behind the tongue.

hyper- A prefix that denotes increased or abnormally raised.

hyperactivity A state of restless movement often associated with pacing and crying; may be the sign of toxicity or encephalitis.

hyperadiposis Excessively fat, *see also* OBESITY.

hyperaemia Increased blood supply; may be an active response when the organ is redder and warmer than normal or passive due to some obstruction in the venous return.

hyperaesthesia State of increased sensitivity to normal stimuli.

hyperaggression Increased response to perceived threat, often furious in nature. Rabies should be considered if the history is not known or there has been a recent sudden change in aggressiveness.

hyperbaric Greater than normal pressure (barometer measures); when applied to oxygenation it may be used during the treatment of disease or inadvertently during anaesthesia.

hypercalcaemia Excess of calcium in the blood, may be one of the signs of overdosing with vitamin D.

hypercapnia Excess of carbon dioxide in the blood, also known as hypercarbia.

hypercortisolism The condition of excess production of cortisol, *see also* CUSHING'S DISEASE.

hyperechoic In ultrasound examination, a tissue or organ reflecting back most of the waves and appearing white, dense tumour tissue being one example.

hyperextension Extension of a limb beyond its normal range, a sinking carpus is an example, *see also* PLANTIGRADE.

hypergalactia Overproduction of milk, may be found in the first few days after birth of puppies or kittens when the mammary glands become overdistended.

hyperglobulinaemia May be an acute phase response to infection with increased globulins in the blood from antigenic stimulation or auto-antibodies.

hyperglycaemia Raised blood sugar level, one possible sign of diabetes mellitus.

hyperkalaemia Elevated levels of potassium in the blood, associated with renal failure, etc. Cats have a characteristic low head carriage if affected.

hyperkeratosis Increased thickness of the stratum corneum, crusting of the nose and foot pads being one of the most obvious signs of zinc deficiency

hypermastia Excessive size of the mammary glands.

hypermetria A high-stepping gait.

hypermobility A loose-fitting joint or unusual mobility when joints are manipulated.

hypermotility, intestinal Increased rate of peristalsis often with fluid and gas sounds, *see also* BORBORYGMUS.

hyperonychia Increased growth of nails often with twisting of the claws.

hyperparathyroidism Oversecretion of parathormone, *see also* RENAL RICKETS.

hyperphagia Abnormal appetite or excessive food ingestion.

hyperplasia Increase in the mass of a tissue or organ (but not a cell increase as in neoplasia).

hyperpnoea More rapid breathing with an increase in the depth of each breath taken as well as the increased rate, *see also* TACHYPNOEA.

hyperproteinaemia Increase in the serum protein content of the blood.

hyperptyalism Increased production of saliva; may be swallowed or may drool from the mouth.

hypersecretion Overproduction of some gland secretion.

hypersensitivity Altered state in which the animal's body reacts in an excessive way to an immune challenge, *see also* ANAPHYLACTIC SHOCK, ATOPY. **Contact hypersensitivity** Response of the skin to direct contact with an antigen in a previously sensitised animal. **Delayed hypersensitivity** The type of response after 24 hours or more, due to T cells reacting with cell bound antigen (known as Type IV). **Flea bite hypersensitivity** Excessive reaction to the protein in the flea's saliva, known also as flea allergy dermatitis or FAD.

hypertension High blood pressure in the arteries. Animals with renal disease may have elevated systemic arterial pressure; cats are three times more likely to suffer than dogs, *see also* RETINAL HAEMORRHAGE.

hyperthermia Body temperature increase to a high level; fatal unless rapid cooling measures can be introduced. Treatment may include immersion in cold water, spirit poured onto the feet or the skin for evaporation, the application of wet towels and a fan directed to increase heat loss by evaporation, ice-cold i/v fluids, cold water enemas, etc., *see also* HEAT STROKE.

hyperthyroidism Overactivity of the thyroid gland. Common in cats; signs include weight loss, aggression and excitement, tachycardia and poor coat.

hypertonic Osmotic pressure greater than another solution; usually refers in fluid therapy to a fluid with a greater 'tension' than blood or tissue fluids.

hypertrophic cardiomyopathy Enlargement of the heart by thickening of the cardiac muscle mass as a response to an increased load; unless treated it is usually followed by dilation and muscle weakening.

hypertrophic pulmonary osteoarthropathy Thickening of limb bones due to some pulmonary disorder, *see also* MARIE'S DISEASE.

hypertrophy Increase in the size of an organ or tissue brought about by an enlargement of cells rather than by an increase in cell number found in neoplasia.

hyperventilation Increased depth of respiration rate; drives off carbon dioxide and can lead to hypocapnia and respiratory alkalosis.

hypervitaminosis Signs of disease produced by injection or by overfeeding vitamins.

hypervitaminosis A Disease which may be caused by cats being extensively fed liver obtained from animals living in sun-rich countries. Seen as spinal disease and stiffness in diseased felines, inability to groom may be one of the first symptoms.

hypervolaemia An increase in the volume of fluid in the circulation, may be produced by over-enthusiastic fluid therapy.

hypha Filament of a fungus, used to help diagnose mycotic infections under the microscope.

hyphaema Blood deposit in the anterior chamber of the eye.

hypnotic A sleep-inducing substance; thiopentone when used as an anaesthetic agent is one example.

hypo- Prefix for less than or below.

hypoadrenocorticism Underproduction of adrenal cortex hormones, *see also* ADDISON'S DISEASE.

hypoandrogenism Deficiency of male hormone production by the body leading to infertility and feminisation.

hypocalcaemia Low level of blood calcium, most likely to occur in the nursing animal, *see also* ECLAMPSIA, LACTATION TETANY.

hypocapnia Reduced level of carbon dioxide in the blood.

hypocarbia *see* HYPOCAPNIA.

hypochloraemia Lower than normal chloride level in the blood, may be the result of repeated vomiting and loss of hydrochloric acid, *see also* ALKALOSIS.

hypochromasia Blood cells that stain less intensely, interpreted as a low haemoglobin content of the erythrocytes.

hypodermic Below the skin but usually used to describe the subcutaneous injection site and for this reason is used sometimes to describe the syringe used for this purpose.

hypoechoic An area discovered on ultrasound examination that does not reflect the waves, indicating a fluid-filled area.

hypogammaglobulinaemia A condition of the new-born animal where maternal immunity has failed to provide the right quantity of protective antibodies.

hypogastric The area of the abdomen below the stomach; the term applies in human anatomy to describe the area of the upper mid-abdomen, similar to cranial abdominal.

hypoglobulinaemia Shortage of globulins in the blood, denotes low immunity status.

hypoglossal Situated below the tongue, most often used for the XIIth cranial nerve that innervates the tongue muscle.

hypoglycaemia Low blood sugar level; may be expected after insulin overdosage.

hypokalaemia Abnormally low levels of potassium in the blood, often associated with renal disease and polyuria.

hypomagnesaemia Low magnesium levels in the blood, causes muscle twitching and tetany.

hypomastia Unusually small mammary glands or a failure of the glands to develop.

hypomelanosis Underdeveloped pigmentation, usually a lack of melanin, *see also* VITILIGO.

hypometria Movement where the foot placement does not reach the intended spot, a form of ataxia.

hypo-oestrogenism Failure of oestrogen secretion or an inability to secrete as is found in the spayed animal.

hypoparathyroidism Disorder produced by the dysfunction of the parathyroid glands or their surgical excision, characterised by a fall in blood calcium, a rise in blood phosphate and eventual tetany.

hypophyseal system Vascular conduction system connecting the pituitary gland with the hypothalamus at the base of the cerebrum.

hypophysis The pituitary gland, so-called from its position on the ventral midline of the cerebral hemispheres and the mid-brain – means an outgrowth (or physis) at the undersurface (base) of the brain.

hypopigmentation Less than normal pigmentation, *see also* VITILIGO.

hypopituitrism Reduced secretion of hormones by the pituitary gland, examples are pituitary dwarfs and diabetes insipidus.

hypoplasia Underdevelopment of an organ or tissue.

hypoplastic anaemia Underdeveloped red cells usually associated with some bone marrow disease.

hypoproteinaemia Lower than normal serum protein level.

hypopyon Deposits of white cells in the anterior chamber of the eye.

hyposensitivity Reduced sensitivity to allergens; usually the aim when using a course of specific vaccines to desensitise a patient.

hypostatic Accumulation of fluid or blood in a dependent part as in stagnant circulation of the lungs, *see also* PNEUMONIA.

hypotension Abnormally low blood pressure, may be the result of fluid or blood loss, or more frequently due to medication.

hypothalamus Part of the forebrain that lies below the thalamus; it has an important function in the control of the autonomic nervous system and the regulation of the pituitary gland.

hypothermia Below normal body temperature.

hypothesis A theory used to explain a group of events, an explanatory argument.

hypothyroidism Underactive thyroid secretion, may be result of drug administration or a lack of pituitary stimulation.

hypotonic Lower osmotic pressure than another fluid such as blood.

hypotrichosis Lack of hair cover or failure of growth from the hair follicles.

hypovolaemic shock Low volume of circulating fluid causing shock.

hypoxaemia Less than normal oxygen tension in the circulating blood.

hypoxia Diminished blood oxygen leads to reduced availability of oxygen to the tissues, a state that must be guarded against during and after general anaesthesia.

hystero- Relates to the uterus.

hysterectomy Surgical excision of the uterus. **Caesarean hysterectomy** Removal of the uterus immediately following hysterotomy to obtain puppies at full term. **Subtotal hysterectomy** Excision of the major part of the uterus but leaving the cervix in place. **Total hysterectomy** Removal of the uterus including the cervix cutting through the anterior vagina.

hysteria A state of excitability where there is a temporary loss of control of movement and normal behaviour.

hysterotomy Surgical incision into the uterus.

I

iatro- Prefix denoting medicine, physician.

iatrogenic Something that results from the medical treatment or surgical technique, usually an adverse reaction through inappropriate medication or an unexpected response.

ichthyosis Skin disease characterised by excessive scaling.

ictal Refers to an acute epileptic convulsion, *see also* PRODROMAL.

icteric Refers to jaundice or the yellow staining of the tissues.

identichip Device implanted subcutaneously that carries a unique number that can be 'read' by the equivalent of a bar-code scanner.

identification Some method of permanent marking or description, *see also* IDENTICHIP, TATOOING.

idio- Prefix used to describe something peculiar to that animal.

idiopathic Disease or condition the cause of which is not known or arises spontaneously.

idiosyncrasy A reaction that is peculiar to that animal or it may be an abnormal susceptibility of that animal to a drug used.

Ig Abbreviation for immunoglobulin, various types (five) from A to M.

iguana Medium-size reptile sometimes kept as a pet. Known to suffer from herpes virus infections.

ile(o)- Prefix indicating the ileum (intestines).

ileal Adjective relating to the ileum.

ileocaecal Relates to the ileum and the caecum as one area.

ileocolic Relates to the ileum and the colon as one area.

ileotomy Operation to incise into the ileum.

ileum The part of the small intestine distal to the jejunum.

ileus Intestinal obstruction due to atony, usually affects the small intestine with a loss of normal peristalsis. Fluid therapy and metaclopromide may be used for treatment, *see also* PARALYTIC ILEUS.

iliac Relates to the ilium bone that forms part of the pelvis.

iliolumbar The region of the lumbar spine and the wing of the ilium.

ilium One of the three bones that make up one half of the pelvis.

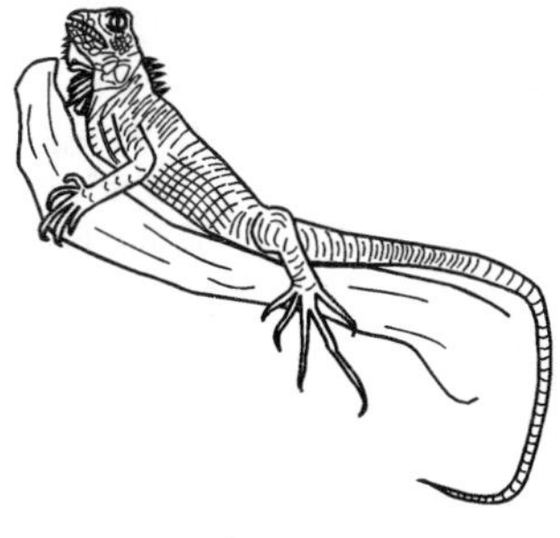

Iguana

illness A disorder where there is variation from the state known as 'good health'.

illumination darkground Method of lighting a microscopic preparation from one side so that the object appears bright against a dark background.

image, X-ray The photo picture produced on X-ray film. The X-ray is essentially a shadow picture caused by different degrees of absorption of the beam by the body tissues interposed between the tube head and the X-ray film.

imbalance Unevenness in response, e.g. a hormonal imbalance.

imbibition Soaking-up a liquid, a method of absorption.

imbrication Method used in surgery to take up excess tissue by folding or pleating it.

immature Not fully developed, yet to advance.

immersion Implies submerging an object in fluid; in microscopy the high power lens is immersed in oil to increase the resolution and magnification (100×) of bacteria, etc.

immobility Lack of or minimal movement.

immobilization The process of making a normally moving part of the body, such as a joint, immobile. Important in fracture repair.

immobilizing drug Medication used to restrain animals without full anaesthesia. Small animal immobilon has been used to give profound and long lasting sedation, medetomidine is preferred as a safer drug for use in the surgery.

immune Protection against infection usually by specific antibodies. There are various forms of resistance to disease usually associated with some form of immunity.

immune deficiency disease A lack of immunity may be present due to virus infection, toxicity or some inherited defect.

immune-mediated thrombocytopenia One form of low platelet count due to antiplatelet antibodies.

immune reaction The response of the body to the presence of antigens.

immune response Specific reaction to antigens resulting in cellular or humoral immunity.

immune system Components of the body responsible for immunity including thymus, bone marrow, lymph nodes, spleen and tonsils, *see also* LYMPHOID TISSUE.

immunity The animal's ability to resist infection and foreign substances that are usually protein in nature. **Acquired immunity** Protection that develops during life following exposure to an antigen but the term also includes the passive transfer of antibody, *see also* SERUM. **Active immunity** Protection that develops directly as a response to an antigen, produced by the body's own cells that remain able to produce more antibody in the future if required. **Cellular immunity** Immunity due to the antibodies on the cell surfaces. Relies on T lymphocytes that are first sensitised by exposure to an antigen. **Humoral immunity** Protection by circulating antibodies formed by specific B lymphocytes. **Maternal immunity** Protection acquired before birth or just after birth by the transfer of immunoglobulins, *see also* COLOSTRUM. **Passive immunity** Temporary protection that may be provided by the injection of antibodies as serum or immunity of the new-born through the mother's blood or colostrum.

immunization The process of stimulating immunity; may be by injection, by the intranasal route, by the oral route or any other method of administering a vaccine.

immunoassay Laboratory method of measuring the level of substances using an antibody–antigen reaction.

immunocompetence Ability to provide protection by mounting an immune response.

immunocompromised The inability to produce a strong protective level; may be the result of virus infection, inherited defect or immunosuppressive drugs used therapeutically.

immunocyte A cell in lymphoid tissue involved in the process of developing immunity.

immunocytoma A neoplasm that may occur anywhere in the body, usually slow growing, *see also* IMMUNOCYTE.

immunodeficiency Failure or deficiency of the immune response, may be inherited or acquired during life.

immunodepression Lower than normal response to infection; lacking circulating antibody and/or cellular immunity.

immunofluorescence Diagnostic test applied to sections of a tissue where fluorescent antibodies attach themselves to an antigen in the tissue for which they have been specifically prepared.

immunoglobulin Special group of serum proteins, the globulin fraction responsible for immunity equivalent to 'antibody'. Divided into IgA, IgD, IgE, IgG, IgM according to their origin and site of action. **Colostral immunoglobulin** The antibody found in the first milk that is ingested by the new-born; IgG can be absorbed unchanged through the gut wall in the first few days.

immunosuppression Inability to mount a normal immune response; may result from infection or a deliberate attempt to modify a disease by using medication.

immunotherapy Method of preventing or treating disease by using an agent to modify the immune response.

impacted An object that cannot be moved; may refer to a kitten or puppy during dystocia or the contents of the anal sacs, etc.

imperforate Lacking an opening; most commonly applied to the new-born animal with a non-functioning anus.

impetigo Superficial bacterial skin infection that usually responds to antibiotics.

implantation (or nidation) The time when the fertilised ova having developed into an embryo becomes attached to the wall of the uterus.

implanting Substance or object inserted into the tissues.

implied (contract) Legal situation, includes when a verbal message is received to request veterinary attention, includes a phone call received – in spite of no written agreement or no verbal negotiation over the likely fee that will be charged to attend to a request.

impotence Inability to penetrate the female whilst the animal is on heat, may be an anatomical or hormonal defect of the opposite sex. In another form there is no discharge of the fluid containing spermatozoa after penetration at the mating has been seen.

impregnation Male activity; usually refers to the act of fertilisation that leads to a pregnancy.

impression smear A preparation of cells or bacteria that can be stained as a way of microscope examination and identification. Taken by pressing a clean glass microscope slide directly on the lesion.

imprinting Behavioural term for the early attachment of a new-born animal to the first available moving object, usually the mother but other attachments are possible.

impulse An uncontrolled action; also refers to the conduction along a nerve tract.

inactivated Refers usually to vaccines where the organism can no longer produce disease but has been treated so that immunity can still be stimulated.

inanimate Lifeless, breathless and almost extinct.

inanition A condition of exhaustion caused by lack of adequate nutrition.

inappetance Poor appetite, reduced food intake; often a sign of disease, *see also* ANOREXIA.

in articulo mortis Term used to refer to the moment death occurs.

inborn Condition acquired before birth, *see* CONGENITAL.

inbred Condition produced as a result of close mating; the risk of recessive genes coming into prominence is increased by such activity.

incarceration Confined or constricted into a small space, sometimes used to describe a hernia.

incidence The frequency with which a certain event occurs, applied particularly to infectious disease or sometimes a genetic defect.

incineration Process of burning, recommended for clinical waste and carcasses, high temperature incineration is essential to destroy some substances.

incipient About to come into existence; used to describe the early stage of a disease.

incision The act of cutting; used surgically to commence an excision or lance an abscess.

incisive Something that will cut sharply, refers sometimes to teeth.

incisive bone The bone that supports the incisor teeth, often called the premaxilla.

incisor The front teeth of the upper and lower jaws.

inclusion body Used in the diagnosis of virus infections; small particles found in the cytoplasm or nucleus infected cells, *see also* NEGRI BODIES.

incompatibility Refers to certain medicaments that should not be used together or at the same time. There may be speedy immune responses if incompatible blood is transfused for example.

incompetence Failure to work properly; usually applies to heart valve disease when backward leakage of blood takes place.

incontinence Inability to control the passage of urine or faeces but commonly means urinary incontinence.

incoordination Clumsy movements, stumbling and a lack of fine control over limb placement, *see also* ATAXIA.

incubate Preparation for growth. May refer to disease, embryo in an egg, or the use of a laboratory incubator for bacterial culture.

incubation Provision for growth and development as for tissue culture or bacteria.

incubation period The time between invasion of the body by organism and the first appearance of the first symptoms.

incubator Container with equipment to provide for optimal growth, may be a laboratory incubator for cultures or a premature baby incubator for rearing puppies.

incurable State of chronic illness where the alleviation of the symptoms is as much as can be provided, *see also* EUTHANASIA, PALLIATIVE.

incus One of the small bones of the middle ear. [L. anvil.]

index Measure or ratio; used in therapeutic index to show how the curative dose relates to the lethal dose.

indication Sign that suggests a certain treatment should be used or the disease has a cause.

indigestion A failure of the normal digestive process; applies mainly to gastric digestion in humans where it equates with abdominal discomfort, *see also* *HELICOBACTER*, MALABSORPTION.

individual reaction Something only a single animal reacts or responds to.

indole A breakdown product of tryptophan, occurs in urine and faeces and is responsible for foul odours.

indolent ulcer An ulcer of the skin or mucous membrane that fails to heal naturally.

induction Term applied in general anaesthesia to the first stage of rendering the animal unconscious.

induction of parturition The artificial starting of the birth process.

indurated Abnormal hardness of the skin or an organ.

indwelling Implies an arrangement that allows a cavity to be occupied for some time as in the use of a urinary catheter.

inert Substance that does not irritate or move.

inertia Feeble or weak muscle contraction, refers to the parturition process where there is some delay before or during birth, often divided into primary and secondary inertia, *see also* DYSTOCIA.

in extremis Implies the patient only has a short time to live.

infantilism Persistence of juvenile behaviour or psychological characteristics into adult life.

infantophagia A disturbance of behaviour where the mother eats the new-born, may be the response to a perceived threat; the over-attentive care by the human may precipitate this in small mammals.

infarct A small area of localised tissue necrosis produced as a result of a failure of blood supply, *see also* THROMBUS.

infarction The formation of the dead tissue following a failure of oxygenated blood supply.

infection Invasion of the body by harmful micro-organisms, after an incubation period when the organisms multiply the symptoms manifest themselves.

infectious canine hepatitis (ICH) Disease caused by adenovirus.

infectious disease Syndrome produced as a result of spreading of microorganisms causing a disease, *see also* COMMUNICABLE DISEASE.

inferior Beneath or below.

infertility Inability of the female to conceive or the male to be able to induce conception.

infestation Restricted to established parasitic diseases, either on the surface or within the body.

infiltration Introduction of a substance into the tissues, includes cancer cells.

infiltration anaesthesia The injection of a local analgesic solution into the tissues to provide anaesthesia.

inflame To light up or redden as if in a fire, or a situation such as a staff/client dispute which may become inflamed, meaning to make it worse.

inflammation A response by the tissues to any harmful stimulus, usually intended to limit the spread of the harm to the rest of the body and to protect the vital organs.

inflammatory response The reaction to a substance that stimulates the tissues – bacterial toxin, trauma, virus, parasite, temperature extreme, radiation, may all cause such a response.

inflation Usually to distend with gas or liquid.

influenza (cat) Term used for an upper respiratory tract infection, often febrile and likely to spread. Specific virus causes, *see also* CALICIVIRUS, HERPES VIRUS.

information technology (IT) The spread of new developments and educational material by electronic communications and other modern methods.

infra- Beneath or below.

infra-orbital Below the orbit, on the floor area of the eye.

infundibulum Any structure that is funnel-shaped. The infundibulum of the brain's hypophysis and the opening of the ovarian tubes that receive the ova after ovulation, are two veterinary examples.

infusion The most frequent use of this word in veterinary nursing is for fluid therapy; usually involves a slow transfer of fluid by gravity into the vein. There is also the pharmaceutical use of the word when a drug is extracted by soaking to obtain its water-soluble active part.

ingesta Food or other substances taken into the body through the mouth.

ingestion Taking in matter by mouth, involves chewing and swallowing, *see also* MASTICATION.

inguinal Area of the body between abdomen and hind leg sometimes called the groin. Important as a site of weakness as the tunnel where the spermatic cord of the male and the round ligament of the female run through the inguinal canal may permit an inguinal hernia to develop, *see also* HERNIA.

inhalant A volatile substance that can enter the body by nose or mouth.

inhalation anaesthetics Volatile agents used in general anaesthesia usually administered by endotracheal tube or face mask.

inhalation pneumonia Gastric contents or other semi-solid substances that enter the trachea by accident and set up disease in the lungs; causes a difficult-to-treat pneumonia.

inheritance Transmission of characteristics from parent to offspring.

inherited disease One that is carried on the genes, from one or both parents.

inhibition Prevention or reduction of activity of an organ. In psychology, a restriction on a certain activity, often controlled by behaviour training.

inhibitor Substance that slows or delays an activity.

initial First or immediate.

injected The appearance of dilated blood vessels as seen on mucous membranes. Popular use of the word is to describe an animal that has been given an injection.

injection Method of administering medication, usually requires a hypodermic syringe and a needle using gentle pressure, *see also* INFUSION.

injury Harm or hurt usually the result of an accident.

inlet, pelvic An anatomical term for the area around the cranial rim of the pelvis, *see also* PARTURITION, PUBIS.

innate Describes a condition or a characteristic present at birth and is inherited from the parents.

inner ear The deepest part of the audio-vestibular system, *see also* OTITIS INTERNA, VESTIBULAR.

innervation The nerve supply of an organ or a tissue area.

innocuous Implies will not produce disease.

inoculation Method of administering a vaccine; a word originally used to describe a method of putting a mild form of disease into the healthy body to provide immunity, *see also* VACCINATION.

inoculum Any substance used in inoculation; originally was for smallpox scabs used for human protection against the disease.

inoperable Description for a surgical situation where further interference will only result in pain and not alleviate the situation.

inorganic Substance not of vegetable or animal origin. Chemically means a non-carbon compound.

inotropic Medication affecting the force of muscle contraction, usually refers to cardiac muscle.

inotropic, positive Medication that increases the force of muscle contraction, includes drugs such as digitalis, dobutamine and enoxamine.

inotropic, negative Medication that reduces the force of muscle contraction, includes beta-blockers and propanalol.

in-patient An animal that is kept in the hospital for more than 12 hours for observation or to ensure nursing care with correct medication or to enforce rest.

input voltage regulator The control on the X-ray machine that ensures constant kV in spite of any fluctuations in the mains supply voltage.

in season Common description of oestrus in the bitch.

insect Small non-mammalian animal that has six legs, an exoskeleton and is often responsible for causing bites or stings.

insecticide Medication intended to kill insects.

insemination The introduction of live sperm into the vagina or uterus to facilitate fertilisation of ova.

insensible water loss Known as inevitable water loss as it is the amount of fluid that leaves the body through the skin and the respiratory tract; it cannot be regulated by the body even at times of water deprivation.

insertion The distal point of attachment of a muscle or tendon to the bone, *see also* ORIGIN.

insidious Describes a disease that develops very slowly, creeping on and is almost imperceptible at first. Any disease is described in this way if it develops unnoticed.

in situ At the normal site or natural position.

insoluble A substance that will not enter into solution; normal solvents are oils, alcohols or water.

inspirate The air inhaled at a single breath.

inspissated Refers to semi-dried pus as found in a long-standing abscess cavity, usually thickened or hardened by evaporation or absorption.

instar A stage in the development of an insect.

instinct That which is inbuilt behaviour as opposed to that learned or acquired during lifetime.

instrument A tool, usually a surgical piece of equipment in veterinary nursing situations.

insufficiency Lacking in quantity or output, usually an organ that is functioning less well than normal. **Cardiac insufficiency** Sub-normal or an inability of the heart to pump, often due to a valve defect or a muscle weakness. **Hepatic insufficiency** Liver disease often precedes hepatic failure and death. **Venous insufficiency** Inadequate venous return to the heart with tissue oedema and visible, distended surface veins.

insufflation Method of introducing a powder or vapour into a structure, used to test patency of tubes, etc.

insulation Protection or layers added for prevention of loss of heat or for the entrance to the body of radiant energy.

insulin Hormone produced in the pancreas by the beta cells of the islets of Langerhans, essential for the regulation of blood glucose levels. Endogenous insulin may have to be supplemented by injections of commercially prepared insulin, *see also* DIABETES MELLITUS.

insulinoma Tumour of the beta cells of the islets of Langerhans, may first manifest itself as hypoglycaemia.

insurance, pet Method of providing for the payment of veterinary fees and other unexpected costs of animal ownership.

integer The complete number not a part or a fraction of a number.

integument The skin; may also refer to a cover of any other organ of the body.

intelligence Intellectual ability; the ability of animals to explore, comprehend or understand, then react accordingly, *see also* COGNITION.

intensification factor Refers to X-ray screens when the exposure needs to be adjusted for the intensification of the image depending on the type of screen in use, *see also* SCREENS.

intensifying screen X-ray screens where calcium tungstate or rare earth phosphors are used to fluoresce on exposure; the image is obtained with a shorter exposure, *see also* X-RAY.

intensity The quantity of X-rays when setting up for a radiograph; the mAs controls the dose rate from the main beam of the X-ray, together with the distance from the tube head.

intensive care Nursing care where all body functions are closely monitored; specialised nursing skills are required for critically ill and immediately post-operative patients.

Intensive care unit (ICU) Dedicated facility with special equipment for monitoring and continuous attention by nursing staff.

intention, first Refers to the manner of healing; this means when a surgical incision is sutured and heals in 5 days without scarring.

intention, second Healing where there is delay due to loss of tissue or infection, *see also* GRANULATION.

intention tremor Sign of nervous disorder, often after a head injury, where the limb or head trembles when the animal tries to perform a normal movement.

inter- Prefix word for 'between'.

interbreeding Reproduction that takes place in a planned but non-pedigree manner, *see also* CROSS BREEDING.

intercalated Something inserted between, e.g. an additional degree during a veterinary degree course.

intercellular Between the cells, as for fluid that is not within the cells and is not in the circulation.

intercostal Between the ribs; a 'space' exists that is filled by muscles but provides a surgical approach to the chest.

intercourse In normal terms refers to speech or a mutual exchange but the term sexual intercourse implies slightly more, *see also* COITUS.

interdigital Between the toes, e.g. an interdigital abscess.

interferon Substance that is produced by healthy cells after they become infected by a virus and are able to produce an inhibitory agent that can be genetically engineered.

interleukins Substances that are involved in haemopoiesis and the immune response. Stimulate the T cells.

interlobar Between the lung lobes or sometimes the liver.

intermandibular The space between the bones of the lower jaw.

intermediate host Refers to the development of some parasites where part of the life cycle involves an invasion of an insect vector or another animal, before the parasite can mature.

intermittent positive pressure ventilation (IPPV) A technique used in anaesthesia to ensure adequate ventilation of the lungs, *see also* VENTILATOR.

internal Within the body but sometimes the word is used in anatomy for a 'medial' structure.

internal fixation Method of fracture repair using plates, pins or wires applied to the bone to minimise movement, *see also* FRACTURE, PINS.

interoestrus A stage in the sexual cycle of cats when there are short periods of non-receptivity.

interosseus tendon Fibrous structure between two bones.

interphalangeal Between the phalanges or the full length of the toes.

interphase Resting stage of the cell division process when the chromosomes are not individually distinguishable.

interpretation, clinical The veterinary surgeon's clinical judgement of the signs, laboratory data and other information such as that supplied by the owner or the veterinary nurse.

interpretation, radiological Reading of X-ray plates and explaining the processes that may be shown.

intersex An individual who shows anatomical characteristics of both sexes, *see also* HERMAPHRODITE.

interstice Small space between tissues or between two body parts.

interstitial Relating to the parts separating the tissue structure.

interstitial cell stimulating hormone (ICSH) Hormone produced by the testes but also known in the female as luteinising hormone when it is produced by the anterior pituitary to stimulate the ovary, *see also* LUTEINISING HORMONE.

interstitial cell tumour An adenoma of the testes in the older dog, often benign but may be associated with peri-anal adenoma.

interstitial nephritis Type of inflammation affecting the cortex and medulla of kidneys, *see also* NEPHRITIS.

intervaginal Between the sheaths, as in tendon inflammatory disorders.

interval Time or space between activity in the body. **Atrioventricular interval** In the heart contraction cycle, measurement can be made on a printout of the ECG; of greatest value is measurement of the PQR time. **P–R interval** Measurement of the PQR times; shows the beginning of atrial activity to the ventricular contraction electrical activity. **QRST interval** The time of the ventricles' electrical stimulation for contraction.

interventricular defect Congenital disease of the heart where the septum is partially absent between the two chambers of the ventricles.

intervertebral disc The flexible cartilagenous plate that occupies the space between successive vertebrae.

intestinal Relates to the intestines.

intestinal atony Cessation or total paralysis of normal peristalsis.

intestinal dilatation Distension of the intestine with gas or fluids, may be associated with an obstruction.

intestinal torsion Twisting of the intestine, may be associated with an old adhesion or a tear of the mesentry.

intestinal tract General term for the tube running between the pyloric sphincter to the anus, *see also* BOWEL, GUT.

intestine The longest part of the alimentary tract. **Large intestine** Includes colon, caecum and rectum. **Small intestine** Duodenum, jejunum and ileum.

intima The inside coat of the blood vessel.

intolerance Inability of the animal to take a particular drug; adverse reactions develop and medication should be stopped or an alternative found.

intoxication Physical state after absorbing poison; medical nursing measures should be applied.

intra- Prefix for inside or within.

intra-articular Within the joint cavity.

intracardiac Within the lumen of the heart.

intracranial Within the skull.

intradermal Within the skin thickness as required for some injections.

intralesional Usually applies to an injection made directly into a localised lesion, *see also* ACRAL, LICK GRANULOMA.

intramammary Within the lumen of the mammary gland, usually some application of medication via the teat canal.

intramedullary Inside the bone medulla, *see also* FRACTURE, FIXATION.

intramuscular (IM) Into the muscle; a common route for a slightly irritant drug injection.

intraocular Within the eye globe.

intraperitoneal Within the peritoneal cavity of the abdomen.

intravascular Inside a blood vessel.

intravascular coagulation The end stage of shock, toxaemia, etc. Recognised when it is difficult to extract a venepuncture sample, *see also* DISSEMINATED INTRAVASCULAR COAGULATION.

intravascular space In fluid therapy this important space is the first distribution point of fluids given intravenously.

intravenous (IV) Within the lumen of the vein. Usually refers to an injection route.

introitus The entrance to a hollow cavity or organ.

intromission The passage of one object into another.

intubation Method of providing an airway by passing an endotracheal tube into the trachea.

intussusception Invagination of a length of small intestine into itself or possibly the large intestine.

in utero Within the lumen of the uterus.

invagination The infolding of a wall or telescoping of a structure. Important activity during the development of the embryo processes.

invasive Usually refers to a rapidly spreading tumour. In surgical procedures, means some activity that will involve entering the body; non-invasive techniques are preferred for many experimental procedures.

in vitro Done in the laboratory. [L. within the glass.]

inventory Catalogue or list of medication, instruments, etc. made during a practice valuation. A safety inventory may be a management tool, *see also* CLINICAL AUDIT.

inversion Turning inwards, term sometimes used for eyelids, *see also* ENTROPION.

invertebrate Animal without a bony spine, includes insects.

in vivo Something happening in the animal. [L. within the living body.]

involuntary Action that takes place without conscious will.

involuntary muscle Plain, visceral or smooth muscle but also includes cardiac muscle.

involuntary nervous system The part of the system concerned with control and homeostasis, *see also* AUTONOMIC NERVOUS SYSTEM.

involution The shrinking of the uterus to its normal size after pregnancy.

iodine Chemical element necessary for life, *see also* THYROXINE.

iodophor Organic iodine compound used as a skin disinfectant.

ion An atom or group of atoms that conducts electricity.

ionizing radiation High-energy radiation such as used in radiotherapy and for diagnostic X-rays.

ipsi- The same.

iridectomy Partial removal of the iris usually at the periphery to promote drainage.

iridencleisis Surgical procedure to trap a sliver of iris in the limbus of the eye to control glaucoma by drainage of aqueous fluid.

iridochoroiditis Inflammation of the iris and the choroid.

iridocorneal angle Part of the anterior chamber of the eye beneath the sclera, where aqueous fluid can drain into the circulation.

iridocyclitis Inflammation of the iris and uveal tract, *see also* UVEITIS.

iridodinesis Trembling of the edge of the iris when the head moves; indicates a partial luxation of the lens so that the iris edge is no longer supported from behind.

iridoplegia Paralysis of the sphincter pupillae of the iris.

iris The pigmented membrane that separates the anterior chamber of the eye from the lens and controls the amount of light reaching the retina.

iris bombe A bulging forward iris.

iris coloboma Defect with a hole in the iris.

iris cyst Small pigmented body, that will sometimes become detached and float freely in the anterior chamber of the eye.

iritis Inflammation of the iris, usually a very painful condition.

iron Elemental substance, essential for the haemoglobin molecule and therefore important in anaemia.

irradiate The application of ionising radiation, *see also* RADIOTHERAPY.

irreducible fracture Bone unable to be placed in its normal position, requires open reduction in many cases.

irreducible hernia Hernia unable to be placed in its normal position by external manipulation requires surgery to enlarge the opening in the muscle wall.

irrigation Fluid flushing, as used in contaminated wounds, etc.

ischaemia Reduced or deficient blood supply.

ischaemic myopathy A disease of cats where aortic embolism occurs causing sudden hind leg paralysis, often associated with advanced cardiac disease (myopathy).

ischiatic Area of the body near the ischium bone.

ischium The area of the pelvic bone that is most caudal; exists as two separate bones anatomically.

islet of Langerhans Endocrine gland tissue situated in the pancreas, *see also* INSULIN.

iso- The same or equal.

isocoria Equal size of the pupils.

isocytosis Equal sized blood cells.

isolation Separate accommodation, usually to prevent the spread of infection.

isoprenaline A drug with an action similar to that of the sympathetic nervous system, dilates the bronchioles and speeds up the heart rate.

Isospora Intracellular protozoal parasite, one of the causes of coccidiosis.

isosthenuria Urine that has the same specific gravity in spite of water deprivation or excessive drinking.

isotonic Equal osmotic strength or tonicity of fluid.

isotope One of many different forms of an element with the same atomic number but a different atomic weight. Used in diagnostic work as tracing devices and in radiotherapy of cancer.

isthmus of oviduct Isthmus means any narrow bridge, but specifically in birds it is the short segment of the oviduct where the egg shell is laid down.

itch The feeling of need to scratch an area, *see also* PRURITUS.

-itis Word commonly used as an ending when an organ or tissue is inflamed.

IU (1) Intra-uterine. (2) International unit.

ivermectin Potent anthelminthic, belongs to the avermectin group of synthetic drugs. Commonly used in small pets and sometimes for treatment of sarcoptic mange but is unlicensed.

Ixodes Genus of ticks; *I. hexagonus* is the common hedgehog tick that is becoming a more frequently found parasite of pets in the UK. Any tick infestation may be called ixodiasis.

J

Jackson cat catheter Urinary catheter designed for male cats, having a luer fitting and a flange so that it can be sutured to the perineum.

Jackson–Rees modification Attachment of a small reservoir bag (with an open end) to a T-piece circuit; modification allows monitoring of respiratory rate (by watching movement of the bag) and facilitates IPPV.

Jamshidi needle Fine biopsy needle.

jaundice Icterus; excess bile pigments in the blood, which are then deposited in the skin, conjunctiva and mucous membranes, giving a characteristic yellow colour. **Haemolytic jaundice** Raised levels of bile pigments in the blood due to excessive destruction of red blood cells, e.g. following incompatible blood transfusions, AIHA, *Haemobartonella*, *Babesia*. **Infective jaundice** Jaundice caused by infective agents such as *Leptospira icterohaemorrhagiae*, hepatitis A, hepatitis B, etc. **Intrahepatic jaundice** Hepatogenous (hepatocellular) jaundice due to inadequate hepatic function, e.g. viral hepatitis, liver cirrhosis. **Obstructive jaundice** Jaundice resulting from obstruction of the bile duct, so that bile is reabsorbed rather than being excreted into the digestive tract; level of obstruction may be within the liver or extrahepatic. **Prehepatic jaundice** Haemolytic jaundice before the liver.

jaw The bones of the face that support the teeth; upper jaw consists of the paired maxillae and the lower jaw the paired mandibles.

jejunum Small intestine from the distal duodenum to the ileum.

Jeyes fluid A cresol-based environmental disinfectant; toxic to cats, *see also* PHENOL.

joint Articulation between two or more bones, usually to allow a degree of movement.

joint ill Infection of a joint; classically in young farm animals where infection spreads haematogenously from the navel.

joint mouse A loose cartilaginous or bony fragment lying within a joint.

joule (J) The unit of work done when a point of application of a force of 1 Newton moves 1 metre in the direction of the force.

jugular Relating to the throat or neck.

jurisprudence The law relating to the legal relationship between a veterinary practice and its clients.

juvenile ataxia Incoordination that becomes apparent during puppyhood; has been reported in several breeds including fox terriers and Jack Russell terriers; may be due to changes in the brain or spinal cord, and some have a genetic component.

juxta- In close proximity; near to.

juxtaglomerular apparatus Renin-secreting cells found close to glomeruli in the kidney.

juxtaposition Next to; side by side.

K

kaliuresis Increased potassium excretion in the urine; occurs with the use of potassium-losing diuretics such as frusemide.

kaolin Aluminium silicate; most commonly available as a powder; when given orally acts as a demulcent and adsorbent, hence its use in cases of diarrhoea; it is also mixed into pastes and used as a poultice.

karyoblast A form of immature red blood cell.

karyogenesis The formation of the nucleus of a cell.

karyolysis The destruction of the nucleus of a cell; a precursor of cell death.

karyon The nucleus of a cell.

karyorrhexis Fragmentation of the nucleus of a cell; this process often precedes karyolysis.

karyotype The chromosome set of an individual animal or species, particularly the number and structure of the chromosomes.

kennel cough Infectious tracheobronchitis; the most common respiratory disease of dogs; usually due to *Bordetella bronchiseptica* and parainfluenza virus infection, although other pathogens have been reported and secondary infection can occur. Frequently arises when groups of dogs are confined together; causes a dry, hacking cough, often finishing with a retch; highly contagious; usually self-limiting but recovery from bacterial infection can be quickened by the use of antibiotics; potentially more serious in elderly or debilitated animals.

keratectomy Surgical removal of the superficial layers of the cornea; diseased tissue is removed along with a margin of healthy cornea; indications include dermoids, pannus, corneal sequestration and neoplasia.

keratin The major protein in hair, hoof and horn.

keratitis Inflammation of the cornea.

keratoconjunctivitis sicca (KCS) 'Dry eye'; inflammation of the cornea and conjunctiva due to insufficient tear production; particularly common in the West Highland white terrier and Cavalier King Charles spaniel; treatment includes frequent use of artificial tears, oral pilocarpine drops or parotid duct transposition. Cyclosporin ointment applied daily may be effective.

keratoconus Conical bulging of the cornea due to thinning of the stromal layer.

keratodermatitis Inflammation and thickening of the skin, with increased deposition of keratin within the epithelium.

keratolytic Agent that softens keratin.

keratoma Benign keratinous neoplasm.

Kessler locking loop suture Suture used in the repair of severed tendons.

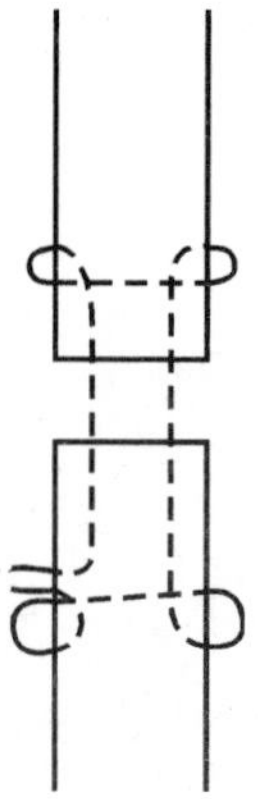

Kessler suture

ketamine Anaesthetic agent that may be given intravenously or intramuscularly; it causes hypertension, increased salivation and muscle relaxation is poor, hence it is most commonly used in combination with other agents to provide balanced anaesthesia.

keto-acidosis The metabolic acidosis arising from increased production of ketones; occurs in the later stages of diabetes mellitus and is a poor prognostic finding.

ketoconazole Antifungal medication.

ketone Organic compounds, mainly acetone, acetoacetic acid and hydroxybutyric acid, that are produced when fat is broken down, e.g. in diabetes mellitus or starvation.

Key–Gaskell syndrome Feline dysautonomia; characterised by dilated pupils, dry mucous membranes, constipation, megoesophagus and lethargy; was first reported in the early 1980s and became a well-recognised condition, but the incidence has since declined; treatment is mainly supportive (fluid therapy, nutritional support, grooming, laxatives/enemas), with recovery in more than 50% of cases, although this may take 2–12 months.

key-hole surgery Surgery performed endoscopically, thus needing only small stab incisions; common in human medicine but rarely performed in small animals; arthroscopic surgery is more common in the horse, and is becoming available for dogs.

kidney Paired abdominal organs that form and excrete urine; also secrete renin and erythropoietic factor; lie just ventral to the spinal column, the right being slightly more cranial than the left; a filtrate is formed as blood passes through the Bowman's capsules in the renal cortex; this filtrate is then collected via ducts and concentrated as it passes through the renal pelvis into the ureter and thus to the bladder.

kilocalorie (kcal) 1000 calories; a measure of energy value, commonly applied to metabolic needs and food stuffs.

kilogram (kg) 1000 grams; a measure of weight.

kilovolt (kV) 1000 volts; a measure of electrical potential difference.

kinesis Movement in response to a stimulus.

Kirschner–Ehmer apparatus External fixation device used for some fracture repairs; consists of metal fixation pins which pass through one (half-pin splintage) or both sides of a limb (full-pin splintage), and connecting bars with clamps; the apparatus is generally well tolerated by animals.

Kirschner wire (K wire) *see* WIRING.

kiss of life Colloquial term for mouth-to-mouth resuscitation.

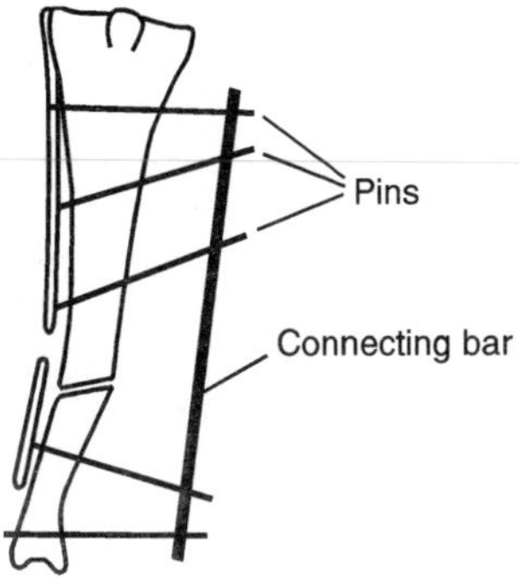

Kirschner–Ehmer apparatus

Klebsiella spp. Family of Gram-negative bacteria associated with respiratory infections and may be opportunistic pathogens in debilitated animals.

Klinefelter's syndrome Genetic abnormality where the male has an additional X chromosome (XXY); affected males are infertile and may have associated abnormalities of external and internal reproductive organs.

knee The human equivalent of the stifle joint.

knee cap Patella, a sesamoid bone.

knocked up Luxation or subluxation of the distal interphalangeal joint; the condition is seen almost exclusively in racing greyhounds and affects the left (inside) forelimb; surgical repair offers the greatest chance of a return to racing.

knot, surgeon's Basic surgical knot consisting of three throws; for the first throw the right end of the suture material is passed over the left, the left passes over the right for the second throw and the final throw is left over right; additional throws may be used to ensure knot security when using suture materials that are liable to slip.

knuckling Weight-bearing on the dorsum of the paw; knuckling denotes neurological deficits and may be due to lesions of the peripheral nerve, spinal cord or higher centres; if the paw of a standing animal is placed in a knuckled over position, the normal response of the animal should be to correctly replace the paw immediately.

Krebs' cycle The citric acid cycle; the final metabolic pathway for carbohydrates and fats; a complex series of enzyme-controlled biochemical reactions that occur within the mitochondria of cells, converting pyruvic acid into carbon dioxide, with the release of energy; this energy can be harnessed by using it to generate adenosine triphosphate (ATP) molecules which can be stored and broken down as required.

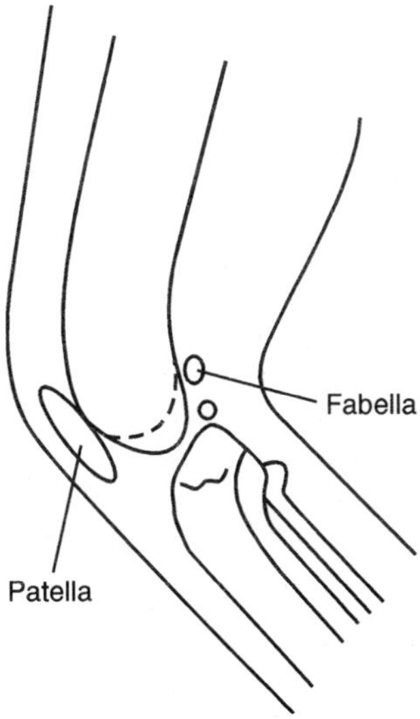

Knee

Kuhnt–Szymanowski operation Ophthalmological surgical technique for the correction of large ectropion defects; a skin flap is reflected below the affected portion of the eyelid, a V-shaped section is removed from the underlying conjunctiva and the defect closed, and the skin flap is then shortened and sutured back into place.

Kuntscher nail Intramedullary pin which is clover-shaped in cross-section; rarely used in small animal surgery.

Kupffer cell Subtype of liver cell which acts as a phagocyte and removes toxins, bacteria and cellular debris from blood entering the liver via the portal vein.

kuru A degenerative disease of the brain in man; due to a slow virus and may be spread by cannibalism.

kyphosis Dorsal (upward) curvature of the spine; usually congenital.

L

labial dermatitis *see* LIP-FOLD DERMATITIS.

labial eczema Dermatosis where the lower lips in the mouth are scaley or crusty, it may be associated with dental disorders.

labile Unstable, prone to change.

labium, pl. labia Lip, or lip-shaped structure.

labour The process of parturition; divided into first stage (cervical dilation), second stage (delivery of the fetus) and third stage (expulsion of afterbirth); in animals producing more than one offspring, the second and third stages may alternate.

labyrinthitis Inflammation of the semi-circular canals (vestibular apparatus) and cochlea of the inner ear; clinical signs include nystagmus, head tilt, circling and ataxia (vestibular signs) and hearing deficits (cochlear signs); often a progression of otitis media, *see also* OTITIS INTERNA.

laceration A jagged wound.

Lack A coaxial anaesthetic circuit where fresh gas flows in the outer sleeve, while exhaled gases flow down the inner tube, *see also* COAXIAL.

lacrimal gland The secretory glands producing tears which then drain via the nasolacrimal duct to the nasal chambers.

lacrimation Tear production; may be increased by any agent that irritates the eyes, and reduced in certain auto-immune conditions and by some drugs, such as salazopyrin, *see also* KERATOCONJUNCTIVITIS SICCA.

lactation Maternal production of milk to feed offspring.

lactation tetany Milk fever, hypocalcaemia causing convulsive spasms, *see also* ECLAMPSIA.

lacteal Lymphatic vessels that run within the wall of the intestine.

lactic acid A breakdown product formed during the oxidation of sugar within cells; lactic acid is then metabolised further to release energy, carbon dioxide and water; when the tissues, particularly muscle, lack sufficient oxygen, lactic acid cannot be fully metabolised and accumulates – an oxygen debt arises, e.g. during strenuous activity; the lactic acid is then metabolised completely when oxygen is available again, e.g. during rest.

lactophenol cotton blue Stain that may be used to demonstrate ringworm spores under the microscope in a hair sample.

lactose The main sugar in mammalian milk; a disaccharide.

lactulose A synthetic disaccharide sugar used in the treatment of hepatic encephalopathy; cannot be digested by mammals, but is fermented by the gut flora; this reduces the intestinal pH and has a purgative effect.

lacuna A depression or pit, e.g. lacunae in cartilage are occupied by chondrocytes.

lagophthalmus Condition where the eyelids do not close properly, due to protrusion of the globe; common in breeds such as the Pekinese and the pug; as the eyelids are important for distributing a tear film over the eye at each blink, the condition leads to corneal ulceration; may be managed medically with artificial tears, though more severe cases may require surgery to narrow the palpebral fissure.

lag screw Orthopaedic technique where a screw is inserted across a fracture, using a large gliding hole in the near cortex and a smaller diameter drill hole in the far cortex; this means that the screw only grips in the far cortex and when the screw is tightened it applies compression across the fracture line.

lamella A thin layer or sheet.

lameness Gait abnormality resulting in a lack of symmetry in the stride pattern; due to pain or mechanical restrictions.

lamina Thin layer.

lamina propria The layer of connective tissue lying beneath the surface of a mucous membrane; blood vessels, lymphatics, glands and nerve endings are located within this layer.

laminectomy Surgical removal of part of the bony neural arch of a vertebra, to allow access to the spinal cord.

laminitis Inflammation of the sensitive laminae within the hoof.

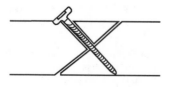

Lag screw

lance Puncture or incise a swelling to allow drainage.

landmark An anatomical site that can be readily visualised or palpated, and acts as a marker to locate other nearby structures.

laparoscope An endoscope used to examine the abdominal cavity and organs.

laparoscopy The technique of visualising the abdomen using a laparoscope.

laparotomy Surgical opening of the abdomen, most commonly performed via the midline.

large intestine The distal portion of the digestive tract, comprising the caecum, colon and rectum.

larva A grub-like stage in the development of some insects and helminths.

larval migrans The development stage in the life cycle of some insects and helminths when larvae migrate through the host's body; visceral larval migrans and ocular larval migrans may cause clinical signs in humans, due to migration of *Toxocara canis* larvae through the body and eye, respectively; this is an important zoonosis, as ocular larval migrans can result in blindness.

laryngeal collapse Collapse of the larynx, leading to airway obstruction, *see also* BRACHYCEPHALIC AIRWAY OBSTRUCTION SYNDROME.

laryngeal paralysis Inability to dilate the rima glottidis due to paralysis of the laryngeal muscles; in the horse the condition is most commonly unilateral, and due to lesions within the left recurrent laryngeal nerve; in the dog, the disease is commonly bilateral and affects older dogs of the large breeds, particularly labrador retrievers and Irish setters. The condition is characterised by worsening stridor, which may eventually affect exercise tolerance and lead to collapse; in early stages the condition may respond to steroids, but when more severe surgery is required to open the airway; the preferred technique is a unilateral arytenoid lateralisation or 'tie-back' procedure.

laryngitis Inflammation of the larynx, often accompanied by alteration in vocalisation.

laryngoscope Instrument with a light source and a tongue depressor, used to facilitate examination of the mouth and larynx; often used to aid intubation at induction of general anaesthesia.

laryngospasm Closure of the rima glottis due to spasm of the laryngeal muscles; may occur during intubation or extubation of cats; prevented by the use of local anaesthetic sprays.

larynx Part of the respiratory tract between the pharynx and the trachea; it is used for vocalisation; the larynx consists of the paired arytenoid and thyroid cartilages and the circular cricoid cartilage, suspended beneath the skull from the hyoid apparatus.

laser Light amplification by stimulated emission of radiation; a devise producing monochromatic light; high-energy lasers are used in human surgery for coagulation and cutting tissues; low-energy lasers are used for physiotherapy; their effects include reducing pain, reducing oedema and improving the blood supply to an area.

latent Not yet apparent, e.g. the latent image on an exposed but not developed radiograph.

lateral Towards the side, away from the midline.

lateral wall resection Surgical technique used to treat chronic otitis externa; the lateral portion of the vertical canal is removed, improving aeration of the deeper structures.

lavage Washing of a cavity or area using large volumes of sterile water, saline, etc.

laxative An agent that increases peristalsis and aids defecation.

lead poisoning Condition seen mainly in puppies; clinical signs include anorexia, vomiting and abdominal cramps, muscle spasms, convulsions and collapse; lead concentrations can be measured in the blood and treatment consists of EDTA injections to chelate the lead.

leads The three electrical wires used when recording an electrocardiograph.

lecithin Phospholipid necessary for the formation of cell membranes.

Legg–Calvé–Perthes disease Aseptic necrosis of the femoral head; occurs in young small breeds of dog, such as West Highland white and Jack Russell terriers; due to impaired vascular supply to the femoral head; signs include lameness and pain on hip manipulation; the treatment of choice is femoral head excision.

leioma Leiomyoma; a benign tumour of smooth muscle.

leiomyosarcoma A malignant tumour of smooth muscle.

Leishmaniasis Infection with the protozoa *Leishmania* spp.; in dogs the parasite causes skin lesions, with dermatitis and alopecia around the muzzle and ears; other signs include pyrexia, lethargy, muscle wastage and hepatomegaly; the diagnosis can be confirmed by blood tests to demonstrate antibodies to *Leishmania*, or by confirming the parasite in biopsies; the condition is spread by the bite of sandflies and is zoonotic.

Leishman's stain An eosin and methylene blue stain used for blood smears.

lens The transparent body between the anterior and posterior chambers of the eye; rays of light passing through the lens are bent and focused onto the retina, *see also* CATARACT, LENS LUXATION.

lens luxation Displacement of the lens from its normal position, due to rupture of the suspensory fibres (*see* ZONULE OF ZINN); the condition is an emergency, as it can rapidly lead to secondary glaucoma which destroys the retina; primary, spontaneous lens luxation is the most common form, particularly in terrier breeds; signs include an aphakic crescent, iridodonesis and pain; surgical removal of the lens is the treatment of choice, *see also* APHAKIC CRESCENT, GLAUCOMA, IRIDODONESIS.

lentectomy Surgical removal of the lens.

leprosy Granulomatous skin disease of the cat, caused by *Mycobacterium lepraemurium*; possibly transmitted via the bites of infected rats.

leptocyte Form of erythrocyte seen in some cases of chronic anaemia; the cell has outer and central zones of pigment, and is sometimes known as a target cell.

leptomeninx, pl. leptomeninges Two delicate, composite layers of membranes covering the nervous tissue of the brain and spinal cord; the pia mater (inner) and arachnoid mater (outer), separated by the subarachnoid space which contains CSF.

Leptospira canicola Aerobic spirochaetal bacterium that can penetrate mucosal surfaces or areas of damaged skin; the kidney is the predilection site for the organism, where it causes an acute interstitial nephritis; clinical signs include depression, vomiting, renal pain and oliguria; the organism may be demonstrated in blood smears, urine sediment, or raised antibody levels may be detected serologically; most animals will respond successfully to antibiotics and supportive fluid therapy; leptospiral antigens are now included in routine dog vaccinations and offer good protection.

Leptospira icterohaemorragiae Bacterium causing Weil's disease, an acute hepatitis, with pyrexia, vomiting, diarrhoea and jaundice; death can occur rapidly in peracute cases; effective vaccination is available.

leptospirosis Zoonotic disease due to infection with *L. canicola* or *L. icterohaemorrhagiae*.

lesion Any abnormality in the gross or microscopic appearance of body tissue resulting from a disease process.

lethal gene A gene that produces a fatal abnormality in the animal.

lethargy Tiredness and lack of energy; a common symptom of many diseases.

leukaemia Proliferation of abnormal white blood cells in the haematopoietic tissues and in the blood; may be sub-typed according to the predominant cell type, e.g. lymphocytic leukaemia; treatment depends on the type of leukaemia and presence of secondary conditions such as nephritis, but is generally based on the use of cytotoxic agents and prednisolone, *see also* FELINE LEUKAEMIA VIRUS.

leukocyte Any of the white cell series or their precursors; the two main divisions are the granulocytes – neutrophils, basophils, eosinophils, and the agranulocytes – lymphocytes and monocytes; granulocytes and monocytes develop from stem cells in the bone marrow, while lymphocytes are formed in the lymph nodes and spleen.

leukocytopenia Abnormally low number of circulating white blood cells; this may be due to overwhelming infection, immunodeficiency, stress and steroid treatment; it is important that a differential cell count is performed to establish exactly which cells in the series are affected and to what degree.

leukocytosis Abnormally high total white cell count; requires a differential cell count to establish exactly which cells in the series are affected; physiological leukocytosis occurs normally during exercise; other causes include infection and inflammation, tissue injury, parasites and neoplastic conditions.

leukodystrophy Rare, metabolic storage diseases that result in accumulation of substrates within the white matter of the central nervous system; occurs occasionally in dogs and cats, affected animals appearing normal at birth, but then failing to grow and developing neurological signs; the prognosis is grave.

leukoencephalomyelopathy Rare neurological disease with degeneration of the white matter of the brain and spinal cord.

levator A muscle that acts to raise its insertion, e.g. levator palpebrae superioris raises the upper eyelid.

Leydig cells The interstitial cells located between the seminiferous tubules of the testes; secrete testosterone.

libido Sexual desire.

lichenification Hyperkeratosis of the skin, with thickening and cracking; a response to chronic self-trauma.

lick granuloma Single skin lesion, usually over the carpus or tarsus, due to licking; may relate to boredom or stress, and can rapidly become a habit; other possible causes include deep underlying infection, joint pain or other skin diseases; most cases respond to modifying the environment, antibiotics and aids such as use of an Elizabethan collar.

ligament Tough, fibrous band joining two bones.

ligate Bind tightly.

ligature Suture material tied tightly around a blood vessel to prevent or control haemorrhage.

lignocaine A local anaesthetic, available as an injection, gel or in a spray.

light beam diaphragm Set of four lead shutters or a cone within the tube head of the X-ray machine, that are used to collimate the primary beam to include only the site of interest; collimating the beam reduces scatter.

limbic Relating to the limbus of the eye.

limbus The sclerocorneal junction.

limp (1) Flaccid. (2) Exhibit lameness.

linea alba The fibrous band running in the midline from the xiphisternum to the pubic symphysis; the internal oblique, external oblique and transverse abdominal muscles insert onto this structure and the peritoneum also attaches in this region; midline laparotomies through the linea alba cause less soft tissue damage than incisions through the musculature itself.

lingual Relating to the tongue.

Linguatula serrata Arthropod parasite causing a severe rhinitis, often with coughing and epistaxis; may require rhinotomy to confirm the diagnosis and remove the parasite, which is, fortunately, very rare.

Linognathus setosus The sucking louse of the dog.

lint An absorbent material used in surgical dressings.

lion jaw *see* CRANIOMANDIBULAR OSTEOPATHY.

lipaemia The presence of large amounts of lipid in the blood stream; lipaemic blood samples can be recognised as on standing the plasma has a milky appearance; may follow a large, fat-rich meal, or be due to liver disease.

lipase The enzyme secreted by the exocrine pancreas for the digestion of fat.

lip-fold dermatitis Chronic inflammation of the lower lip in breeds such as spaniels; saliva collects in deep lip folds, with secondary infection and ulceration; may respond to clipping the hair, antibacterial washes and corticosteroid cream; more severe cases may require surgical ablation of the fold.

lipid Any substance that can be extracted with fat solvents.

lipofuscinosis Deposition of brown lipid pigments in internal organs.

lipoma Benign tumour of adipose tissue.

lipomatosis Presence of excessive fatty deposits in the body, often as discrete nodules.

lipoprotein Complex formed from lipid and protein molecules; in the blood most lipids are carried as lipoprotein particles of varying sizes.

liquid nitrogen Form of nitrogen stored at a very low temperature; used for cryosurgery, *see also* CRYOSURGERY.

liquid paraffin Oily liquid used as a laxative or enema. An inert mineral oil.

***Listeria* spp.** Gram-positive bacteria.

litmus paper A paper containing an indicator that turns red in acidic solutions and blue in alkaline solutions.

litre Measure of liquid volume; 1000 ml (2.2 pints).

litter All the offspring born to a bitch or queen at a single pregnancy.

liver The largest organ in the body, lying caudal to the diaphragm and close to the stomach; functions include the secretion of bile, formation and storage of glycogen, stores and filters blood, metabolism of fat, protein and many drugs, and storage of vitamins A, D, B_{12} and iron.

liver enzymes Undertaking many metabolic processes, liver cells possess a wide range of enzymes and several are used as laboratory markers for liver damage; enzymes that may be measured to assess liver damage include aspartate aminotransferase (AST), alanine aminotransferase (ALT) and gamma-glutamyl transferase (γGT); these enzymes do not give any indication of liver function, however, and other tests, such as bile acids, should be used to assess this aspect.

liver function tests Laboratory tests that assess liver function; the standard test was bromosulphaphthalein clearance, but this has been superseded by bile acids assays.

livid Having a purple/blue colour.

lobe Division of an organ, separated by fissures, e.g. lobes of the liver.

lobectomy Removal of a lobe of an organ.

lobule Subdivision of a lobe.

local anaesthetic A preparation that blocks the sensory conduction pathways (and motor pathways to some degree) in peripheral nerves; injectable solutions may be used to infiltrate around an area or block a specific nerve, thus desensitising the entire area served by that nerve, or in specific techniques such as epidural anaesthesia; sprays are used to desensitise mucous membranes, e.g. for intubation; topical gels are also available, but have little use in veterinary practice; some injectable preparations also contain adrenaline to prolong the duration of action; local anaesthetics without adrenaline should be available in the anaesthetic emergency drugs box and they may be given by intracardiac or intravenous injection in cases of cardiac arrest as they have anti-arrhythmic effects.

local immunity Active or acquired immunity to a disease with the production of immunoglobulins at a specific site in the body, usually the site of entrance of the organism, e.g. intranasal kennel cough vaccine produces a localised immunoglobulin (IgA) response in the tissues lining the nasal cavity.

localise Pinpoint or limit to a defined area.

lockjaw *see* TETANUS.

locomotion Movement; normal locomotion requires coordinated functioning of the CNS and locomotor systems.

locus The location on a chromosome occupied by a single gene.

loin The region along the side of the abdomen between the last rib and the pelvis.

long-acting Having an extended duration. Formulation used for antibiotics, hormones, etc. Known as LA preparations.

longissimus system A group of overlapping epaxial muscles, running along the dorsal and lateral aspects of the spine from the ilium to the head; action is to extend the spine and provide lateral flexion.

longitudinal In the direction of the long axis of the body.

longus system A group of overlapping hypaxial muscles located ventral and lateral to the vertebral column; main action is to flex the spine.

loop diuretic Drug that promotes urine production by acting on the loop of Henlé, e.g. frusemide; such diuretics also promote potassium loss and may cause hypokalaemia in the long term.

loop of Henlé Part of the nephron – the functional unit of the kidney – extending from the proximal tubule in a loop that dips deep into the

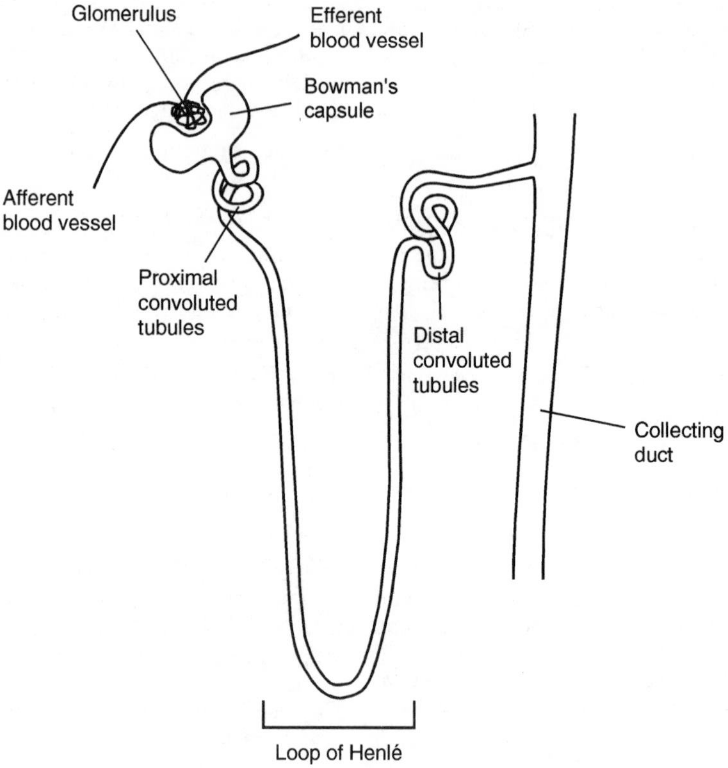

Loop of Henlé

renal medulla, rising towards the cortex again and the distal tubule; this loop allows resorption of water and its integrity is important for the correct functioning of the counter-current mechanism.

lordosis Congenital skeletal deformity with excessive downward (ventral) curving of the spine.

louse, pl. lice Arthropod ectoparasites living on the skin surface; host-specific; they are just visible with the naked eye, have three pairs of legs and either biting (broad, e.g. *Trichodectes canis*) or sucking (narrow, e.g. *Linognathus sertosus)* mouth parts; the eggs (nits) are anchored to hairs and the life cycle takes approximately 4 weeks; signs include scratching and pruritis.

lower motor neuron Ventral horn cell; the efferent nerve cell having its body in the ventral horn of the grey matter of the spinal cord, and an axon that exits the spine and runs in a spinal nerve to innervate a specific group of muscle fibres or a gland; lesions affecting the lower motor neuron typically cause a flaccid paralysis with reduced or absent reflexes, *see also* UPPER MOTOR NEURON.

lubricant Agents such as liquid paraffin, petroleum jelly and K-Y jelly, which aid in insertion of rectal thermometers, obstetric procedures, etc.

Luer The standard fitting on the end of a syringe, where the needle attaches.

Lugol's iodine An iodine/potassium iodide aqueous solution used as part of the Gram bacterial staining method.

lumbar Relating to the region around the lumbar vertebrae.

lumbosacral disease Cauda equina syndrome; pain and neurological deficits due to pressure on the nerve roots running in the cauda equina through the lumbosacral region of the spine; possible causes include vertebral stenosis, intervertebral disc disease, tumour, discospondylitis, etc; decompression of the cauda equina (e.g. dorsal laminectomy) may be beneficial but the primary cause must also be addressed.

lumbosacral plexus Nerve plexus ventral to the lumbosacral spine, formed by the spinal nerves L4–S2; this plexus gives rise to the nerves of the hind limb (sciatic and femoral nerves).

lumen The space within a hollow organ or tube.

lung Paired intrathoracic organs where oxygenation of the blood occurs across the walls of alveoli, *see also* ALVEOLUS, RESPIRATION.

lung lobe torsion Twisting of a lung lobe, leading to inadequate perfusion and aeration of alveoli; associated with chylothorax and other pleural effusions; may be diagnosed by radiography and bronchoscopy; requires surgical removal of the affected lobe.

lungworm Nematode parasites that live in the airways; host specific; when larvae hatch they are coughed up and swallowed, and are passed in the faeces, *see also AELUROSTRONGYLUS ABSTRUSUS, CAPILLARIA AEROPHILA, FILAROIDES OSLERI.*

lupus Immune-mediated, multisystemic disease characterised by an auto-immune haemolytic anaemia, thrombocytopenia, nephritis, erosive skin lesions, polyarthritis and other signs. Laboratory tests may confirm high levels of antinuclear antibody; the prognosis is guarded but treatment may be attempted with cytotoxic drugs and immunosuppressive doses of corticosteroid, *see also* DISCOID LUPUS ERYTHEMATOSUS, SYSTEMIC LUPUS ERYTHEMATOSUS.

luteinisation Formation of a corpus luteum from the granulosa cells of the Graafian follicle, following ovulation, *see also* CORPUS LUTEUM.

luteinising hormone (LH) Interstitial cell-stimulating hormone; hormone produced by the anterior pituitary gland; it causes ovulation and subsequent formation of a corpus luteum in the female; in the male it promotes the secretion of testosterone by Leydig cells in the testes.

luteolysis Regression of the corpus luteum, under the influence of naturally occurring prostaglandin.

luxation Dislocation of a joint so that there is no contact between the articular surfaces; usually the result of trauma, but congenital deformities and growth plate damage may also lead to luxation.

Lyme disease Inflammatory joint disease in man caused by the spirochaete *Borrelia burgdorferi*; disease is transmitted via tick bites and has been reported in dogs in the UK and more commonly in USA.

lymph Clear filtrate that bathes all cells; the fluid is collected into lymphatic vessels and flows through lymph nodes to be returned to the venous circulation via the thoracic ducts; the only cells normally found in lymph are lymphocytes.

lymphadenectasis Dilated enlargement of a lymph node.

lymphadenitis Inflammation of a lymph node.

lymphangiectasis Dilation of lymphatic vessels.

lymphangiogram Radiographic technique where contrast agent is introduced into lymphatic vessels.

lymphangitis Inflammation of lymphatic vessels.

lymphatic Relating to lymph nodes or vessels.

lymph node Small organs located along lymphatic vessels, e.g. submandibular, prescapular, popliteal and mediastinal; the nodes have a fibrous capsule surrounding sinuses through which the lymph filters.

lymphoblast Immature lymphocyte.

lymphocyte Small cell in the white cell series, formed mainly in the spleen, thymus and bone marrow; the cells have intensely staining nuclei, with little cytoplasm. Lymphocytes are divided into two types: B lymphocytes are short-lived and involved in antibody responses to infectious agents; T lymphocytes are long-lived and are responsible for cell-mediated immunity.

lymphoid tissue Any tissue resembling lymph node or lymphatic tissue.

lymphoma Neoplastic disease characterised by proliferation of lymphoid tissue; clinical signs associated with solid tumour masses depend on the site – if lymphoid tissue is developing at several sites it is termed 'multicentric'; systemic effects of lymphoma cells include anaemia, thrombocytopenia, hypercalcaemia and DIC.

lymphoproliferative disease *see* LEUKAEMIA, LYMPHOMA, MYELOMA.

lymphosarcoma Malignant invasion of other tissues, e.g. intestinal wall, by lymphoid tissue.

lyophilisation Freeze-drying; common process in vaccine production.

lysis Breakdown of cells.

lysosomal storage disease Disease arising due to a lack of a specific lysosomal enzyme; that enzyme's substrate accumulates within cells, eventually disrupting cell function; storage diseases are rare, but the majority affect the CNS; the prognosis is grave; specific diseases include gangliosidosis, globoid cell leukodystrophy, mucopolysaccharidosis and ceroid lipofuscinosis, *see also* LYSOSOME.

lysosome Intracytoplasmic membrane-bound vesicle containing hydrolytic enzymes that are secreted by the cell.

M

MacConkey An agar jelly used in bacteriology cultures, for distinguishing between lactose fermenting bacteria (such as *E. coli*) seen as red colonies and the other enteric bacteria that produce pale colonies.

McMaster technique Method of measuring the number of parasitic eggs in a faeces sample, involves using a special counting chamber. The eggs counted in a gram of faeces can be estimated using the 10× objective of the microscope.

macaque Member of Old World monkey group. The monkey genus is *Macaca*.

macaw One of the larger parrots, usually with bright plumage and bare face patches.

maceration Method of breaking down tissues by soaking. In obstetrics the word is used for the breakdown of a dead fetus in the uterus.

macroblast An abnormally large erythrocyte with the nucleus still present.

macrocyte An abnormally large erythrocyte, seen in macrocytic anaemia.

macrognathia Abnormal growth of the jaw, leads to overshot or undershot condition.

macrolide An antibiotic group that includes tylosin and erythromycin.

macromastia Abnormal development and size of the mammary glands.

macrophage A single nucleus phagocytic cell, part of the reticulo-endothelial system of the tissues, *see also* MAST CELL.

macroscopic The overall appearance as seen with the naked eye.

macula The most sensitive part of the human retina rich in cones; it does not have an equivalent in animals. The word is sometimes used for a grey spot on the cornea, often after a scar forms following injury.

macule A flat circumscribed area of skin.

mad itch Condition where the animal chews at itself to relieve an irritation; in farm animals is associated with the virus causing Aujesky's disease.

mad cow disease Popular description for bovine spongiform encephalopathy (BSE); the disease is of interest as it has been blamed for spongiform encephalopathies in other animals including the domestic cat, *see also* KURU.

Magendie's foramen An opening in the roof of the fourth ventricle of the brain that allows the passage of cerebrospinal fluid.

maggots The larvae of Dipteran flies; occasionally cause the death of rabbits when they invade areas of soiled skin, eating down into the flesh.

Magill circuit Anaesthetic delivery system, consists of a corrugated hose and reservoir bag; an expiratory valve at the end of the tube nearest the patient allows for the expulsion of waste gases as the animal breathes out. Used in animals over 7 kg.

magnesium Mineral element, required for both bone structure and for metabolic controls (phosphokinases, acetyl CoA). The salts such as magnesium sulphate are used for poulticing or as a saline laxative; struvite calculi have a complex structure that includes magnesium, *see also* CALCULI.

magnetic resonance imaging (MRI) Method of scanning using diagnostic equipment usually only found at specialist centres. Computer analysis of high-frequency radio waves passed through the body allows for imaging of tissues and organs, especially the brain.

magnification Any apparent increase in size as by using a microscope or in radiography the image increases depending on the distance of the object from the cathode.

Maine coon cat Breed of cat noticeably larger and longer haired than other domestic varieties, colours vary.

mal French word for illness or disease. **Grand mal** A form of epileptiform convulsion where there is loss of consciousness and major limb and jaw movements occur. **Petit mal** A mild seizure that may be no more than a vacant stare and a reluctance to move. Term taken from human epilepsy when there are brief spells of dissociation and both posture and balance are maintained.

malabsorption Refers to a reduced rate of absorption of the contents of the small intestine. The malabsorption syndrome is also seen as semi-formed faeces, loss of fluids and electrolytes and a degree of weight loss.

malacia Abnormal softening of tissues, *see also* OSTEOMALACIA.

malar Refers to the cheek area; commonly a malar abscess denotes an upper molar tooth root infection, *see also* ZYGOMATIC BONE.

Malasezzia Parasitic micro-organism; a yeast found in moist skin areas often causing pruritus and hair loss. Previously known as *Pityrosporon.*

male Denotes the masculine sex. Characterised by spermatozoa production for mating.

male sex hormones Those produced by the gonads – testosterone being produced by the interstitial (Leydig) cells.

malformation Any variation from normal anatomical structure, often congenital or acquired during early growth.

malignancy Indicates a neoplastic tumour; multiplying cells invade and destroy the tissues from which they originate, may also spread to other sites of the body.

malleus Small bone of the ear, known as the 'hammer' ossicle.

malnutrition State of under-nourishment as seen in starvation cases but also in patients suffering from malabsorption syndrome.

malocclusion Describes the condition of the teeth where one tooth does not meet the tooth of the opposite one in the jaw. A common defect in dwarf rabbits and it may have a genetic or a nutritional cause.

Malphigian Named after an Italian anatomist, for structures in the kidney capsule and the skin layers.

malunion Lack of healing after a bone fracture, often due to excessive movement, infection or non-alignment of fractured pieces of the bone.

mammillated Constructed like a mammary gland, the term is used for any nipple-like protrusion of the body.

mamma General term for the milk-secreting mammary glands characteristic of the mammalian species for nutrition of the new-born.

mammal One of the vertebrates that belongs to the class Mammalia; another characteristic in addition to milk production is the growth of body hair.

mammary Adjective of milk-producing gland of the female.

mammary abscess Usually an abscess is only found in the early stages of lactation in the bitch; if it bursts a large amount of necrotic matter comes out in the form of pus and with treatment resolution occurs in a matter of days.

mammary gland The milk-producing gland, usually described as a modified sweat gland. Bitches average five pairs and queens four pairs. The glands are not always arranged in pairs.

mammary tumour Neoplasm, invariably malignant in the cat; although common in the unspayed bitch where a large proportion are not malignant if removed in their early stages.

mandible The bone that forms the lower jaw; the left and right sides are fused at the symphysis, *see also* RAMUS.

mandibular symphysis The semi-fibrous junction between the two halves of the lower jaw mandibles; a weak point as fractures in cats are quite common after head trauma.

mange A traditional word used to describe parasitic skin disease; multiple origins of infection, each parasite needing different treatment according to the life cycles. **Demodectic mange** Chronic skin infection caused by *Demodex.* **Ear mange** Parasitic infection of the ear, mainly found in cats, caused by *Otodectes*. **Sarcoptic mange** Very pruritic or sometimes chronic scaly infection caused by *Sarcoptes.*

manipulation Method of moving joints to relieve stiffness, involves the forceful but passive movement of a joint beyond its normal angle of movement.

manubrium Part of the sternal cartilages: the most cranial (first part), it is adjacent to the clavicles of the cat, *see also* CLAVICLE.

Marburg disease Named after the university town in Germany where the infection was first recognised, it is a fatal virus disease of humans who have contracted an infection from green monkeys. Laboratory workers and visitors to certain areas in Africa are those likely to be at risk.

Marek's disease A disease of chickens due to one of the herpes viruses, also called neural lymphomatosis. It achieved distinction as one of the first tumours to be recognised to have a virus as its cause.

Marie's disease A disease of dogs seen as a thickening of certain bones of the skeleton often as the result of some intrathoracic or intra-abdominal mass, *see also* CHRONIC PULMONARY OSTEOARTHOPATHY.

mask In veterinary anaesthesia implies a soft rubber cone that can be applied to the face of a dog or cat to provide a near gas-tight seal to facilitate the induction of gaseous anaesthesia. Masks may also be used to filter the human's expired air during a surgical procedure or to remove harmful bacteria from the inhaled air of persons involved in such tasks as dental hygiene or carrying out some laboratory procedures.

masking down Considered a less than satisfactory method of inducing anaesthesia using a volatile agent, it involves applying a mask to the face of a preferably premedicated animal, until enough anaesthetic gases reach the lungs to induce anaesthesia. Unfortunately this technique is stressful and increases pollution in the theatre with anaesthetic agents.

massage Method of manipulation of body tissues to promote a sense of well-being, known to have a therapeutic effect in humans but not often used in veterinary conditions in small animals. **Cardiac massage** Specific treatment used in cardiac arrest where blood is propelled by the hand of the operator from the atria to the ventricles; pressure may be applied to the heart through the rib cage or by direct heart compression after opening the thoracic cavity, *see also* RESUSCITATION.

mast cell Specialised cell most often recognised in subcutaneous tissues, facilitator of many allergic reactions. On degradation, the cells release histamine as well as heparin and other inflammatory agents. Mast cell tumours occur most often in the younger dog's skin, growing quite rapidly, and must be identified histologically to confirm that the growth is benign.

mastectomy Surgical removal of one or more mammary glands.

mastication Process used in digestion to reduce food particles to a size where the digestive juices can act more quickly; involves mainly the molar teeth that have a grinding action to pulverise the food.

mastitis Inflammation of the mammary tissue, most frequently the result of bacterial infection of the overfull gland or when there has been stagnation of the milk secreted.

mastoid bone One of the bones in the skull that forms part of the middle ear.

materia medica Implies the study of the drugs in use for pharmacy, their actions and effects on the body.

mattress suture Method of surgical repair where additional strength or compression of tissue may be needed.

maturation Development to a point where it is complete, especially used in physiology for the follicle in the ovary or in cell division when the number of chromosomes may be halved, *see also* MEIOSIS.

maxilla Bone of the upper jaw area.

maximum permissible dose (MPD) Legal amount of radiation to which personnel may be exposed.

Mayo scissors Surgical instrument for cutting tissues, designed with narrow but rounded blunt points to allow for safe use, may be straight or half-curved in shape.

meatus A passage way or opening as in external auditory meatus, the urethral meatus is the external opening of the urethra.

mebendazole Therapeutic drug group with low toxicity principally in use for the broad-spectrum anthelminthic effect.

mechanism of labour Process leading to the normal birth of the offspring; three stages are usually described, *see also* PARTURITION.

medetomidine Agent causing deep and dose-related sedation, useful when facilities for full anaesthesia are limited by time or staffing. An α_2 agonist licensed for companion animal use; is very safe but gloves may have to be worn by nurses when administering the product. May be used with propofol to reduce the total dose used. After an IV dose, 5 minutes delay is essential before giving the propofol.

medial Towards the mid-line; opposite to lateral.

medial canthus Term used to describe the inner corner of the eyelid – the angle at which the upper and lower eyelids meet.

medial pterygoids Muscles in the head for mastication; the lateral pterygoids are responsible for side to side chewing movements of the lower jaw.

median nerve One of the forelimb nerves supplying the caudal aspect of the foot.

median plane The longitudinal division of the body into two equal halves.

mediastinum The connective tissue partition or septum separating the two sides in the thorax. The structure ensheaths the heart, trachea, aorta, oesophagus and thymus gland.

medical records Essential documents, may be hand-written or kept on a computer. Records may be asked for in legal cases and must be retained for at least 3 years and preferably longer.

medication Substances administered by mouth, applied to the body or introduced into the body for the purpose of treating a disorder.

medicine (1) Any substance used as a remedy for disease. (2) A general word used for the non-surgical treatment of animals, e.g. the Department of Medicine and Surgery or as in veterinary medicine.

medium (1) A substance such as broth or agar used to culture living organisms. (2) In radiography to denote a contrast substance to delineate hollow organs – a contrast medium.

medroxy progesterone Long-acting form of progesterone, not a corticosteroid; sometimes called MPA if acetate is included in the name.

medulla The innermost portion of an organ often surrounded by the cortex.

medulla oblongata The part of the hind brain above the spinal cord, contains the centres for the control of respiration and cardiac function.

medullated (myelinated) nerve fibre Nerve fibres surrounded by myelin sheaths.

mega- (1) Large size or giant proportions. (2) Denotes a million.

megacolon Medical disorder of a dilated large intestine, most commonly seen in older cats, may be a sequel to pelvic fracture. Lack of exercise and house training leads to older animals retaining faeces and eventual loss of the defecation reflexes. Surgical treatment to reduce the size of the colon may be necessary.

megakaryocyte A giant cell in the bone marrow, creates the blood platelets.

megaoesophagus Disorder of the proximal alimentary canal with atonic muscle, recognised on X-ray by a dilated oesophageal tube; it may be first reported as the regurgitation of food and sometimes signs of inhalation pneumonia will also be present.

meibomium glands Sebaceous glands in the eyelid responsible for producing the lipid component of the tears that protect the cornea.

meibomium cyst A retention cyst often seen as a rounded prominence near the edge of the eyelid, *see also* CHALAZION.

meiosis Cell division when the number of chromosomes in the nucleus is halved. The process is necessary in the production of ova and spermatazoa.

melaena Blood in the faeces, recognised as blackish faeces often with a red tinge on their edges, the consistency may be softer and slimier than normal.

melanin Normal pigment of the body that accounts for the dark colour of the skin, the iris and the coat of the animal.

melano- Prefix for black pigmentation or the deposition of melanin.

melanoma Tumour that has a high proportion of melanin deposited in it; despite the -oma name, some may be aggressively malignant, so all such tumours should not be ignored but require veterinary examinations. May be found anywhere on the skin, in the eye or in the mouth or the perineum.

melanosis Condition of 'blackening', may be called melanoderma as the end stage of chronic inflammation of the skin. A specific problem is corneal melanosis when blindness may result from a series of slow to heal eye ulcers.

melatonin A hormone derivative of serotonin produced in the brain; it may be associated with sleep and certain depressive states in humans although the role in animals is not clear.

membrana nictitans Commonly known as the 'third' eyelid, the nictitating membrane has the function of lubricating and clearing the corneal surface of the eye, *see also* HORNER'S SYNDROME.

membrane A thin layer of tissue that covers a body surface, *see also* FETAL MEMBRANES.

menace reflex An eyelid response when a hand is used to threaten the dog or cat's eyes, used to look for cerebral injury or the ability of the retina responding as a protective reflex.

menadione The synthetic form of vitamin K, it is used most commonly for the treatment of warfarin or other poisoning by an anticoagulant.

Mendelian inheritance Normal method of hereditary characteristics being passed from generation to generation.

mening- Relating to the membranes covering the brain and the spinal cord.

meningioma A neoplasm affecting the brain or spinal cord when a benign growth places pressure on the nervous tissue often causing unusual neurological signs.

meningitis An inflammatory condition of the meninges, often the result of bacterial infection; cerebrospinal fluid may have to be collected to find out the cause of the illness.

meniscus (1) A disc-like structure, especially relevant to injury to the stifle joint where tearing of the attachment of the menisci will add to joint instability. (2) Refers to the concave surface of a column of liquid in a glass tube as when laboratory fluid measurements are needed.

merchandising Recent introduction of marketing into the veterinary scene; usually includes all those non-medicinal products that are retailed or otherwise promoted by the veterinary practice.

mercury poisoning Toxic state caused by the unintentional absorbtion of mercury compounds; results in gastric irritation, fatal kidney and liver damage.

merozoite Development stage of protozoal parasites such as *Coccidia.*

mésalliance Polite description for the unintentional mating of the female with an undesirable male. Frequently the cause of a request to prevent pregnancy developing, *see also* MISMATING.

mesencephalon The midbrain area; fluid flows through the mesencephalic aqueduct from the forebrain to reach the fourth ventricle, *see also* CEREBROSPINAL FLUID.

mesenteric Relating to the suspensory ligaments of the abdominal viscera known as the mesentery.

mesh, surgical Net substances or mesh grafts used in surgical repair when there has been tissue loss or weakness, *see also* HERNIA.

mesial Another word for midline or medial. Also used in dental terminology to describe the inner surface of the tooth.

mesocephalic heads The breeds of dogs and cats that have the most 'normal' skull shape, *see also* BRACHYCEPHALIC, DOLICHOCEPHALIC.

mesoderm One of the three developmental layers of the embryo, responsible for future connective tissue formation – blood vessels, lymphatics, pleura and peritoneum as well as liver, kidneys and spleen.

mesometrium Suspensory ligament of the uterus covered on both sides with peritoneum but important blood vessels running down it may needing ligation during surgical operation, *see also* BROAD LIGAMENT.

mesosalpinx Mesentery carrying the ovarian tubes adjacent to the ovarian bursa.

mesosternum The body or central part of the sternum, *see also* STERNEBRAE.

mesothelioma Malignant tumour within the thorax derived from cells of the mesothelium.

mesothelium The single layer of cells that lines serous membranes, *see also* ENDOTHELIUM, EPITHELIUM.

mesovarium Suspensory structure that attaches the ovaries to the posterior pole of the kidney capsules; part of the broad ligament but contains the ovarian artery and vein that may be a source of haemorrhage during 'spaying'.

metabolic Relates to the mainly internal functions of the body.

metabolic acidosis Physiological state due to alkali loss as in diarrhoea or accumulation of carbonic acid, *see also* ACID.

metabolic alkalosis An abnormality of the acid–base mechanism that occurs infrequently but results from loss of acid or accumulation of alkalai, e.g. vomiting or after the excessive transfusion of fluids.

metabolic rate Measure of the body energy processes, also the BMR (basal metabolic rate) is the minimal output of the resting animal which can be measured.

metabolic toxins Substances that damage the normal functions, e.g. phenols, histamine and the ketone bodies produced in acidosis.

metabolic water The involuntary production of water by the body as part of the utilisation of ingested food.

metabolism The total amount of chemical and physical processes taking place in the body at one time. **Basal metabolism** The minimal amount of energy needed for the body to function in a total resting state.

metabolite An end product of some metabolic action in the body.

metacarpus Skeletal structure beyond the carpus or 'wrist' of the foreleg; consists of four parallel small bones that help to form the foot. The innermost digit has several miniaturised bones that can be removed after birth, *see also* DEWCLAWS.

metacestode Developmental stage in the life cycle of the cestode tapeworm parasites of some animal hosts.

metoclopramide Medication used for its central effect in suppressing vomiting.

metaldehyde poisoning Poisoning from slug bait; it is now less frequent since the composition of the pellets has been revised; death occurs from respiratory failure following a period of incoordination, hyperaesthesia and convulsions.

metamyelocyte Cell found during the development and maturation of granulocyte (white) cells, the stage before a band neutrophil.

metaphase Second stage of cell division when the nuclear membrane breaks down, then followed by anaphase, *see also* MITOSIS.

metaphyseal osteopathy Severe lameness in growing puppies associated with painful joints and raised body temperature, *see also* BARLOW'S DISEASE.

metaphysis The part of the bone shaft between the diaphysis and the epiphysis region of growth plates in immature animals, situated between the two diaphyses.

metastasis Spread of tumour cells often into other organs or structures distant from the primary site, *see also* NEOPLASM.

metatarsus Bones of the hind limb, distal to the distal row of tarsal bones; four in number connect to the phalanges.

metazoonosis Type of disease transmitted from invertebrates to vertebrate hosts includes blood parasites such as *Babesia, see also* TICK FEVER.

methaemoglobin Oxidation of haemoglobin which prevents the transport of oxygen to tissues, this toxic damage to erythrocytes such as nitrite poisoning causes signs such as dyspnoea and muddy-coloured mucous membranes.

methanol Known as wood alcohol, can cause permanent blindness, by brain injury, *see also* METHYLATED SPIRIT.

methionine Amino acid important in metabolism, may be used therapeutically in the treatment of paracetamol poisoning.

methohexitone Anaesthetic agent twice as potent as thiopentone and similarly is made up as a solution from the dry powder. Short acting and considered suitable for greyhounds, etc. occasional violent recovery stages have led to its replacement by other agents such as propofol.

methoxyflurane Anaesthetic agent based on a halogenated ether; it is environmentally friendly and safe for very small patients.

methylated spirit A mixture containing ethyl alcohol and methyl alcohol with petroleum hydrocarbons. As little as 10 ml of pure methyl alcohol will cause blindness in humans if ingested.

methylcellulose Substance used as a bulking agent in the treatment of constipation and sometimes in liquid form as a lubricant jelly.

metoestrus Stage of the oestrous cycle when the corpus luteum is still active in the ovary, includes the time up to the development of false pregnancy in the bitch, *see also* PSEUDOPREGNANCY.

metric units of measurement Adopted for all scientific work but not fully used in the USA, etc. The system of measurement with the metre as the basic unit (of length), *see also* SI.

metronidazole Synthetic compound mainly used against Gram-negative organisms and protozoa.

microbiology The study of bacteria, viruses, fungi and protozoa.

micrococci Very small bacteria, micrococci are mainly Gram-positive, found in soil and water.

microcoria Smaller than normal pupils, often a congenital defect found soon after the eyes open at 10 days.

microcyte Red blood cell that is smaller than normal, often associated with certain anaemias including those due to iron deficiency (microcytic anaemia).

microdontia Underdevelopment of the teeth.

microfilaria Development stage of worms of the *Filaroidea* family that are residing in the blood. Produced by adult heartworms in dogs, their presence can be detected by fresh blood smears, *see also* HEARTWORMS.

microflora Small organisms that may be found residing in the mouth or the intestines, includes bacteria, viruses, protozoa and fungi.

microglia The parts of the central nervous system cellular structure that are not nerve cells but may have a phagocytic action.

microgram One-millionth of a gram or one-thousandth of a milligram, written as: μg.

microhaematocrit Instrument to centrifuge small quantities of blood in capillary tubes to measure PCV.

micrometer Instrument to measure length or size of small structures, *see also* MICROSCOPE.

micron Smallest unit of measurement in light microscope measurement, one-thousandth of a millimetre, written as μm.

micro-orchidia Underdeveloped or very small testes. Not necessarily infertile but associated with lower libido of the male.

micro-organism Small organisms, includes bacteria, viruses, protozoa, fungi and algae.

microphallus Smaller than normal penis; may be a hindrance when attempting to catheterise neutered male cats.

microphthalmos Very small eyes; often a congenital defect, may be associated with entropion and epiphora.

micropipette Laboratory instrument for measuring minute quantities of fluid.

microscope Instrument for magnification and measurement divided into electron and light types, only the light microscope is available in most practice laboratories; known as a compound microscope it may have binocular eye pieces. The purpose is to magnify very small objects and measurement may be possible using a measuring scale in the eyepiece. A moving stage with a micrometer adjustment can be used to locate objects. **Binocular microscope** Instrument with two adjustable eyepieces; contains the ocular lenses mounted in each eyepiece. **Compound microscope** Regular microscope with lenses in the eyepiece and the objective to increase the magnification. An advance on the older simple microscope. **Electron microscope** Superior method of magnification using electrons to produce the magnified image. **Scanning electron microscope (SEM)** Used to view the surface of the object which first has to be coated with a fine metallic substance so the electrons can then produce an image. **Transmission electron microscope (TEM)** More complex method where the beam of the electrons crosses an ultra-thin slice of the tissue.

Microsporum Fungus causing one form of ringworm of dogs and cats; *M. canis* will infect either cats or dogs. Distinguished by hyphae with conidia and under ultraviolet light some 50% of samples fluoresce apple green unlike *M. gypseum*, *see also* WOOD'S LAMP.

microsurgery Delicate surgical work that includes the repair of blood vessels and nerves, involves dissection under the microscope.

microteeth The type of forceps ends used in ophthalmic surgery on forceps used to grip the most delicate eye structures.

microtome Laboratory equipment for making the very thin slices of tissue for biopsy and histological studies.

microvascular Involving small blood vessels, as in the techniques to restore blood supply to organs in microsurgery.

microvillus Small folds or finger-like projections to increase surface area and aid absorption in the small intestine epithelium.

micturate The action of emptying the bladder, similar to urination.

midbrain The part of the brainstem that carries nerve tracts from the cerebrum to the hind brain but does not include the pons or the medulla. Contains the visual and auditory centres.

middle ear The non-visible part of the ear in the tympanic bulla of the skull's temporal bone, it contains the three small bones that connect the ear drum to the inner ear, the

Eustachian tube connects to the throat, *see also* AUDITORY, EAR.

midges Small biting insects, responsible for acute dermatoses and 'hot spots' in dogs.

midline Refers to the central approach as in abdominal incision through the linea alba.

migration Movement from an original site, of ova, metal inserts, microchips, etc. Also refers to protein electrophoresis separation process, *see also* ELECTROPHORESIS.

miliary Refers to particles the small size of a millet seed when describing a nodule or skin lesions, *see also* DERMATOSIS.

milk The fluid of the mammary glands used to nourish the newborn.

milli- One-thousandth of a part, symbol is 'm'.

milligram One-thousandth of a gram, used in medication calculations for dose-rate per kg body weight, symbol 'mg'.

millilitre One-thousandth of a litre, symbol 'ml'. Equivalent to the older 'cc' measurement of a cubic centimetre of water.

millimetre One-thousandth of a metre, symbol 'mm'.

millimole One-thousandth of a mole, the measure of osmolarity, *see also* FLUID THERAPY.

mineral Group term for essential elements such as iron and calcium; can also include the trace elements such as cobalt.

mineralocorticoid Corticosteroid produced by the adrenal cortex that controls water and salt balance, *see also* ALDOSTERONE.

mineral oil Term used in USA for the product liquid paraffin derived from petroleum refining; light and heavy grades are available.

minimal inhibitory concentration (MIC) A figure used in measuring the effectiveness of antibiotics, etc.

minimal lethal dose (MLD) A standard used when testing the safe use of drugs and correct dose rates for therapeutics.

miotic Substance that constricts the pupils.

misalliance Popular term when a bitch or queen becomes mated by a casual or undesirable male. In polite circles may be called mésalliance.

miscarriage Popular term for unexpected termination of a pregnancy, *see also* ABORTION.

mismating, *see* MISALLIANCE.

Misuse of Drugs Act 1971 States the rules for the possession of 'controlled drugs'.

mite Any small crawling insect but does not include ticks. May cause direct parasitic disease or allergic responses, *see also* DERMATOPHAGOIDES, MANGE.

mitochondria Particles in the cell known as organelles; the mitochondria release energy from food and store it in the cell, *see also* ADENOSINE TRIPHOSPHATASE.

mitosis Stage of cell division when cells duplicate themselves and the nucleus doubles the number of chromosomes before two new cells split.

mitotane Substance used to cause atrophy and necrosis of the adrenal cortex, used therapeutically in Cushing's syndrome; as a carcinogen care in its handling must be observed, *see also* CHEMOTHERAPY.

mitotic figure Condition of the nucleus chromosomes when the cell is about to divide. High numbers of mitotic figures in a tissue indicate neoplasia.

mitral Shaped like a bishop's hat – tapered like a mitre. Describes the two valves at the entrance to the left ventricle, *see also* HEART VALVE.

Mittendorf's dot Opacity of the posterior lens capsule where the hyaloid artery was attached during the embryonic development of the eye.

mixed mammary tumour One of the commonest neoplasms of the older bitch, resulting from tumour growths of the epithelium, the gland tissue and other connective tissue; frequently found not to be malignant if removed early enough.

moist One of the commonest descriptions of an acute skin lesion; serum oozes through the inflamed epithelium.

moist dermatitis Superficial localised skin response often the result of insect bite or other allergic response.

moist lung sounds Fluid effusion into the bronchii, often with a productive cough when mucus is expectorated.

moist heat sterilisation Describes 'sterilisation' by boiling water, now replaced by steam under pressure sterilisation, *see also* AUTOCLAVE.

molar (1) The area of teeth that fill the posterior part of the upper and lower jaw, *see also* TEETH. (2) Describes the molecular content of a solution; the molarity of a volume of a solution is important in fluid therapy.

mole (1) Common term for a black pigmented skin tumour; melanotic warts are usually non-malignant, *see also* MELANOMA. (2) The unit in the SI system for the amount of a substance: one mole of a compound has a mass equal to its molecular weight in grams, symbol 'mol'.

molecular Relating to the composition of molecules; molecular biology is used in many investigative procedures in the laboratory.

Moller–Barlow's disease *see* BARLOW'S DISEASE, METAPHYSEAL OSTEOPATHY.

moniliasis Infection with the small yeast-like parasite *Candida*.

monitor An instrument that may record pulse, respiration or bag movement as an indication of respiratory function. The word can also be applied to the actions of the person overseeing the patient.

monitor lizard Larger reptile occasionally kept as a pet; exercise is important as they would normally have to hunt for their food so may become adipose, with a fatty liver, if in captivity.

monoblast Precursor cell for the monocyte, its appearance in the blood suggests some leukaemic disorder.

monochromatic Single colour, used when describing dyes in microbiology. The same word may be used to describe animal vision – a human with complete colour blindness is a 'monochromat'.

monoclonal An antibody produced artificially from a cell clone and thus has a very pure single type of immunoglobulin. Used frequently in many laboratory investigations.

monocular Using one eye, a single eyepiece as in the basic microscope.

monocyte One of the granulocytes of the white cell series, they are phagocytic cells larger than the others in the series. A persisting monocytosis indicates some chronic disorder.

monofilament suture Synthetic material consisting of a single thread, favoured for its strength and lack of capillary action in tissues, *see also* BRAIDED SUTURE.

monoplegia Paralysis of one limb.

monorchid The presence of only one testis in the scrotum, the 'hidden' testis may be small and soft in the inguinal canal or entirely within the abdomen.

monosaccharide Single sugar substance such as glucose and fructose.

monozygotic twins Arising from two fetuses that developed from a single egg.

monster A fetal abnormality, seen as a congenital defect of the abdomen, the limbs or face.

morbid Death-like, diseased or a pathological state.

morbillivirus One of the virus groups that includes canine distemper and the similar condition of wild seals.

moribund Dying, usually without hope, so simple nursing care is all that is needed prior to death.

morphine Opioid drug with strong analgesic properties, narcotic and addictive in humans.

morula Early stage of the development of the zygote as a solid ball.

mosquito forceps Name used to describe very fine forceps, *see also* HAEMOSTATS.

motility Ability to move as in the propulsion of intestinal contents, in small organisms activity is often the result of flagella or the tail of the sperm.

motions Popular term for the products of bowel evacuation, *see also* FAECES.

motor neuron Nerve fibril that will cause muscle movement.

motor nerve Part of the nerve trunk that runs from the spinal cord to the muscle or other effector organ; dysfunction may lead to rigidity or muscle weakness.

mould Fungi that are seen as fluffy growths on substances, often decaying matter. Cause of some inhaled allergies.

mouth Orifice in the head used for ingesting food, vocalisation or for respiration in times of distress, *see also* BUCCAL.

mouth-to-nose respiration First-aid procedure for inflating the lungs with human exhaled air containing additional carbon dioxide as a respiratory stimulant. Equivalent to the 'kiss of life' in human first aid.

mucin Glycoprotein or polysaccharide used by the body where lubrication is needed.

mucocele, salivary Distension under the tongue or in the angle of the jaw containing saliva from abnormality or duct leakage, *see also* RANULA.

mucocutaneous junction Relating to the areas where the skin joins the intestinal tract or other mucous membrane.

mucocutaneous system Name used in dermatology when disease affects the skin or the mucosa, *see also* ALOPECIA, PRURITUS, PYODERMA, SEBORRHOEA.

mucolytic Substance that reduces the viscosity of secreted mucus and may allow coughing to remove mucus quicker.

mucometra The state of the uterus that may occur in metoestrus when fluid or 'uterine milk' accumulates in the lumen of the uterus. An ascending or a blood borne infection may cause the rapid development of disease, *see also* PYOMETRA.

mucopurulent Description of any discharge from the body when infection causes pus to be mixed in with mucus.

mucosa Alternative word for mucous membrane.

mucous The adjective that describes anything that is like mucus or a tissue that secretes mucus. A mucoid internal surface that has some or many goblet cells can cover the surface with a mucus film so that lubrication and protective factors are valuable.

mucous membrane Protective lining to the body cavities; some are ciliated to move the mucus along with waves of propulsion.

mucus The protein substance produced by the goblet cells of the epithelium.

müllerian duct Embryonic paramesonephric first stage that forms the uterus, vagina and ovarian tubes or remains as a remnant in the male prostate.

multi- Prefix denoting very many.

multicentric More than one place of development as in multicentric lymphoma where numerous lymph nodes enlarge simultaneously.

multifactorial More than one cause of a condition.

multigravida An individual who has been pregnant at least twice.

multilocular ranula Outpouchings filled with saliva that may develop after injury to the salivary duct. The fluid pouches grow between the more rigid structures in the neck and lower jaw area.

multi-organ failure (MOF) Generalisation in a diseased state indicating the rapid deterioration of a patient and anticipated death.

multiparous Having had at least two separate pregnancies and births with viable kittens or puppies, etc.

murine Relating to the mouse or rat family. Murine typhus causes human disease and deaths.

murmur A noise in the cardiac area, caused by fluids passing a slack or leaking weak heart valve. Regurgitation of blood occurs to some extent. Anaemic murmurs can be heard when the blood lacks viscosity. Variants may describe the murmur sound as in machinery and musical, whilst the location is the usual description as with aortic or mitral.

muscle Contractile tissue that controls locomotion and movement; divided into three types: smooth, cardiac and voluntary.

muscular dystrophy A degeneration of muscular tissue due to faulty nutrition. In humans a genetic cause affects certain young males; the most common form is Duchenne dystrophy. A similar hereditary disorder may occur in golden retrievers.

musculoskeletal Organ system of the body comprising the bones and their attached muscles responsible for the support and propulsion of the animal.

mutant Change in the genetic composition may occur spontaneously or after damage to the genes from chemicals, radiation or from some viruses.

mutation Process of an alteration in the DNA; usually harmful but sometimes by introducing novel characteristics the individual competes for survival better and characteristics may be transmitted to the next and subsequent generations.

mutilation Harmful change to the body; docking, dewclaw removal and ear cropping are examples often quoted, as the original reason for these procedures has largely been forgotten.

muzzle (1) The part of the face surrounding the nostrils. (2) A device to cover the head and stop the mouth opening so that the muzzled animal cannot bite.

myasthenia gravis Disorder of muscle tissue where there is a lack of acetylcholine production or a loss of acetylcholine receptors at the motor end plate, leading to muscle weakness, exercise intolerance and megaoesophagus.

mycelium Strands of fungal tissue that make up the main visible part of the organism.

Mycobacteria Genus of rod-like bacteria, characterised by their 'acid-fast' staining character of the capsule where the dye is not removed by an acidic solution.

Mycoplasma Small organisms that lack a rigid cell wall, may be found in respiratory tract infections and have been associated with canine distemper. *M. felis* is found in many equine cough infections but it can also be a cause of conjunctivitis in cats.

mycosis Indicates a disease produced by fungus.

mydriasis Dilated pupils often suggest blindness, but may be induced by drugs used to 'rest' the pupil or allow for a thorough ophthalmoscope examination of the lens and fundus. Mydriasis may indicate a neurological or glaucoma disease, *see also* GLAUCOMA.

myectomy Removal or excision of a muscle.

myelin Fat-like substance that covers nerve fibrils; myelin in sheaths is produced by the Schwann cells that lie wrapped around the axon of the nerve.

myeloblast Bone marrow precursor cell responsible for granulocytes, occasionally may appear in the peripheral blood.

myelocyte An immature form of a granulocyte, may differentiate into an eosinophil or a polymorph.

myelogram X-ray picture after myelography, using the method of introducing a contrast medium into the subarachnoid space around the spinal cord.

myeloid (1) Refers to the bone marrow. (2) Used as an adjective relating to the spinal cord. (3) May mean like a myelocyte cell.

myeloma Neoplasm of the bone marrow usually diagnosed from haematology and bone marrow biopsy.

myelopathy (1) Pathological disease of the bone marrow. (2) Any functional change or degenerative condition of the myelin in the spinal cord.

myelopathy of the spinal cord Specific and progressive degenerative disease of German shepherd and other large breeds, *see also* CHRONIC DEGENERATIVE RADICULOMYELOPATHY.

myiasis Infestation with fly maggots; rabbits with the cutaneous form can die quickly from toxins absorbed by the subcutaneous blood vessels.

myocardial degeneration Myocardial disease is the early stage of potential heart failure, *see also* MYOCARDIOPATHY.

myocardium The muscle of the heart, the middle and strongest layer of the three that make up the heart wall, *see also* ENDOCARDIUM, PERICARDIUM.

myocardiopathy Progressive degenerative condition of heart muscle, usually leads to death.

myocarditis An inflammatory disease of the heart muscle, the result of an infection – viral or bacterial.

myoclonus Repeated small contractions of voluntary muscle groups that persist even when the animal is asleep, often the result of a virus infection, *see also* CHOREA.

myoglobin Substance in the muscle for oxygen transport; similar in structure to the haemoglobin in the blood.

myometrium Smooth muscle tissue of the uterus between the endometrium and the peritoneal outer cover.

myopathy Any disease of a muscle; some are inherited as in the golden retriever breed, some may result from bacterial infections. Myopathies are usually bilaterally symmetrical but often only one muscle group may be affected such as in cardiac myopathy.

myorrhaphy Repair of a muscle by suturing.

myosin The most common protein of muscle tissue, has the ability to contract, *see also* ACTIN.

myositis Inflammation of body muscle, usually with pain and lameness if a leg is affected. **Atrophic myositis** A chronic progressive disease usually affecting the dog's jaw muscles; eventually makes it impossible to open the mouth by more than a few centimetres. **Eosinophilic myositis** A specific disease of the German shepherd dog usually associated with an eosinophilia in the blood picture. Treatment with steroids is possible but the cause is unknown.

myotonia Refers to a state where active contraction of the muscle persists after voluntary effort or stimulation has stopped. Muscle stiffness and spasm may be acquired or have a hereditary basis as in chows, Great Danes and Staffordshire bull terriers.

myringitis Inflammation of the ear drum, *see also* OTITIS MEDIA.

myringotomy An operation to incise the ear drum to create an artificial opening for drainage. Not in common use in animal surgery.

myxo- Prefix denoting mucus or mucoid.

myxoedema A clinical sign of hypothyroidism in people. In animals it may occur in dogs with a thickening of the skin and contribute to the 'tragic' expression.

myxomatosis A virus infection of rabbits characterised by swollen head and closed eyes with profuse oculo-nasal discharges. Rabbits appear grotesque with swelling due to subcutaneous lumps mainly around the head and genitalia. Mortality rate is near 100%.

N

n.a.d. Abbreviation used during a clinical examination to denote that no abnormality was detected; it does not rule out the possibility of any 'hidden' disease.

naevus Term used to describe a small red area of the skin, popularly known as a birth mark.

nail (1) Keratin structure covering for the claws of an animal. (2) Intramedullary device used in internal fixation of bone structures.

nail-bed infection Infection at the base of the nail, *see also* PARONYCHIA.

nalidixic acid Medication once used for urinary infections; inhibits DNA synthesis.

naloxone Antagonist substance used to reverse the effect of opiates in the narcotic drugs group; an antidote for morphine.

nandralone Anabolic steroid used therapeutically; has androgenic properties as well.

nanogram The smallest weight measurement, weighing one-thousand-millionth of a gram (10^{-9} g).

nanometre The size of a millimicron, one-thousand-millionth of a metre (10^{-9} m).

naproxen Non-steroidal anti-inflammatory drug (NSAID) used in humans; can be fatal if accidentally swallowed by a dog as it causes gastric haemorrhage, vomiting and melaena.

narco- Prefix that implies a sleep situation or drug-induced stupor.

narcosis State of diminished consciousness or complete unconsciousness.

nares The external nostrils; as the opening to the nasal cavity. Narrowness of the two openings is a problem in brachyocephalic breeds.

nasal Relates to the nose.

nasociliary Anything in the area of the base of the nose, the eyes and the eye brows.

nasogastric tube A fine tube inserted into the stomach through the nose, used for oral fluid administration.

nasolacrimal The tear duct drainage apparatus that runs to the nose, includes the two ducts draining the eye, the lacrimal sac and the nasolacrimal duct.

nasopharynx (rhinopharynx) The part of the pharynx craniodorsal to the soft palate communicating to the nasal cavity.

nates Anatomically the buttocks.

National Council for Vocational Qualification (NCVQ) A central government organisation set up in the 1980s for moderating and supervising training in many areas of work, including veterinary nursing and animal care courses. The RCVS is the sole awarding body for Veterinary Nursing Scottish/National Vocational Qualifications (VN S/NVQs).

natural A term widely used when describing treatment or medication, implies that it occurs in nature unaffected by mankind.

nausea A feeling of sickness, often associated with brain stimulation, *see also* VESTIBULAR DISEASE.

navel The umbilical cord attachment point of the abdomen, *see also* UMBILICUS.

near-far-far-near suture Method of suturing that gives a flattened figure-of-eight, used to relieve tension on the wound edges, *see also* MATTRESS SUTURE.

nebula A mild corneal opacity not affecting vision; the same word is used for a very small healed ulcer opacity in the cornea.

nebuliser An instrument for making a spray; used in oxygen administration to moisten the gases; also used to give medications directly to the respiratory tract.

neck The anatomical area between the skull and the thorax around the cervical vertebrae. The same term is used for any constricted area such as in bones, teeth or the cervical area of the uterus.

necropsy Alternative word for a post-mortem examination, *see also* AUTOPSY, POST MORTEM.

necrosis Death of cells or tissue.

needle A pointed object either with a hollow centre to use for injections or as a solid rod used in suturing or possibly for acupuncture. **Acupuncture needle** A very fine long object for inserting into the skin at the points deemed to relate to the condition under treatment. **Aspiration biopsy needle** A hollow needle to which suction can be applied to obtain a core of biopsy material. **Needle holders** Variety of patterns in use by surgeons to place needles accurately when suturing skin or other tissues. **Hypodermic needle** An injection needle originally used for drugs placed beneath the skin, now in general use for any injection or aspiration needle.

negligence A legal term that implies there has been a lack of care and attention resulting in harm to the patient, but in law if a person has observed normal procedures and there has been adequate supervision, there should be little or no risk to the veterinary nurse working on veterinary premises.

Negri bodies The name of the inclusion bodies recognised under the microscope in nervous tissue – the brain. They are diagnostic of rabies.

nemaline myopathy A rare disease of cats, probably hereditary, that causes twitching. Seen at ages 6–15 months, it may progress to a generalised muscular atrophy. Named after the presence of nemaline rods in the skeletal muscles.

nematode Any one of the group of roundworms; the body is not segmented and tapers to a point at both ends, *see also* ASCARID, ROUNDWORM.

neo- Prefix for something new.

neonatal The period immediately after birth has occurred, usually in the first week.

neonatal jaundice The yellow coloration of the new-born animal, may be due to haemolysis of its own blood or liver failure.

neonate Used to describe the newborn puppy, kitten or similar animal that is in the stage of not surviving without its mother or similar intensive care.

neoplasm New growth; used for cancer or any type of condition with abnormal cell production.

neostigmine Medication used for its response in producing a parasympathetomimetic effect.

nephro- Prefix indicating something in the kidney system or the body area in the abdomen under the lumbar muscles.

nephrectomy Surgical operation to remove a kidney.

nephritis A well-used term for inflammation of the kidney; many such conditions would be better called a nephrosis, *see also* GLOMERULONEPHRITIS.

nephron The active filtering unit of the kidney. Composed of glomerulus, Bowman's capsule, proximal and distal convoluted tubules and a loop of Henlé.

nephrosis Refers to any kidney disease but it usually implies a degenerative condition rather than an infectious disease.

nephrotic syndrome Condition with loss of protein in the urine often with a fall in albumin in the blood, subcutaneous oedema and ascites; an end-stage disease often the result of a glomerulonephritis.

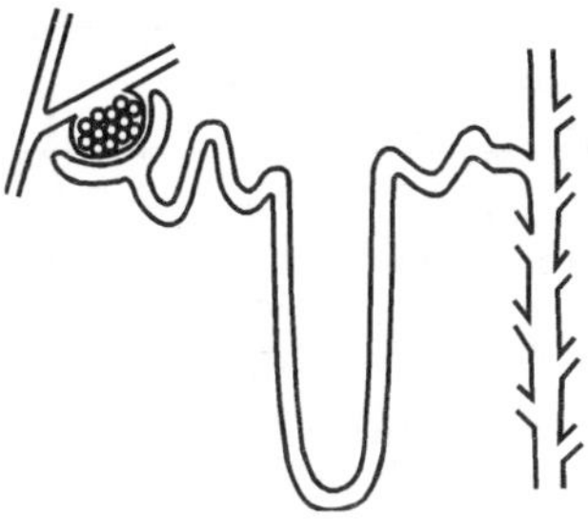

Nephron

nerve Collection of nerve fibres, a conducting structure of the body where impulses are carried between effectors, receptors and the whole of the central nervous system. May be divided into motor, sensory and mixed nerves.

nerve block Method of local analgesia using specific substances to stop nerve transmission, resulting in a loss of sensation or movement of a part of the body. An epidural injection may be used or local infiltration.

nettle rash Papular-like eruption of the skin vesicles may be present, *see also* URTICARIA.

neural Relating to a nerve or nerves.

neuralgia Pain, often severe, following the course of a nerve, *see also* TRIGEMINAL NEURALGIA.

neuropraxia Temporary loss of nerve function, may be caused by pressure on the nerve from an intervertebral disc, numbness and weakness result.

neuraxial anaesthesia Anaesthetic injections within the spinal canal, *see also* EPIDURAL.

neurilemmoma (Schwannoma) Type of tumour of the peripheral nerve: may be found first as a benign nodule under the skin. Arises from the Schwann cells that normally produce the myelin to coat the axon.

neuroglia Connective tissue of the nervous system, the packing material around neurons.

neuroleptanalgesia A form of chemical restraint close to general anaesthesia. Various combinations of analgesics and neuroleptics may be used.

neuromuscular junction The junction of the nerve ending and the muscle it innervates at the specialised motor end plate.

neuron A specialised cell to transmit nervous impulses; may be unipolar, bipolar or multipolar depending on the position of the dendrites through which nerve impulses enter the cell. Afferent and efferent neurons carry impulses to or away from the cell.

neuropathic bladder A non-functioning bladder where catheterisation may be necessary; can be the result of spinal trauma or sometimes associated with bladder neoplasia.

neuropathy Any abnormal condition characterised by inflammation and degeneration of the peripheral nerves. **Diabetic neuropathy** Diseased state of sensory nerves, more common in human diabetics than dogs or cats. **Giant axonal neuropathy** Hereditary disease of German shepherds; develops when young and is first seen in the hind legs progressing to ataxia and mega-oesophagus.

neurotmesis Partial or complete severance of a nerve as may occur in aural ablation surgery affecting the facial nerve – a neurotomy.

neurotoxin An exotoxin produced by bacteria that damages the nervous system – tetanus is the most common example.

neuter Common expression for a procedure that renders a pet incapable of breeding, *see also* CASTRATION, SPAY.

neutropenia A low white cell count, *see also* AGRANULOCYTOSIS.

neutrophil A granulocyte, one of the white cell series, frequently referred to as a 'polymorph' or leukocyte because of the shape of the nucleus.

Newcastle disease A notifiable disease of poultry and other birds. Acute infections are sudden with a high mortality rate; mild cases show respiratory, intestinal or nervous symptoms with a drop in egg production and an increase in soft shell eggs. Birds can be vaccinated from a day old with live Newcastle disease (ND) vaccine. Revaccination after 14–21 days is necessary.

niacin One of the vitamin B group, it is an essential component of two enzymes NAD and NADP involved in the oxidation/reduction system of carbohydrate, protein and fat.

nicotinamide adenine dinucleotide (NAD) A co-enzyme, *see also* NIACIN.

nicotinamide adenine dinucleotide phosphate (NADP) A co-enzyme, *see also* NIACIN.

nictitans gland Anatomical structure in the 'corner' or medial canthus of the eye that secretes lubricating mucus to protect the cornea.

nictitating membrane The so-called 'third eyelid' that has a protection function and on its inner surface has lymphoid tissue as well as mucous producing glands, *see also* MEMBRANA NICTITANS.

nidation Known as 'egg-nesting' or the implantation of the fertilised egg in the endometrium at the very earliest stages of pregnancy before the fetal membranes develop.

night blindness Popular name of progressive retinal atrophy where dogs see less well in the half-light of dusk; observed particularly in gun dog breeds with PRA where the dog misses moving animals. Was first made publicly aware when the Irish setter breed had PRA identified in the 1950s as a dominant gene inherited disorder that was then bred out of British stock, *see also* PRA, RETINAL DYSPLASIA.

nipple Any small protuberance; usually used as an alternative name to teat; the orifice from which milk is obtained in lactating mammals.

nit Diminutive word; refers to the egg of the louse that can be found adhering to the hair shaft, only just visible to the naked eye.

nitrofuran One of the synthetic antibacterial substances used for treating urinary and respiratory tract infections now superseded by more advanced medication.

nitrogen balance Measurement of the body's ability to absorb and process protein from the diet and excrete nitrogenous waste products mainly in the urine.

nitroimidazoles A group of synthetic substances used against protozoa including *Giardia*, *see also* METRONIDAZOLE.

nitroscannate An anthelminthic used against tapeworms.

nitrous oxide Anaesthetic gas used in circuits mainly for its analgesic properties; it has a diluting effect on oxygen as a carrier gas. Less popular since the potential health hazard to staff in the operating theatre was recognised. Cannot be used in closed anaesthetic circuit.

NMDA receptor antagonist Drugs used for the control of pain.

NOAH A trade-organisation National Office of Animal Health, the UK national body that represents manufacturers of veterinary products, etc.

Nocardia A group of soil bacteria, Gram-positive acid-fast staining, associated with non-healing nodules and ulcers on dogs' legs.

nociceptive Noci- is a prefix for harmful, the word describes nerve fibres, endings or pathways concerned with the conduction of pain.

noct- Indicates a night-time occurrence or activity. Noctambulation describes an animal that moves about at night.

node Any small grouping or protuberance of tissue may be called a node. **Atrio-ventricular (A–V) node** The point in the heart muscle where cardiac fibres lying between the septa of the atria delay the impulse originating in the S–A node. Waves of electrical activity then spread from the A–V node to the ventricles. **Lymph node** Part of the defence mechanism of the body where lymphoid tissue is grouped at strategic points to filter or otherwise deal with infections, etc. **S–A node** The sino-atrial node, an area of specialised cardiac tissue situated on the wall of the right atrium, is where the electrical impulse originates to set the heart rhythm, *see also* BUNDLE OF HIS. **Nodes of Ranvier** Points along the nerve fibres where there are gaps in the myelin sheaths. Ionic exchanges take place to reinforce the nerve impulses.

nodule A smaller collection of tissue than a node, a term often used to describe small lumps in the skin, etc.

non-accidental injury (NAI) A term used in nursing where it is believed that injuries to the body may be the result of the activity of 'carers' of the patient. Similar situation in animals may be due to abusers and other deviants.

non-invasive tumour A benign tumour or a tumour that does not spread locally nor by metastasis, *see also* BENIGN.

non-protein nitrogen (NPN) Sources of nitrogen that are not proteins. Urea and ammonia are two examples.

non-specific Indicates there is no one recognisable cause or it may be used to show that the effect of the condition is general, throughout the body, rather than specific to 'target' areas.

non-steroidal anti-inflammatory drug (NSAID) Chemical compounds that have a similar effect to cortisone in suppressing inflammation; they work by suppressing prostaglandins and have activity against pain (analgesic) and fever (antipyretic) as well as their anti-inflammatory effect.

non-union fracture Term used where fractured bone ends fail to unite; may be due to excess movement, insufficient blood supply or infection at the ends of the bone.

noradrenaline (norepinephrine) One of the two hormones secreted by the adrenal medulla, with a sympathomimetic effect, *see also* ADRENALINE.

norethisterone A progesterone-like hormone produced synthetically, *see also* PROGESTOGEN.

normoblast A development stage of erythrocytes; they still have nuclei, having developed from the erythroblast; found in certain anaemias like the reticulocytes that are one further stage in the red blood cell's development, *see also* ERYTHROGENESIS.

normocyte An erythrocyte that is normal in size, structure and function.

nose Anatomical structure of the head carrying the external nares.

nose pad Also known as rhinarium, it was thought to be of use in identifying dogs similar to finger prints used in humans. It is a thick keratinised structure free of body hair, surrounding the external nares, usually kept moist by the tongue.

nosocomial pneumonia Lung infection acquired during hospitalisation; it may be fungal or bacterial; associated with the lowered resistance of inpatients of a veterinary hospital. Gram-negative infections may be a problem, e.g. *Pseudomonas*.

nostril External openings of the upper respiratory tract; muscular activity can dilate or close the size of the openings especially in the rabbit.

notch A depression, usually on a bone surface. **Acetabular notch** The indentation on the medial surface of the rim of the acetabulum or 'cup' of the hip joint. **Cardiac notch** The area of the thorax where the lungs do not obscure the heart sounds, used when auscultating the heart during a clinical examination. **Vertebral notch** The area at the base of the vertebral arch above the centrum that gives room for nerves to run through an intervertebral foramen.

notifiable disease One of a number of listed diseases that have to be reported to statutory authorities such as the Ministry of Agriculture in the UK. Usually they are zoonotic diseases, although some large animal diseases are reportable because of the economic losses.

notochord A stage in the embryonic development of the skeletal system, its main interest in veterinary nursing is that remnants become the nucleus pulposus of the intervertebral discs, *see also* INTERVERTEBRAL DISC.

notoedric mange A fairly uncommon type of mange, found on the head of cats especially in and around the ears and caused by *Notoedres cati.*

noxious stimuli One that causes pain; may be used when testing for nerve paralysis in the feet, etc.

nuchal Describes the area of the neck or the crest; the head is supported by the nuchal ligament that runs from the occipital bone of the skull and the neural spine of the axis bone to the first thoracic vertebra's neural spine.

nucleic acids The genetic material of the cell nucleus; chromatin fibres consist of long-chain molecules of DNA and associated protein, *see also* DEOXYRIBONUCLEIC ACID, RIBONUCLEIC ACID.

nucleolus, pl. nucleoli Found inside the nucleus of the cell; a spherical structure responsible for the manufacture of ribosomes.

nucleus, pl. nuclei The control centre of the cell contains the chromosomes and one or more nucleoli.

nulliparous Not having given birth to any young.

nurse A person who has undergone professional training and is qualified and authorised in his/her country to practise nursing.

nursing process An individualised problem-solving approach to the patient care and nursing. It should involve four stages: assessment, planning, implementation of the plan and evaluation of the care.

nutrient That which nourishes, usually a food; includes water, minerals and vitamins.

nutrition A state when substances are taken into the body from the alimentary canal that leads to the correct function of cells and promotes life. Scientific study of this process and the interaction of components for optimal health is of importance to all those caring for animals. **Intravenous nutrition** Feeding by the intravenous route includes crystalloids, colloids and various protein, carbohydrate and fat emulsions, often with additional vitamins. **Parenteral nutrition** Feeding by routes other than by mouth, mainly by the intravenous route but also the subcutaneous and the intraperitoneal route may be used.

nylon Synthetic plastic substance used for suture and other forms such as mesh for surgical repair. Monofilament nylon is used more frequently than braided nylon.

nymph Juvenile form of some insects, ticks, lice and mange mites, being of special interest in nursing animals.

nystagmus Unusual flicking movement of the eyeballs. Most easily recognised by using the ophthalmoscope to examine the fundus. May be due to disorders of the parts of the brain controlling the eyesight and the balance. **Congenital nystagmus** Present from birth, 'wandering' may be a sign of blindness as the retina can never 'fix' on one distant spot or may be from a benign injury to the nerve pathway to the brain. **Horizontal nystagmus** The side-to-side movement most often seen in the cat or dog with vestibular disease. The fast component always 'kicks away' from the side of the brain where there is a lesion; then this is followed by a more slow return phase. **Jerk nystagmus** One of the signs of vestibular disease. **Labyrinthine nystagmus** Jerking movement due to disturbance to the labyrinth or the adjacent vestibular nucleus. **Pendular nystagmus** Appears as a to-and-fro eye movement where there is no fast phase. **Rotatory nystagmus** More violent movement of the eyeball usually indicates more severe brain damage. **Vertical nystagmus** Rapid eyeball movement on a vertical axis, more severe brain damage is suggested than with horizontal nystagmus.

nystatin An antibiotic substance usually applied in the form of an ointment in the treatment of yeast and fungal infections.

O

obedience training System for training dogs usually involving the owner in the training and with giving rewards in the form of praise and food. Methods used make the dog a better companion as well as being able to compete in tests at shows etc.

obesity A condition of excessive fat accumulation that is detrimental to health.

object–film distance In radiography, the distance between the object being X-rayed and the film, usually the closer the better.

objective Refers to the lens situated at the lower end of the microscope closest to the object being examined.

obligate parasite One that spends all its time on or inside the host and has no free-living adult existence.

oblique Slanting; a radiographic view where the beam is aimed at the object passing through at an angle may be described this way, or a fracture where the broken ends are at about a 45° angle to the perpendicular.

oblique muscle Refers to the muscles running diagonally across the abdomen, known as the internal oblique and the external oblique.

obsessive compulsive disorder (OCD) A behaviour pattern that develops most frequently in confined animals; repetitive actions often are performed for no obvious reason, *see also* AGGRESSION, STEREOTYPIC.

obstetrics The branch of science concerned with care in pregnancy, the birth process and the immediate post-parturient weeks. In veterinary terms it is often limited to dealing with problems during birth, *see also* DYSTOCIA.

obstetric ultrasound Scanning in the first trimester for the confirmation of viable fetuses; scanning is performed also after dystocia, *see also* ULTRASOUND.

obstipation Refers to a severe form of constipation.

obstruction The condition of being blocked; may occur in the intestines, the uterus, the bladder or the respiratory tract. **Intestinal obstruction** Severe disease characterised by vomiting, complete loss of appetite with gas seen on X-ray. Commonly due to a foreign body, neoplasia or severe constipation. **Urethral obstruction** Calculi are the most frequent cause, *see also* UROLITHIASIS.

obtund Dull or deadened; a description used for brain-damaged puppies or kittens after anoxia at birth. The sense of smell may be obtunded in an adult animal after brain injury.

obturator From obturate, to stop up; used to describe the muscles and a foramen in the floor of the pelvis. The obturator nerve that passes through the opening may be damaged in parturition where the fetus is oversized.

occipital bone Flat bone at the caudal aspect of the skull, carries the occipital condyles for articulation with the first cervical vertebra. Between the condyles is the foramen magnum.

occiput The area at the back of the skull.

occlusion (1) Closing off a vessel or similar. (2) In dentistry the tooth surfaces between the upper and lower sets.

occlusive dressing Impervious wound dressing designed to concentrate a topical application so it will be absorbed through the skin or to protect a wound from outside contaminants.

occult blood 'Hidden' blood is evidence of haemorrhage from a gastrointestinal ulcer or damage to an internal organ from parasites or neoplasia.

occupational exposure standard (OES) A measure of inhalation of anaesthetics such as nitrous oxide or halothane.

ocular Relates to the eyes or to vision.

ocular reflexes Nervous system tests to ascertain the function of the eye and the eyelids, *see also* CONSENSUAL LIGHT REFLEX.

oculocardiac reflex A potentially dangerous response to manipulating the eye with a slowing of the heart; the bradycardia may lead to death unless corrective measures are taken.

oculomotor The muscle movement of the eyeball is by six muscles and the cranial nerve III is also involved in eye position and the size of the iris.

odonto- Relating to the teeth. Odontology is another term for dentistry.

odontogenesis The formation of the teeth whether temporary or permanent dentition.

odontoid Any bony process thought to resemble tooth, especially the odontoid peg of the axis bone.

oedema Excessive accumulation of fluid in the body, usually in the tissues and the body cavities, *see also* ASCITES, ANASARCA, HYDROTHORAX.

Oedipus complex Repressed sexual feelings of a child for the parent of the opposite sex and sometimes rivalry with the same sex parent; made famous by Freud, has no veterinary equivalent due to the earlier independence from the dam.

oesophageal Relating to the tube connecting pharynx to the stomach used as in oesophageal stethoscope, etc.

oesophagoscope Instrument to inspect the interior lining of the oesophagus especially an obstruction, may be a rigid or a fibre-optic instrument.

oesophagostomy Surgical procedure to open the oesophagus with an incision through the neck or via a thoracotomy, usually to retrieve a foreign body.

oesophagus Part of the alimentary canal lined with mucous membrane with striated muscle to propel food to the stomach especially used by animals floor feeding.

oestradiol Natural female hormone responsible for receptivity to the male during the oestrous cycle; formed in the follicle of the ovary but also some is produced by the adrenal cortex.

oestriol One of the weaker female sex hormones; like oestrone produced by the ovary.

oestrogens The group of steroidal sex hormones responsible for female behaviour and preparing the lining of the vagina, etc. for coitus and the reception of fertilised eggs. In the male oestrogens may be produced by the testes retained in the abdomen, *see also* SERTOLI CELL TUMOUR.

oestrous cycle The repetitive changes in behaviour and the reproductive tract separated by short or long times without sexual activity. The secretion of hormones from the pituitary and negative feedback are responsible for female breeding patterns which vary with the species. Note that primates have the equivalent of a menstrual cycle which is a different way of preparing the lining of the uterus for the reception of fertilised eggs.

oestrus The noun that describes the most receptive part of the breeding cycle in animals. Adjective, oestrous.

-oid Suffix indicating like something else, *see also* SARCOID.

oil contamination A major problem for animals in coastal and any inland waterway where fuel oil may be spilt. Domestic pets may be contaminated through oil spilt in garages and motor repair yards.

ointment A pharmaceutical description of a cream or stiff paste, semi-solid and greasy; usually insoluble in water but easily removed by licking, *see also* OCCLUSIVE DRESSING.

old dog encephalitis (ODE) Degenerative brain disorder of dogs, sometimes associated with canine distemper virus, *see also* ENCEPHALITIS.

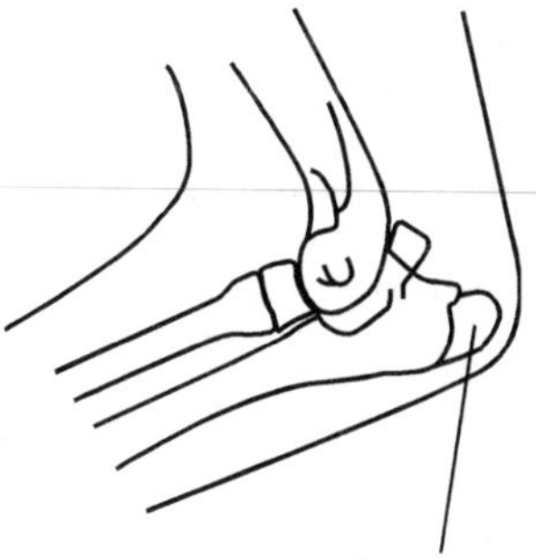

Olecranon process of elbow

olecranon The bony projection at the head of the ulna, helps to stabilise the elbow joint.

olfaction The process of smelling, olfaction is important in hunting animals to locate food sources.

olfactory nerve The first cranial nerve originates from the olfactory bulb and the cerebrum caudally.

oligo- Prefix, means few or scant in number.

oligaemia Shortage of circulating blood, *see also* DEHYDRATION, PACKED CELL VOLUME.

oligogalactia Sparse or insufficient milk secretion, a problem in nursing bitches and queens.

oligosaccharides Simple sugars formed into chains of 3–10 monosaccharide molecules

oliguria The production of an unusually small quantity of urine. If fluid is available to drink it is a sign of renal damage.

Ollulanus tricuspis Worm that occurs in the stomach of foxes, some cats and pigs.

-oma Term for a growth or tumour.

omental leaf A method of attaching part of the omentum to the intestine or the prostate to provide an increased blood supply and more antibodies to an area of weakness or bacterial contamination.

omentopexy Method of fixation of the omentum to a site such as an enterotomy to improve the repair potential and bring a rich supply of blood containing white cells and antibodies.

omentum Anatomical structure in the cranial abdomen arising as a fold in the peritoneum but its lace-like structure allows it to pass anywhere in the abdomen: it can be used to assist surgically in repair. **Greater omentum** The fold that arises from the greater curvature of the stomach that can be stretched as far as the pelvic cavity. **Lesser omentum** Small structure attaching the duodenum to the shorter and inner concave stomach surface known as the lesser curvature.

omniverous Having a wide range of animal and plant origin foodstuffs to feed on.

omphal- Word stem for something relating to the umbilicus, *see also* NAVEL.

omphalocele A hernia, when an abdominal organ protrudes through the unclosed umbilicus in the new-born animal. Emergency repair is called for, *see also* UMBILICAL HERNIA.

onco- Prefix, refers to a cancer or a tumour.

Onchocerca A parasite spread by microfilaria when flies bite the host; affects deer, cattle and horses; not known in small animals.

oncogene A gene in viruses and mammalian cells that can cause cancer.

oncology The study of tumours and cancers.

oncovirus Virus that may cause cancer, *see also* LEUKAEMIA.

on heat Terminology for pro-oestrus combined with oestrus in the bitch's breeding cycle; breeders incorrectly perceived a raised body temperature as an indication that the bitch was receptive to the male.

ontogeny The developmental time of an individual from the fertilised egg to maturity.

onych- Prefix that relates to the nail.

onychectomy The excision of a claw or a nail in its nail bed. Carried out in domestic cats for social reasons.

onychomycosis A fungal infection such as ringworm affecting the claws.

oo- Prefix relating to the egg or ovum.

oocyst A resistant stage in the life cycle of organisms such as *Coccidia*, *see also* COCCIDIOSIS.

oocyte An immature egg in the ovary undergoes meiosis to become the ovum. The maturation of the oocyte after its release from the ovary is necessary for successful fertilisation.

oogenesis The production of mature eggs in the ovary from oocytes that develop in the fetus; eventually the cells lining the Graffian follicle mature at the time of ovulation.

oophorectomy Alternative word for the surgical removal of the ovaries, as in spaying.

opacity A lack of transparency to light as found in a corneal opacity.

opaque The inability to see the other side of a structure or situation; part of the body may be opaque to X-rays which is called radiopacity, *see also* CATARACT.

open angle glaucoma Raised pressure in the anterior chamber of the eye when there is no blockage of the drainage channel by the iris, but there is some defect in the drainage mechanism.

open pyometra Disease of the female reproductive tract where blood, mucopus or green to yellow thick purulent matter originating in the endometrium is discharged from the vulva, *see also* OVARIOHYSTERECTOMY.

open wound An injury that is exposed to the air and thus subject to contamination and infection, *see also* ABRASION, INCISION, LACERATION, PUNCTURE.

open rooted teeth Those that continue to grow throughout life as found in rabbits and herbivorous rodents.

operable Term used by surgeons for a condition where there is a justifiable chance of a full recovery or a clinical judgement that the situation will be improved by undertaking a surgical procedure.

operation Action performed on the body with the hands and the use of surgical instruments.

operculum The covering to an opening, the plug of mucus that covers the cervical canal during pregnancy.

ophidian Member of the snake family.

ophthalm(o)- Relating to the eyes.

ophthalmencephalon Nerve tissue that includes the retina, the optic nerves and the visual cortex of the brain.

ophthalmia Inflammation of the eye especially the conjunctiva; the term is antiquated. Horses suffered with periodic ophthalmia or 'moon blindness'.

ophthalmia neonatorum Conjunctivitis occurring in the newborn animal; previously thought to be due to infection within the vagina during the birth process.

ophthalmologist A person who has made a specialised study of eye disorders and their correction.

ophthalmoscope An instrument projecting light onto the eye and into the fundus so that the structure can be examined; lenses are used to focus at various depths of the orbit structures.

-opia Indicates a defect of the eye or vision.

opiate A morphine-type substance to induce sleep, provide analgesia or sedate an animal.

opistho- Prefix, indicates backwards, dorsal or posterior direction.

opisthotonus Relates to posture where the head, neck and spine are arched back as seen in toxaemias and other neurological problems.

opportunistic An organism that happens to take advantage of a 'niche' to multiply in becoming pathogenic. May be a sequel to immunosuppression.

Opsite A sterile disposable drape used for preparation of a sterile field for the surgeon to operate in.

optic Concerned with the eye or vision and sight.

optic chiasma Part of the eye structure at the base of the brain where the optic nerves cross like an X, allowing fibres to distribute to both sides of the brain and to both eyes.

optic disc (papilla) Colourless spot in the fundus where all the nerve fibres collect before leaving the orbit to form the optic nerve, accompanied by blood vessels; examination is important in the diagnosis of PRA.

optic nerve The second cranial nerve originates in the sensory receptors of the rods and cones; the nerve is entirely sensory with the motor component absent; the autonomic nervous system controls the pupils.

oral The mouth, as when suggesting the route of communication; unwritten rules are oral traditions. Some medicines should be administered by the oral route.

oral administration The most common method of administering therapeutic substances, *see also* PER OS.

oral cavity The area inside the mouth behind the lips.

orbicularis oculi The muscle that closes the eye.

orbicularis oris The muscle that closes the mouth.

orbit The cavity in which the eyeball lies; the bony orbit of the skull is made of several bones.

orchi- Prefix, denotes the male's testis or testicle.

orchidectomy Castration, or the removal of male gonads; in some European countries 'castration' would also include female neutering as in the UK 'spay' operation, so this term is more specific.

orchiectomy Alternative term for excision of the testes.

orchitis Inflammation of the substance of the testis.

orf Viral infection of sheep; it is a zoonosis as persons may develop nodules on their hands that should resolve spontaneously.

organ Independent structure composed of various tissues to fulfil a specific function.

organ of Corti The spiral sense organ within the cochlear of the ear.

organ of Jacobson A taste or sense organ (vomeronasal) that communicates between the roof of the mouth and the nose in rabbits.

organism An individual plant or animal, often microscopic.

organelles Small microscopic structures inside the cell but not part of the nucleus, includes mitochondria, lysosomes, reticular structures and the Golgi complex.

organochloride Chemical substances previously widely used for skin parasite control; their use is much restricted because of toxicity problems in the food chain.

organophosphate Chemical compounds used for internal and external parasite control; recently fallen out of favour or much restricted in their use because of nerve toxic changes, *see also* ACETYLCHOLINE.

orgasm The climax of sexual excitement; some pet owners describe seeing this in animals, but it is not known to occur during animal breeding.

orientation Obtaining a sense of place or direction, important in surgical technique.

orifice An opening in any anatomical area of the body, *see also* OSTIUM.

origin Usually the beginning of anything, but anatomically the muscle origin is the fixed attachment of the proximal part, *see also* INSERTION.

ornithosis Disease of birds that is zoonotic, *see also* CHLAMYDIOSIS, PSITTACOSIS.

oro- Prefix for the mouth.

oropharynx The cavity of the mouth beyond the soft palate, into the pharynx chamber and up to the hyoid bone.

orphan virus A term for a recently discovered or emerging virus that has no specific disease known to be caused by it.

ortho- Prefix, straight or normal.

orthodontics The branch of dental science concerned with malocclusions and providing straighter teeth.

orthopaedics The science of correcting deformities of the skeleton often by operating on joints or bones, *see also* BONE.

orthopnoea Breathlessness, with the ability to have a normal breathing pattern only whilst standing or if the thorax is lifted up.

Oryctolagus cuniculis *see* RABBIT.

Ortolani's sign Test used in human infants for hip joint laxity by lifting the head of the femur out of the acetabulum; a click can be felt or heard on return into the joint cavity, *see also* HIP DYSPLASIA.

os (1) Describes the oral area or any body opening, *see also* MOUTH. (2) Word for a bone, *see also* HIP.

oscheitis Inflammation of the scrotum, may be caused by chemical scalds or trauma.

oscillating saw A rotating saw that regularly reverses its direction of cut so it will not harm underlying structures when cutting.

oscilloscope Traditional name for a cathode ray tube or 'screen' in computers.

oscillotonometry Method of measuring blood pressure in animals by attaching a special cuff with a sensor to the tail or a limb.

Oslerus osleri Species of tracheal worm of dogs previously known as *Filaroides osleri*, named after the Canadian surgeon Sir William Osler.

-osis Word for a generalised disorder or disease state, *see also* NEPHROSIS, ORNITHOSIS.

osmolarity The osmotic power of a solution expressed in osmoles per litre of solution (osmolality is per kg solution), *see also* HYPERTONIC.

osmosis The passage of fluid or 'solvent' from a low concentration liquid to a high concentration one, *see also* SEMI-PERMEABLE MEMBRANE.

osmotic pressure The pressure by which water is drawn into a solution through a semi-permeable membrane; the greater the concentration or strength, the larger the pressure.

osmotic diarrhoea An important cause of fluid loss from the body when osmotic substances are present in the intestinal lumen; the result of a digestive failure or villus atrophy, *see also* MALABSORPTION.

osseous A bony structure. Most often applied to a type of bony substance.

ossicle A bony nodule, especially the three that form a chain across the middle ear.

ossification The process of producing, by osteoblasts, the bone normal in the growing animal; if pathological the results may be seen on X-ray as bony slivers appearing in tendons near their insertions.

ostectomy Cutting away part or all of a bone, an osteotome may be used.

osteitis Inflammation of a bone, *see also* PERIOSTITIS.

osteoarthritis A degenerative disease of joint cartilage where damage to the underlying bone may cause pain and immobility.

osteoarthropathy Disease of the joints and the bone, *see also* DEGENERATIVE JOINT DISEASE.

osteoblast A cell that forms bone.

osteochondroma A benign but slow-growing tumour of long bones.

osteochondrosis A developmental disease of articular cartilage with poor differentiation during growth of the long bones, principally the elbows, shoulders and hocks, *see also* ELBOW DYSPLASIA.

osteochondritis dissecans (OD) The disease where the thickness of the cartilage becomes so great that slivers of cartilage form flaps or become detached and ulcerated areas of the cartilage remain; may be seen as defects on X-rays of young dogs. Part hereditary, part environmental.

osteoclasts Cells that remove bone.

osteocytes Cells in the bone matrix within the lacunae, responsible for bone integrity; form part of the Haversian system, *see also* LAMELLA.

osteodystrophy Disease of bone during its development and growth. **Nutritional secondary osteodystrophy** Seen in growing puppies and kittens when there is a lack of available calcium, often due to feeding an all meat diet or excess cereal in the diet when phytates 'lock up' the calcium. **Canine hypertrophic osteodystrophy** A condition occasionally seen in rapidly growing larger breeds of dog where there is lameness from swollen joints, *see also* BARLOW'S DISEASE. **Renal secondary osteodystrophy** Disorder seen in advanced kidney disease when phosphates are retained and calcium is withdrawn from the bones especially from the lower jaw, *see also* RUBBER JAW.

osteogenesis The formation and development of bone.

osteoma A benign bone tumour.

osteomalacia A disease of the skeleton caused by inadequate intake of bone-forming elements in the diet or a deficiency of vitamin D, *see also* RICKETS.

osteomyelitis Inflammation of the bone, usually a deep-seated and persisting infection; involves both the cortex and the medulla. Caused by infection or by trauma, foreign bodies or surgical implants.

osteon The basic unit of bone consisting of the Haversian canal and the Volkmann canal in the concentric lamellae of compact bone as found in the cortex, *see also* CORTEX, HAVERSIAN SYSTEM.

osteopathy Any disease of bone in the skeleton. **Craniomandibular osteopathy** Specific disorder of the West Highland white terrier and similar terrier breeds with enlargement of the skull bones and lower jaw, often limiting the width of the

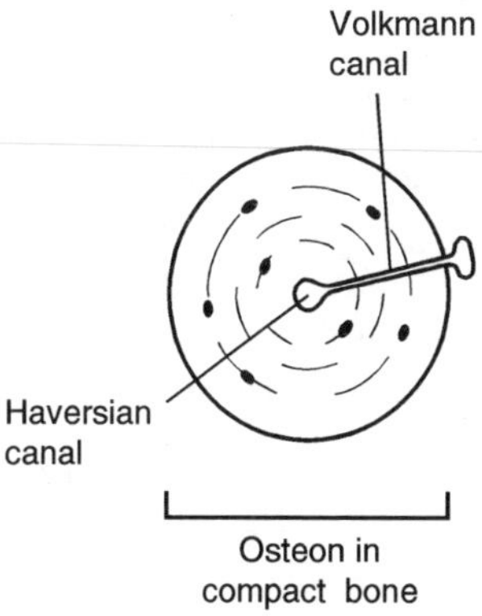

Osteon in compact bone showing Volkmann canal

mouth opening. **Secondary hypertrophic osteopathy (Marie's)** Disease associated with neoplasia and lung changes where the peripheral limb bones swell due to periosteal bone deposited especially above the carpal region.

osteophyte Spicule of bone seen on X-ray near a joint capsule; a sign of osteoarthritis, *see also* EXOSTOSIS.

osteoporosis A loss of bone density, resulting in bones that are brittle and liable to fracture.

osteosarcoma Malignant bone tumour; secondaries (metastases) are common and the lungs should always be radiographed before treatment is given.

osteotome Surgical instrument for cutting bone.

osteotomy Surgical procedure that involves the removal of bone. **Bulla osteotomy** Removal of the tympanic bulla to drain the middle ear, used in the treatment of otitis media. **Pelvic osteotomy** One of the possible treatments for hip dysplasia where the pelvis is realigned to stabilise the hip joint.

ostium A specialised opening such as the ostium abdominale where the oviduct from the uterus opens into the abdominal cavity, but within the ovarian bursa.

-ostomy Description of any operation where a surgical opening is made often to allow drainage, *see also* URETHOSTOMY.

ostrich Bird with long legs and long neck, farmed commercially for meat, leather and its feathers. Herbivores; males can run very fast before attacking intruders to their paddocks. Females are more docile but easily frightened.

oto- Prefix, relates to the ear.

otitis General term for ear inflammation.

otitis externa Inflammation of the outer ear tube and pinna; may be detected by violent shaking, scratching with the back leg and the head held down on one side.

otitis interna Inflammation extends to the balance centre, *see also* COCHLEAR.

otitis media Middle ear infection; may follow otitis externa or infection from the throat via the Eustachian tube.

otoacariasis Infestation of the ear canal with mites, *see also* *OTODECTES.*

Otobius lagophilus Species of tick that may be found on rabbits.

Otodectes cynotis Species of mite found not infrequently in cats' ears, and when present in the dog's ear usually causes severe irritation.

otolith (otoconium) Part of the balance mechanism of the inner ear; calcium carbonate particles float in fluid in the macula of the utricle and saccule of the inner ear.

otorrhoea Any discharge from the ear, usually a sign of otitis externa.

otoscope Instrument for examining the outer ear canal and the tympanic membrane, *see also* AUROSCOPE.

ototoxic Substances used medicinally that can damage the balance or the hearing centres of the ear. Streptomycin is an example of an antibiotic toxic to the VIIIth cranial nerve.

outbreeding Planning a mating to have as few common ancestors in recent generations as possible; it may be a way of breeding out an undesirable trait or reducing recessive gene problems that have resulted from close or inbreeding.

outcome The end result, as after head trauma in a road accident; the eventual degree of recovery can not always be predicted.

out-patient Attending on a daily basis, an alternative to hospitalisation as an 'in-patient'.

output, cardiac The aortic blood flow may be measured with Doppler equipment; regurgitation occurs if valves do not close completely in systole.

ova Describes the eggs as released from the follicle either by spontaneous or induced ovulation, *see also* FERTILISATION.

ovari(o)- Prefix, relating to the ovary, often used as a surgical operation prefix.

oval window The communication from the outer ear to the middle ear covered by the tympanic membrane.

ovarian Adjective, part of the ovary.

ovarian bursa Membranous layer of peritoneum that almost envelopes the ovary of the bitch, assisting the eggs released from the follicles being wafted into the oviducts.

ovarian cycle The reproductive cycle, controlled by the hormones of the pituitary and the ovary.

ovarian cyst Structure like a very large follicle in the ovary, often associated with excess oestrogen production and one form of pyometra.

ovariohysterectomy The surgical operation to remove all of the uterus and both ovaries, commonly known as spaying.

ovary, pl. ovaries The endocrine glands of the female, also responsible for release of ova to perpetuate the genes after male fertilisation. There are two ovaries in the abdomen normally found in the area of the kidneys.

overdeveloping An uncommon film fault if automatic processors are used. Indicated by a uniform darkening of all of the film or 'development fog'.

over-the-counter (OTC) medicines Non-prescription medicines; some may not have undergone safety evaluation especially if of herbal nature. General sales list (GSL) medicines will all have been subjected to scrutiny and are therefore safest, dispensing rules must be observed by nurses.

over-the-needle catheter A type of cannula used in fluid therapy; a cut down on the vein may be needed to prevent the catheter being dragged back by the animal's skin during insertion.

overdose (OD) Usually an accidental act of drug administration, caused by misreading the instructions on the label or in some cases miscalculating an animal's weight, *see also* POISONING.

overexposure In radiography a lack of definition or all over greyness of the plate may be due to incorrect technique; the areas covered by metal markers still remain white in overexposure faults, *see also* OVERDEVELOPING.

overhydration Undesirable complication of fluid therapy; fluid may accumulate in the lungs and pulmonary oedema reduces respiratory function; a moist cough may be the first sign during the administration of intravenous fluids.

overriding fracture Complex fracture in which the ends of the bone overlap each other; reduction is essential before fixation of the fracture.

overshot jaw State of the mouth when the lower jaw is short so that the maxilla protrudes and the teeth of the upper jaw are in advance of the teeth of the lower jaw.

oviduct Delicate structure connecting the fimbria in the ovarian bursa to the lumen of the uterus; of importance as it is the site for fertilisation of ova, *see also* FALLOPIAN TUBE.

oviparous Refers to an egg-producing reptile or to birds.

ovoviviparous Refers to the birth of living offspring from an egg in the body, in certain reptiles, lizards and some amphibians.

ovulation The release of ova (or a single ovum) from the follicle in the ovary. Spontaneous in the bitch but induced in the female cat by the mating procedure with the male, *see also* OESTROUS CYCLE.

ovum Egg, carries the genetic material of the mother that after fertilisation allows for an embryo to form.

oxalate calculi Concretions that may form in the urinary tract composed of calcium oxalate, characterised by sharp knife edge to the 'stones' often causing haematuria. Diet changes make these more common than struvite calculi in cats.

OXF Anticoagulant used in specimen containers for glucose estimation; the potassium oxalate with sodium fluoride kills the cells preventing further oxidation of the glucose in the sample.

oxygen Colourless gas in common use for anaesthetic circuits as a carrier and a life support agent. High pressure cylinders are black with a white top in UK.

oxygen saturation A measure of tissue oxygen availability; the haemoglobin content can be measured in the laboratory.

oxygen therapy Any form of administration by oxygen cage, mask or tent to relieve hypoxaemia in shock or after blood loss.

oxyhaemoglobin The carriage of oxygen from the lungs to the body tissues is dependent on the ability of the haemoglobin in the red blood cells to make up this molecule.

oxytetracycline Broad-spectrum antibiotic widely used in veterinary medicine.

oxytocic Any medication that aids contractions of the uterus.

oxytocin Hormone produced by the posterior pituitary responsible for contraction of the smooth muscle of the uterus and also for milk let-down in the lactating female.

Oxyuris Parasitic worm, mainly of equines. Nurses may be asked about 'pinworms' that are causing itching and tail rubbing in ponies but the worms do not infect dogs and cats. The smaller animal pets have oxyurid parasites: *Passalarus ambiguus* in the rabbit, or *Syphacia obvelata* in the hamster, *see also* THREADWORMS.

P

P-wave The electrical wave on the ECG trace that occurs before the QRS complex and represents depolarisation of the atria; in the normal trace every QRS complex should be preceded by a P-wave.

pacemaker Small electrical device implanted under the skin, with electrodes that run to the heart, to control the heart beat.

Pacheco's disease Cause of sudden death in psittacine birds, due to a marked fatty hepatitis.

pachy- Prefix denoting thickening.

pachydermia Thickening of the skin.

pachymeningitis Inflammation and thickening of the dura, which is otherwise known as the pachymeninx.

Pacinian corpuscle Encapsulated sensory mechanoreceptor found in the skin; sensitive to deformation; consists of a number of capsular layers wrapped around a sensory nerve ending.

paediatrics The branch of medicine dealing with disease in children; in the veterinary sphere it may be used to describe disease in young animals.

PAF Platelet aggregating factor.

pain An unpleasant physical and emotional experience, associated with potential or actual tissue damage.

packed cell volume (PCV) The percentage of the circulating blood volume that is taken up by cells, as opposed to fluid; PCV can readily be determined in the laboratory by spinning a blood sample at 5000–10 000 r.p.m. for 5 minutes. The red and white blood cells will settle to form a solid column, the platelets will form a cream-coloured band above this (the buffy coat) and the straw-coloured plasma will be on the top. A raised PCV may indicate dehydration; a low PCV indicates shock, anaemia, excessive re-hydration etc., *see also* BUFFY COAT, HAEMATOCRIT.

palatability A measure of how much an animal likes a food.

palate The structure that forms the roof of the mouth, separating the oral and nasal cavities; is in two parts, the more rostral hard palate is formed by the horizontal parts of the palatine, maxillary and incisive bones; this is continued caudally as the soft palate, a flap of muscle covered by mucous membrane, *see also* CLEFT PALATE, PALATORRHAPHY.

palatine Relating to the palate, e.g. the palatine arteries.

palatoglossal Relating to the palate and tongue.

palatorrhaphy Surgical repair of a congenital cleft palate or acquired break in the palate; involves carefully mobilising the soft tissues around the defect and suturing them in place.

palliative Symptomatic treatment that will improve quality of life, but will not cure the underlying disease, e.g. adequate pain relief for animals that are terminally ill.

pallor Paleness, lack of skin colour.

palmar The undersurface of the front paws, as in the human palm, *see also* PLANTAR.

palmigrade Abnormal stance where the caudal aspect of the carpus contacts the ground; causes include carpal hyperextension injuries in animals that have fallen from a height, carpal luxation, etc.

palpable Able to be detected by touch, e.g. palpation of superficial lymph nodes, such as the prescapular and popliteal.

palpate Investigate by touch; a cornerstone of clinical examination.

palpation Careful investigation using the hands; commonly used for pregnancy diagnosis in the bitch at 28 days post-mating, the time when any conceptuses are most likely to be palpable.

palpebral Relating to the eyelids.

palpebral fissure The opening of the eye; the gap between the upper and lower eyelids.

palpitation Sudden rapid pounding of the heart.

pampiniform plexus The tortuous plexus formed by the testicular vein, lying within the mesorchium just proximal to the testis.

pan- Prefix meaning across, throughout.

pancarpal arthrodesis Surgical fusion of all the levels of carpal joint, i.e. the antebrachiocarpal, intercarpal and carpometacarpal joints; the treatment of choice for most carpal hyperextension injuries; technique involves removal of all articular cartilage, packing the joints with cancellous bone graft and rigidly fixing with a bone plate.

pancreas Both an endocrine and exocrine gland, lying close to the stomach and duodenum; the exocrine acinar cells secrete amylase, lipase and trypsinogen into the duodenum via the pancreatic ducts. The endocrine function is carried out by the β-cells of the islets of Langerhans, that secrete insulin into the blood stream, *see also* DIABETES MELLITUS, EXOCRINE PANCREATIC INSUFFICIENCY, PANCREATITIS.

pancreatitis Inflammation of the pancreas; causes anterior abdominal pain and affected animals may adopt a 'praying' stance; may recur in bouts, and can lead to EPI and/or diabetes mellitus, *see also* DIABETES MELLITUS, EXOCRINE PANCREATIC INSUFFICIENCY.

pancuronium bromide (Pavulon) A potent non-depolarising neuromuscular blocking agent; standard doses provide about 20 minutes blockade, and the effects can be reversed with neostigmine.

pancytopenia Reduction in the number of all cells (red, white and platelets) circulating in the blood, e.g. due to bone-marrow suppression.

pandemic An infection that spreads across a whole country, or even the world, e.g. influenza can be pandemic.

panleukopenia Abnormally low numbers of all the circulating white blood cells (neutrophils, eosinophils, basophils, lymphocytes), *see also* FELINE INFECTIOUS ENTERITIS.

panniculitis Inflammation of the subcutaneous fat, to form hard nodules that may drain out onto the skin surface. The condition is usually idiopathic, but may be secondary to bacterial and fungal infection; single lesions may be surgical excised, multiple lesions usually respond to steroids.

panniculus reflex The skin twitch response; when the skin along the trunk is pinched, or the hair coat lightly touched, the animal responds by twitching the skin of that region. The reflex is brought about by the cutaneous trunci muscle and is particularly well developed in the horse and cow, where the muscle continues into the neck and across the loins. Used during the diagnosis of intervertebral disc protrusion.

pannus (1) A chronic progressive keratitis and vascularisation of the cornea; most common in the German shepherd dog; aetiology is unclear but an auto-immune component is likely; most cases respond to topical steroids or cytotoxic agents. The disease is likely to re-occur; severe cases require superficial keratectomy, *see also* UBERREITER'S SYNDROME. (2) Growth of hyperplastic synovial membrane across the articular cartilage of a joint; the result of chronic joint inflammation; the cartilage is destroyed by degradative enzymes released from synoviocytes and inflammatory cells; synovectomy may be required.

panophthalmitis Inflammation of the eyeball and all its contents.

panosteitis Inflammation of intramedullary tissues, as a sequel to focal areas of fat necrosis; a common cause of pain and lameness in young dogs of the large breeds. It most commonly affects the humerus, but is also found in the radius, ulna, femur and tibia; has a characteristic radiographic appearance, with mottled thumb-print lesions; may reoccur in bouts and cause a shifting lameness, but responds well to analgesics and has a good prognosis.

pansteatitis Discolorations and inflammation of fat deposits within the body; due to high intake of unsaturated fats in the diet, and inadequate levels of the antioxidant vitamin E; rarely seen, but occurs in cats who are fed solely on fish; signs include pyrexia, lethargy, hyperaesthesia and pain on handling, and a stiff gait; treatment involves correcting the diet and supplying vitamin E.

pant Rapid, shallow breathing; a normal body response in the dog to hyperthermia, as evaporation from the upper respiratory tract helps cooling; may also occur in shock. In contrast, mouth breathing in the cat is always abnormal and is a sign of severe respiratory distress.

pantothenic acid Part of the B vitamin complex, *see also* VITAMIN B.

panzootic Affecting all the animals within a given area.

papilla, pl. papillae A nipple-like bud; describes anatomical structures with this form, e.g. the optic papilla where the optic nerve enters the eye.

papillary muscle The muscular columns that attach the chordae tendinae to the walls of the ventricles of the heart, preventing the atrio-ventricular valves from everting.

papilloedema Swelling of the optic disc.

papilloma Benign neoplasm of stratified squamous epithelium; a small, pedunculated growth, often referred to as a wart.

papilloma virus Virus causing warts, *see also* PAPILLOMATOSIS.

papillomatosis The growth of many benign papillomas, predominantly on the limbs, head and in the mouth, usually due to viral infection; spontaneous recovery occurs in most cases; surgical removal may be required, depending on the exact location of the growth.

papular Having papules.

papule Small, solid, raised skin nodule; may be a precursor to a pustule if infection becomes established.

para- Prefix meaning near to, through or beside.

paracentesis The aspiration of fluid, usually from the abdomen; an area in the midline at the lowest point of the abdomen should be prepared aseptically; the tap can usually be performed with a hypodermic needle, and requires minimal restraint or sedation, *see also* FELINE INFECTIOUS PERITONITIS.

paracetamol A widely available human analgesic; other licensed veterinary products are preferred for animals. Care is required if paracetamol is given to animals by their owners as it can be hepatotoxic.

paracrine Hormone effects that are limited to a localised area.

parafollicular cells Cells in the thyroid gland that produce calcitonin, the hormone that lowers levels of blood calcium, *see also* CALCITONIN, PARATHORMONE.

parainfluenza virus A myxovirus causing acute upper respiratory disease, *see also* KENNEL COUGH.

paralysis Complete loss of function of an area of the body; when applied to a limb, the term means that the animal is unable to make any stepping movements, even if aided; the most common cause of paralysis is disc disease, *see also* INTERVERTEBRAL DISC DISEASE, LARYNGEAL PARALYSIS, PARAPLEGIA, PARESIS, QUADRIPLEGIA, TETRAPLEGIA.

paralytic ileus Tympany and stasis of the intestines, owing to a lack of the normal peristaltic waves; may occur after intestinal surgery or if there has been severe distension of the gut, *see also* ILEUS.

parameter A vital sign that should be monitored regularly in hospitalised patients, to chart their progress, e.g. temperature, pulse rate, respiratory rate.

paramyxovirus An RNA-virus causing Newcastle disease – a notifiable disease mainly of pigeons; common signs include diarrhoea, upper respiratory sounds, poor plumage and nervous signs; a vaccine is available but not compulsory.

paranasal sinuses The large sinuses which are extensions of the nasal chambers and are located within the bones of the skull; there are maxillary and frontal sinuses, that are subdivided into communicating compartments.

paraneoplastic syndrome Syndromes associated with neoplasia, but not directly due to the space-occupying effects of the primary tumour or metastases; includes hormonal, neurological and metabolic imbalances leading to hypercalcaemia, Marie's disease, glomerulonephropathy, DIC, etc. Paraneoplastic neuropathies can occur.

paraphimosis Constriction of the prepuce around an engorged penis, so that the penis cannot be retracted back into the prepuce; common in the dog; surgical correction or manipulation under anaesthesia may be required if the penis cannot be replaced; if neglected, gangrene of the tip may result.

paraplegia Paralysis of the hind limbs.

paraprostatic cyst Large, fluid-filled sacs that develop in the tissues adjacent to the prostate; may be a precursor of prostatic hypertrophy; usually requires surgical drainage/removal or marsupialisation.

paraquat A weedkiller, whose toxic effects include vomiting, lethargy and progressive respiratory distress due to marked interstitial oedema, leading to death within 3–10 days. There is no specific antidote, but support therapy may be tried.

parasite An organism that lives on the surface of (ectoparasite) or within (endoparasite), another organism.

parasitology The scientific study of parasites, their life cycles and the diseases they may cause.

parasympathetic nervous system Part of the autonomic nervous system that has a craniosacral outflow and produces involuntary effects such as slowing the heart, pupil constriction and peristalsis, *see also* AUTONOMIC NERVOUS SYSTEM, SYMPATHETIC NERVOUS SYSTEM.

parasympatholytic A drug, such as atropine, that reduces the effects of the parasympathetic nervous system.

parasympathomimetic Drugs such as acetylcholine and pilocarpine, that act to increase the effects of the parasympathetic system.

paratenic host A species that is not the normal host for a parasite but that may be used opportunistically by the parasite.

paratenon The connective tissue immediately surrounding a tendon.

parathormone One of the hormones secreted into the blood stream by the parathyroid glands; it acts to elevate blood calcium levels by increasing resorption from bone and uptake from the gut, while promoting renal phosphate excretion, *see also* CALCITONIN.

parathyroid glands The four small glands situated close to the lobes of the thyroid gland; they secrete parathormone and calcitonin, to provide regulation of blood calcium levels.

paravertebral anaesthesia The injection of local anaesthetic solution adjacent to the spinal nerves where they emerge between the transverse processes of the lumbar vertebrae. The technique is used in cattle to provide analgesia over the abdomen to allow procedures such as rumenotomy and Caesarean section.

parenchyma The tissue substance of a gland.

parenteral Any route of drug administration that does not involve the gastrointestinal tract, e.g. subcutaneous, intramuscular, intraperitoneal, intravenous.

paresis Muscle weakness with neurological deficits, but the animal can still make coordinated walking movements if the body weight is supported, *see also* PARALYSIS.

parietal Close to the body wall, e.g. the parietal pleura is applied to the inner wall of the chest, while the visceral pleura covers the lung tissue.

paronychia Inflammation of the nailbeds, often with ulceration; may be caused by bacteria, fungi, or diseases such as demodecosis and pemphigus.

parotid salivary gland Salivary gland located at the base of the vertical ear canal.

parous Having produced live offspring, *see also* MULTIPAROUS, PRIMIGRAVIDA, UNIPAROUS.

partial carpal arthrodesis Surgical fusion of the intercarpal and carpometacarpal joints, sparing the antebrachiocarpal joint, where most of the movement occurs, *see also* PANCARPAL ARTHRODESIS.

parturition The process of giving birth.

parvovirus A small DNA virus that causes acute gastroenteritis in many species; the canine parvovirus is thought to have mutated from the feline form; it causes severe vomiting and diarrhoea, which can be fatal in young pups. The virus is resistant to many disinfectants, and can spread rapidly through susceptible populations; faecal and serological tests can be used to confirm the diagnosis; the virus can also replicate in heart muscle, causing an acute myocarditis and sudden death; a component of multivalent canine vaccines, that offer effective protection against the disease.

passerine Term used to describe birds that perch.

passive movement Gentle flexing and extending of the limb joints, with the animal in recumbency; part of physiotherapy and important in the nursing of paraplegic patients.

***Pasteurella* spp.** Group of Gram-negative bacteria causing respiratory disease and septicaemia in many species. *Pasteurella multocida* is associated with cellulitis and infection from dog and cat bites or scratches.

patella The knee cap; a sesamoid bone within the tendon of the quadriceps muscle mass.

patellar ligament The ligament running from the distal pole of the patella, inserting on the tibial crest.

patellar luxation Displacement of the patella; a congenital abnormality, with a genetic component in many breeds; in the toys and terriers, particularly those with bow legs, such as the Staffordshire bull terrier and Jack Russell, the displacement is medial and is often associated with displacement of the tibial crest too. In the labrador retriever and other large breeds, it is most often lateral; affected animals show signs of intermittent or persistent hind leg lameness; surgical treatment involves sulcoplasty (deepening of the trochlear groove), releasing the joint capsule on one side and tightening it on the opposite side and transplanting the tibial crest back to its correct midline position.

patent Open, having a lumen.

patent ductus arteriosus (PDA) Failure of the ductus arteriosus to close within the first few days after birth, thus allowing left-to-right shunting of blood from the aorta to the pulmonary artery; clinical signs include poor growth, exercise intolerance, rapid heart rate and a machinery murmur; surgical ligation of the duct via a thoracotomy is the treatment of choice.

pathogen Any living micro-organism that can cause disease, e.g. bacteria, viruses, protozoa.

pathogenicity The ability to cause disease.

pathognomonic A finding that is specific to a certain disease;

presence of this finding allows the disease to be diagnosed, e.g. hyperkeratosis of the pads and nose in cases of distemper.

pathology The scientific study of the cause and effects of disease.

PDH (1) Pituitary-dependent hyperadrenocorticism, *see also* CUSHING'S SYNDROME. (2) Police dog handler.

pectinectomy Surgical removal of a portion or all of the pectineus muscle; used as a treatment for hip dysplasia in young dogs; is thought to relieve tension on the joint capsule of the hip, and thus reduce pain.

pectus excavatum A rare congenital abnormality of the chest wall, where the caudal sternebrae and xiphisternum curve inwards towards the spine.

pedal reflex The withdrawal or flexor reflex; when the animal is placed in lateral recumbency and the toe or web is pinched, the foot should be withdrawn from the noxious stimulus.

pedicle A stalk.

pedicle graft A portion of skin and underlying subcutaneous tissue that retains an attachment to the body (and a vascular supply) via a pedicle of tissue; the skin flap can be transposed and used to close tissue defects.

pediculosis Infestation with lice, *see also* LOUSE.

pedigree The family line or ancestry of an individual.

peduncle A stalk or pedicle.

pellagra Name for vitamin B complex deficiency in man.

pelvis The girdle of bone connecting the lumbosacral spine to the hind legs; two symmetrical halves, each comprising the ilium, ischium and pubis; organs contained within the pelvis include the bladder (when empty or partially filled), non-gravid uterus and rectum.

pemphigus An auto-immune complex, characterised by the formation of skin vesicles; diagnosis is confirmed by immunohistochemical staining of biopsy material from the blisters; treatment is based on immunosuppression with glucocorticoids; adjunctive therapies such as gold salts or cytotoxic drugs may also be used.

pemphigus erythematosus Bullous lesions appear over the nose and ears; made worse by sunny weather and may be confused with the solar dermatitis seen in breeds of dog such as the collie and German shepherd dog.

pemphigus foliaceous The most common auto-immune skin disease, affecting mainly the head and feet, although lesions may occur elsewhere.

pemphigus vegetans Rarest form, with the formation of crusts and scabs.

pemphigus vulgaris The second most common form of pemphigus, with vesicles appearing around the nailbeds and at mucocutaneous junctions.

penicillin A bacteriocidal antibiotic originally derived from *Penicillium* spp. mould but now made synthetically.

penile Relating to the penis.

penis Part of the external genitalia of the male and the organ of copulation; it is composed of erectile tissue that becomes engorged with blood prior to mating; the urethra runs through the penis. In the non-erect state, the penis is retained within the prepuce; in the cat the penis is caudally directed when not engorged and carries papillae on the surface, *see also* MICROPHALLUS.

pentobarbitone sodium A barbiturate commonly used for euthanasia, although it has also been used at lower concentrations as an induction agent or in the treatment of status epilepticus.

penumbra The area of half-shadow or blurring around the edges of an object that is placed within a beam of X-rays. Penumbral blurring on the finished radiograph can be minimised by using a small focal spot, *see also* FOCAL SPOT.

pepsin One of the key digestive enzymes; secreted as the precursor, pepsinogen, by the chief cells of the gastric mucosa, pepsin hydrolyses the peptide bonds in ingested proteins.

pepsinogen The precursor of pepsin, *see also* PEPSIN.

peptide A compound containing two or more linked amino acids.

peptone Soluble peptides, often added to bacterial culture media.

per Through, via or most.

peracute Having an extremely rapid onset.

percuss Tap with the hand or a percussive instrument to determine the density of a part.

percutaneously placed gastrotomy (PEG) tube An enteral feeding tube placed directly into the stomach via the abdominal body wall; can easily be made by modifying a Foley catheter. For placement, the animal has to be anaesthetised, and an endoscope is required; the tube is well tolerated and can be left *in situ* for several weeks.

perforation An abnormal opening.

peri- Prefix meaning around, in the region of.

perianal Around the anus.

perianal fistula Blind-ending, necrotic tracts opening to the skin around the anus; occur almost exclusively in German shepherd dogs, *see also* FURUNCULOSIS.

periapical abscess An abscess that develops around the root of a tooth, usually necessitating removal of the tooth to allow drainage, *see also* MALAR.

periarticular Around a joint.

pericardial effusion Collection of fluid within the pericardial sac; causes include spontaneous haemorrhage, bleeding from haemangiosarcomata, infection and oedema fluid from congestive heart disease. The effusion leads predominantly to right-sided heart failure; pericardiocentesis is required to type the fluid and drain the pericardium; if there is recurrence of idiopathic effusion, a window may be surgically cut in the pericardium to allow drainage.

pericarditis Inflammation of the pericardium.

pericardium The double-layered (visceral and parietal layers) membranous sac that encloses the heart and the start of the great vessels.

perichondrium Limiting membrane covering cartilage (but absent across the articular surface of cartilage in joints).

perilymph The fluid contained within the scala tympani and scala vestibuli of the inner ear, *see also* EAR, ENDOLYMPH.

perimysium The fibrous membrane around skeletal muscle fibres.

perinatal The period around birth, covering the first 2 or 3 days.

perineal The region around the perineum.

perineal hernia Rupture of the perineal musculature (the pelvic diaphragm) allowing protrusion of fat and abdominal contents. The urinary bladder may also retroflex into large perineal hernia defects; often associated with chronic straining, e.g. prostatic hypertrophy, constipation; males are far more commonly affected than females; requires careful surgical replacement of the contents and closure of the defect; castration is also recommended in the male animal.

perineum The region extending from the ischium, between the hind legs to the pubis; includes the anus, vulva and scrotal sac.

perineurium The connective tissue sheath around nerve fibre bundles.

periodontal membrane The tough fibrous membrane anchoring a tooth to the gum.

periodontitis Inflammation of the periodontal membrane; usually due to the build up of plaque and calculus within the pockets around the tooth, and the start of gingivitis; if left untreated the gums will recede and the tooth will eventually be lost.

periople The outer layer of the hoof.

periorbital Region around the eye.

periosteal proliferative polyarthritis (PPP) An erosive polyarthritis seen in the cat; in addition, there is marked proliferation of bone spreading away from the joints; it affects mainly the tarsal and carpal regions; diagnosis is confirmed by radiography.

periosteum The tough, fibrous membrane that surrounds the outer surfaces of bones; important as the blood supply to the outer third of the cortex runs in the periosteum, which is also rich in nerve endings.

periostitis A bone disorder where there is inflammation of the periosteum, the outer cover of the bone. Dental periostistis may be due to tooth infection.

peripheral Away from the centre.

peripheral nervous system (PNS) The cranial and spinal nerves that run from the brain and spinal cord to the other parts of the body; most nerves are mixed, carrying sensory information towards the CNS, motor information away from the CNS and also carrying fibres from the autonomic nervous system.

peristalsis The coordinated muscular contractions that sweep along the gastrointestinal tract to mix the food and move it along the tract.

peritoneal dialysis Injection of relatively large volumes of fluid into the abdomen, and withdrawal of the fluid after allowing time for waste products in the blood to diffuse across the peritoneum into the fluid.

peritoneum The membrane lining the inner wall of the abdomen and covering the viscera, *see also* EPIPLOIC FORAMEN.

peritonitis Inflammation of the peritoneum; a painful abdominal condition.

perivascular Around a blood vessel; it is important that irritant intravenous substances, such as thiopentone or vincristine, are not injected into perivascular tissues by accident, as they can cause tissue necrosis.

permanent teeth Teeth present in an adult mouth, *see also* TEMPORARY.

permeable Able to allow molecules through.

pernicious Indicates a fatal disease, such as pernicious anaemia.

peroneal Relating to the fibula.

per os Via the mouth.

perosis A nutritional disease of young birds where there is shortening of the limb bones and displacement of tendons; possibly due to manganese deficiency, but may be exacerbated by poor flooring and overcrowding.

peroxide H_2O_2; a bleaching agent; may be used diluted to flush abscesses, but can be toxic to tissues.

persistent hyperplastic primary vitreous (PHPV) Congenital condition affecting the vitreous body, where the fetal blood supply to the lens fails to regress; fibrovascular tissue forms on the posterior surface of the lens, which may cause blindness if extensive. An inherited defect in the Dobermann and Staffordshire bull terrier.

persistent right aortic arch (PRAA) Congenital abnormality in the formation of the aortic arch, so that the aorta lies on the right of the trachea and oesophagus rather than to the left; this creates a ring around the oesophagus as the ligamentum arteriosum passes round to the pulmonary artery. The signs of oesophageal constriction become apparent at weaning when solid food is regurgitated; surgical sectioning of the ligamentum may resolve the problem, although some degree of oesophageal dysfunction may remain.

pervious urachus Congenital defect due to failure of the urachus to close and regress after birth; urine dribbles constantly from the umbilicus; surgical correction is required.

pessary A medicated vaginal suppository.

petechia, pl. petechiae A tiny area of haemorrhage.

pethidine An opiate analgesic, about one-tenth as potent as morphine; may also be used as a premedicant, and has some spasmolytic properties; a controlled drug.

petit mal Minor epileptiform seizure, without loss of consciousness; may be a transient lack of awareness of surroundings, *see also* EPILEPSY.

Petri dish A shallow plastic dish with a lid; used in the laboratory as bacterial culture plates, etc.

petrissage A kneading movement used in massage.

petroleum jelly A commonly used lubricant gel.

-pexy Surgical fixation.

Peyer's patches Aggregates of lymphoid tissue within the wall of the small intestine.

pH A scale used to measure acidity, ranging from 0 (most acidic) to 14 (most alkaline), with 7 being neutral; may be measured with probes, or more roughly with colour change strips based on litmus paper, *see also* LITMUS PAPER.

phacoemulsification The use of low frequency ultrasound to break down a cataract so that it can be removed with minimal disturbance to the eye.

phaeochromocytoma A rare tumour of the chromaffin cells of the adrenal medulla, giving rise to signs such as weakness, vomiting, diarrhoea, tachycardia and PU/PD.

phagocyte A scavenger cell that can ingest bacteria, foreign material and other cells.

phagocytosis The processes of ingestion and digestion of substances by phagocytes.

phalanx, pl. phalanges A toe.

phallus Penis.

pharmacodynamics A study of the therapeutic effects an individual drug has on the body.

pharmacokinetics A study of the absorption, distribution, metabolism and excretion of an individual drug.

pharmacology The study of drugs, their effects and uses.

pharmacy A place where drugs are dispensed.

pharyngeal Relating to the pharynx.

pharyngostomy Creation of a surgical opening into the pharynx via the skin of the throat region; most commonly to allow placement of a feeding tube; iatrogenic damage can be caused during this procedure, and the tube is poorly tolerated by patients.

pharyngostomy tube A feeding tube surgically placed into the pharynx, *see also* PHARYNGOSTOMY.

pharynx The cavity at the back of the mouth leading to the oesophagus and trachea; divided into the (lower) oropharynx and (upper) nasopharynx.

phenobarbitone A sedative anticonvulsant used in the control of epilepsy, *see also* EPILEPSY.

phenol A group of potent disinfectants, toxic to cats.

phenotype The outward appearance of an animal, reflecting the genetic make up, *see also* GENOTYPE.

phenylbutazone The standard non-steroidal anti-inflammatory drug (NSAID); used widely for chronic locomotor diseases, such as osteoarthritis, and as an analgesic.

phenytoin An anticonvulsant used to treat epilepsy.

pheromone A hormone secreted by an individual that causes a change in the sexual behaviour of a second member of that species; may play an important role in courtship rituals. Used therapeutically to stop 'spraying' by cats.

phimosis Narrowing or constriction of the prepuce, *see also* PARAPHIMOSIS.

phlebitis Inflammation of a vein.

phlegm Excessive amounts of mucus produced from the respiratory tract.

phospholipid A lipid molecule containing phosphorus; such molecules are important constituents of cell membranes.

photophobia Avoidance of light; associated with painful ophthalmologic conditions such as glaucoma and uveitis.

photoelectric effect Generation of electricity from the action of light.

photoreceptor A cell that is sensitive to light, e.g. the rods and cones of the retina.

photosensitisation Sensitisation of the skin to the effects of sunlight.

photosynthesis The process plants use to build complex molecules from water and carbon dioxide, using chlorophyll and driven by the action of sunlight.

phototaxis Movement of an organism in response to a light stimulus.

phrenic Relating to the diaphragm.

phthisis bulbi A shrunken, blind eye.

phylum A taxonomic division used in the classification of plants and animals.

physiology The study of how the normal body functions.

physiotherapy Physical treatments designed to speed healing and recovery.

physis The epiphyseal plate, or growth plate; the cartilage zone at the epiphysis of long bones, that allows lengthening of the bone in immature animals, *see also* ENDOCHONDRAL OSSIFICATION.

pia mater Literally 'tender mother'; the innermost of the three meningeal layers, a delicate membrane that is closely applied to nervous tissue of the brain and spinal cord.

pica Depraved appetite.

picornavirus Group of small RNA viruses that includes feline calicivirus.

pigment Coloration.

pill A small round object, *see also* TABLET.

pilocarpine Parasympathomimetic drug used to treat intestinal stasis and atropine overdosage, *see also* PARASYMPATHOMIMETIC.

pilo-erection Raising of hairs due to the action of pilo-erector muscles; the hair coat may stand on end to trap an insulating layer of air to prevent excessive loss of body heat in cold environments. The same effect is used when animals 'raise their hackles' to make themselves appear bigger and more threatening.

pinch graft Skin grafting technique where a punch is used to collect numerous 4–5 mm diameter plugs of skin from a clipped donor site; the plugs have the subcutaneous fat trimmed away and are then pressed into small pockets cut into the recipient site.

pineal gland Pine-cone shaped structure within the midbrain; exact function remains poorly defined, but it influences growth and seasonal patterns of behaviour.

pin fitment The arrangement of pins and pinholes that allows only the correct gas cylinder to be fitted to the port of an anaesthetic machine.

pinioning Surgical removal of one wing tip in young birds, to prevent flight; it is permanent, unlike clipping of flight feathers.

pinna The external ear flap.

pinocytosis The process by which a cell forms invaginations along its outer membrane; the invagination forms a vesicle that gets pinched off, trapping external molecules that are then taken into the cell.

pins Metal implants used for internal fracture fixation; the pin is inserted into the medullary cavity of the fractured bone; pinning is best used for long, oblique fractures; although in man the pin is commonly removed after fracture healing, in animals the pin is usually left *in situ*.

pinworm *see* OXYURIS.

piperazine A common worming preparation formerly used to treat ascarid infestations.

pipette A piece of laboratory equipment for accurately measuring out volumes of fluids; mouth pipettes should no longer be used, due to the possible danger of swallowing toxic chemicals.

pituitary dwarf Congenital abnormality of the anterior pituitary which fails to secrete sufficient levels of growth hormone; affected animals are stunted and retain their soft, juvenile hair coat; most commonly affects German shepherd dogs, where it is inherited as an autosomal recessive trait. Seen in Siamese and exotic cat breeds also.

pituitary gland An endocrine gland, also known as the hypophysis, lying ventral to the optic chiasma on the base of the brain. The pituitary is divided into two lobes, separated by Rathke's cleft; the anterior lobe (adenohypophysis) secretes growth hormone, prolactin, thyroid stimulating hormone, follicle stimulating hormone, luteinising hormone, adrenocorticotrophic hormone and lipotrophin; the posterior lobe (neurohypophysis) secretes oxytocin and antidiuretic hormone (vasopressin), *see also* HYPOTHALAMUS.

placebo A harmless substance given as a medicine and commonly used in drug trials as a comparator for the active treatment. In man there may be a placebo or psychological effect associated with taking medication, even if it contains no active drug – this effect is not seen in animals.

placenta The highly vascular membranous structure that allows attachment of the developing fetus to the uterine wall; the placenta allows the transfer of nutrients and oxygen from the mother to the fetus, and the transfer of fetal waste products in the opposite direction, *see also* AFTERBIRTH.

placentation The formation of the placenta into one of three types, depending on the distribution of the chorionic villi, i.e. diffuse (mare, sow), cotyledonary (ruminants) or zonary (dog, cat).

placing reflex The normal reflex when an animal is held up and brought towards the edge of a table, so that the limbs are extended, ready for weight-bearing; visual placing may be tested in this way, and tactile placing can be tested by covering the animal's eyes with your hands during the test.

plane A surface, real or theoretical, along which any two points can be joined by a straight line, e.g. a transverse plane cuts across the long axis of the body at right angles and the median (vertical) plane cuts the body into two equal sides.

plantar The undersurface of the paws on the hind legs, *see also* PALMAR.

plantigrade Abnormal stance where the hock and caudal aspect of the metatarsus contacts the ground; causes include rupture of the common calcaneal tendon and tarsal luxation, *see also* PALMIGRADE.

plaque The sticky film that builds up on the teeth, eventually hardening to form tartar; the initial film consists of a mixture of saliva, food debris and bacteria; plaque formation leads to periodontitis and may necessitate descaling.

plasma The fluid component of the blood, including the clotting proteins; may be obtained by taking a blood sample into an anticoagulant and spinning it so that the cells settle out. The fluid therapy of choice to treat haemorrhagic shock, but rarely available in sufficient quantity in practice, *see also* SERUM.

plasma cell Cell that is stimulated to secrete specific antibody, in the presence of the trigger antigen; derived from B lymphocytes.

plasma proteins Albumin, globulins and other enzymes, clotting factors, hormones and carrier proteins normally found within the blood; commonly measured as 'total protein'. Commonly increases in total protein are associated with dehydration, immune-mediated and chronic disease; hypoproteinaemia may be caused by liver disease, nephrotic syndrome, burns and protein-losing enteropathies.

plasmid A length of DNA that carries a number of non-essential genes and can be transmitted from one bacterium to another; this can have clinical implications, for example, if the plasmid codes for antibiotic resistance.

plasminogen A precursor of plasmin, a potent fibrinolytic enzyme.

plaster of Paris (PoP) Powdered calcium sulphate, derived from gypsum; it is used to coat white openwove bandage which then hardens when wetted; used to make casts and splints. The material is cheap, easy to apply and can be removed with plaster shears; setting time is long, allowing time to construct complex casts; disadvantages include the long setting time (during which the animal should not bear weight on the cast), the heavy weight and the fact that the cast must be kept dry, or it will soften.

plastron The ventral surface of chelonians, such as the tortoise and terrapin; the plastron is made from a number of keratin shields or scutes.

platelet Thrombocyte; small cell fragments found in the circulation, derived from megakaryocytes; platelets stick to areas of damaged endothelium and, in conjunction with fibrin, form a clot.

plate out Laboratory technique for preparing colonies of bacteria by streaking them across the surface of a shallow culture plate, using a platinum loop, and then incubating the plate (usually at 37°C for 24–48 hours); the loop is sterilised between each of the streaks, gradually reducing the concentration of bacteria so that separate colonies can be grown; different patterns are required if the plate is to be used for antibiotic sensitivity testing, *see also* PETRI DISH, PLATINUM LOOP.

platinum loop A fine wire loop with a handle; used for plating out bacteria for culture; the loop can be repeatedly sterilised by holding it in the hottest part of a Bunsen flame until it glows red.

platyhelminth A flat-worm or fluke, *see also* TREMATODE.

pleotrophic Exhibiting varied shapes and forms.

pleura The serous membranes lining the thoracic cavity; the parietal pleura is closely applied to the inner surface of the chest wall, while the visceral pleura covers the lung tissue. There is a small, fluid-filled space between, which means that the lungs follow the movements of the chest wall during respiration.

pleural effusion Collection of fluid in the pleural space between the visceral and parietal layers of the pleura; the fluid may be a transudate, exudate, blood, pus, chyle or associated with neoplasia. Clinical signs include progressive dyspnoea, with tachypnoea and unwillingness to remain in lateral recumbency; radiography usually confirms the diagnosis, and paracentesis is used to type the fluid; affected animals require careful handling and should not be stressed unnecessarily.

plexus A network of blood vessels or nerves, *see also* BRACHIAL PLEXUS, LUMBOSACRAL PLEXUS, PAMPINIFORM PLEXUS.

plication Surgical technique making tucks or folds in a tissue or organ to make it smaller.

***Pneumocystis* spp.** Group of bacteria that cause pneumonia; may occur as opportunistic pathogens in immunocompromised animals.

pneumocystogram The introduction of air as a radiographic negative contrast agent into the bladder; may be used to demonstrate calculi, tumours, etc.

pneumonia Inflammation of the lung tissue; causes include bacterial or viral infection, allergy, aspiration of gastric contents, paraquat poisoning.

pneumomediastinum The presence of free air within the mediastinum of the chest; usually a result of damage to the trachea.

pneumoradiography The use of air as a negative contrast agent.

pneumothorax The presence of free air within the thoracic cavity; usually the result of trauma to the thoracic wall, but may also result from tracheal rupture, over-inflation of the lungs during IPPV, lung lobe torsion, etc.

pododermatitis Inflammation of the skin around and between the toes; causes include demodectic mange, hookworm and grass seeds, *see also* INTERDIGITAL CYST.

poikilocyte Irregular, pear-shaped or 'tear-drop' shaped erythrocyte seen in some cases of chronic anaemia.

poikilotherm A cold-blooded animal; having a body temperature that varies according to the environmental temperature.

poison A harmful or toxic substance; possible sources of poisoning include insecticides, rodenticides, weedkillers, paints, anti-freeze, plants such as yew, rhododendron and deadly nightshade, fungi, heavy metals, bites and stings, drug overdosage or misuse of human medicines for animals. Clinical signs vary according to the type of poison; first-aid measures include administering an emetic if a non-corrosive poison has been ingested, giving mild purgatives, removing skin contamination and administering specific antidotes if appropriate. Information on the toxic effects of drugs and how to treat them can be obtained in the UK from the regional Poisons Information Centres (Belfast, Cardiff, Dublin, Edinburgh, London), although the centres primarily deal with cases of human poisoning.

polioencephalomyelitis Inflammation of the grey and white matter of the brain; a rare condition in animals, of undefined aetiology.

poly- Prefix meaning many.

polyamide Nylon; synthetic, non-absorbable suture material; high tensile strength and fair knot security although the larger diameters can be stiff to handle and difficult to tie, low tissue reactivity, ends of suture may irritate; widely used as a skin suture.

polyarteritis nodosa Inflammation of a number of small arteries, with distension and bulging of the vessel walls; an auto-immune condition that may also be associated with a polyarthritis; rare.

polyarthritis Inflammation of several joints.

polyarthritis/polymyositis syndrome Inflammation of joints and muscles; a rare syndrome reported in dogs; affected animals have a stiff gait and muscle atrophy may be marked; thought to be immune-mediated; treatment with prednisolone and cytotoxic drugs may be tried.

polychromasia Varied pattern of staining; term used to describe the staining of immature red blood cells.

polycystic Containing many fluid-filled cysts; used to describe multiple cysts in the kidney, for example.

polycythaemia Increased number of circulating red blood cells, *see also* PACKED CELL VOLUME.

polydactyl Having more than the normal number of toes; a common congenital deformity in the cat and usually of no clinical significance.

polydipsia Increased thirst; a common clinical sign, and often associated with polyuria. The causes include dehydration, hyperthermia, restricted access to water, diabetes insipidus, diabetes mellitus, renal disease, liver disease, pyometra, Cushing's disease, Addison's disease, hyperthyroidism, etc.

polydioxanone Synthetic monofilament suture material (PDS); high tensile strength, handles well and ties good knots; removed by hydrolysis, retains up to half its strength for 30 days and takes 180 days for complete absorption; widely used for internal sutures where strength is needed; more expensive than catgut.

polyester Braided, synthetic, non-absorbable suture material; may be coated; very high tensile strength, moderate ease of handling and knot security.

polyglactin Coated, braided, synthetic, absorbable suture material (Vicryl); strong, with good knot security and handling; absorbed by hydrolysis; shorter lasting than polydioxanone.

polyglycolic acid Braided, synthetic, absorbable suture material that may also be coated (Dexon-Plus); strong, with good handling and knot security; absorbed by hydrolysis; shorter lasting than polydioxanone.

polymeric diets Balanced liquid diets that can be used for meal replacement; due to their small particle size they can be fed through fine diameter nasogastric tubes.

polymorph Adult neutrophil, *see also* LEUKOCYTE, NEUTROPHIL.

polymyopathy Any disease affecting multiple muscle groups; may be inflammatory, degenerative or metabolic; associated with conditions such as Cushing's disease and hypothyroidism; specific inherited myopathies have been reported in the labrador and golden retriever and some spaniel breeds, an idiopathic form occurs in cats, *see also* MYAESTHENIA GRAVIS, POLYMYOSITIS.

polymyositis Inflammation of several muscles; associated with diseases such as toxocariasis (visceral larval migrans), clostridial infection and toxoplasmosis.

polyneuritis Inflammation of nerves.

polyneuropathy Widespread nerve disorder affecting sensory then motor nerves, may be immune-mediated. May be associated with neoplasia, *see also* PARANEOPLASTIC SYNDROME.

polyoestrous Having more than one breeding season per year.

polyp Benign, pedunculated growth arising from a mucous membrane, e.g. nasal polyps may enlarge behind the soft palate in the cat, causing increasing dyspnoea and nasal discharge; treatment is usually surgical removal.

polypeptide A chain of three or more linked amino acids.

polyphagia Increased appetite.

polypharmacy Use of several drugs to treat a condition; the drugs may be given separately, or may be available within the same product; this approach should be based on careful clinical judgement as it may be effective but associated with increased risk of developing resistance.

polyploid Having more than twice the usual haploid number of chromosomes in a cell, e.g. triploid cells have three times the haploid number, *see also* DIPLOID.

polysaccharide Large carbohydrate molecule consisting of several linked simple sugars; starch, glycogen and cellulose are all examples.

polysome Group of ribosomes linked by a molecule of RNA; the ribosomes move along the RNA strand to synthesise a specific protein, *see also* RIBONUCLEIC ACID.

polytocous Normally producing more than one offspring, e.g. a litter.

polyunsaturated fatty acid (PUFA) A fatty acid containing more than one double bond.

polyuria Increased production of urine; often associated with polydipsia; causes include diabetes insipidus, diabetes mellitus, use of diuretics, etc., *see also* POLYDIPSIA.

polyvalent Term used to describe a vaccine that contains more than one antigenic agent, e.g. combined 'flu and enteritis vaccine for cats.

pons Part of the brainstem; the bridge of tissue between the medulla oblongata and the midbrain; a major relay centre.

popliteal Relating to the calf region of the hind leg, behind the stifle, e.g. popliteus muscle, popliteal sesamoids, popliteal lymph node.

porous Containing pores or minute openings that will allow molecules to pass through.

porphyria Elevated levels of circulating porphyrins, usually due to a metabolic defect; excess porphyrins are excreted via the urine and faeces. Urine colours are unusual.

portal Relating to the venous blood system that takes blood rich in dietary nutrients from the intestine to the liver.

portfolio Defined as a receptacle or case in the form of a large book cover for keeping loose sheets of paper and drawings. A portfolio is required to be kept by the student veterinary nurse to record evidence of practical knowledge and competence.

portocaval The portal vein that drains blood from the spleen, stomach and the anterior mesentry. It connects to the posterior vena cava after the blood has passed through the liver by a short vein, also spelt portacaval.

portocaval shunt Abnormal anastomosis between the hepatic portal vein and the caudal vena cava; usually congenital, but may be acquired following liver cirrhosis. Blood is diverted away from the liver, affecting the metabolism of many products. The clinical signs include weight loss, lethargy, stunted growth and nervous signs (hepatic encephalopathy) that are often most pronounced soon after feeding; laboratory tests show low plasma urea, but elevated ammonia and bile acids; portal angiography is required to accurately localise the shunt; surgical partial ligation of discrete, extrahepatic shunts may be possible, although intrahepatic shunts may be more difficult to locate and correct, *see also* PORTOSYSTEMIC SHUNT.

portosystemic shunt Any vascular anastomosis between the portal vein and the systemic circulation; most commonly due to a patent ductus venosus. The ductus venosus carries fetal blood from the gut and placenta to the vena cava; although the duct runs through the liver, blood bypasses the hepatic sinusoids; this duct usually closes within a few hours of birth.

position Spatial relationship between the spine of the fetus and the birth canal; positions may be dorsal, ventral, right or left lateral, *see also* POSTURE, PRESENTATION.

positive pressure ventilation Controlled techniques for pushing air into the lungs of patients who cannot breathe for themselves, *see also* INTERMITTENT POSITIVE PRESSURE VENTILATION.

post mortem After death; usually an autopsy or examination to find out the cause of death.

posterior Towards the rear; the caudal surface.

posterior chamber The caudal chamber of the eye, behind the lens; contains the vitreous body and the light-sensitive retinal layers.

post-hibernation anorexia (PHA) Common condition in tortoises who have drawn upon body protein reserves during hibernation; affected animals should be kept at 25–30°C, stomach tubed twice a week and given a recovery diet and multivitamins.

post-operative Occurring after surgery.

post-partum Occurring after birth.

post-prandial After a meal.

posture Position of the fetal limbs, e.g. forelimbs extended, *see also* POSITION, PRESENTATION.

potassium Dietary mineral and intracellular electrolyte. Deficiency causes muscle weakness, and may arise following severe diarrhoea, vomiting, end-stage renal disease, prolonged fluid therapy or the use of potassium-losing diuretics. Excess (hyperkalaemia) occurs in Addison's disease, acute renal failure and use of potassium-sparing diuretics; elevated levels of potassium can be cardiotoxic and lead rapidly to cardiac arrest, so prompt treatment with intravenous fluids to dilute the potassium is required, *see also* ADDISON'S DISEASE.

potentiated sulphonamide Group of broad-spectrum antibiotics.

Potter–Bucky A type of moving grid housed within the radiography table and used when tissue more than 10 cm thick is being radiographed; as the grid moves rapidly during the exposure, grid lines are blurred and do not appear on the fixed radiograph, *see also* GRID.

poultice A paste (often kaolin-based) that is applied to an area to draw out infection; used more widely in large animal medicine than for small animals.

povidone iodine An iodophor skin disinfectant and surgical scrub solution.

PRA Progressive retinal atrophy, a disorder causing loss of sight. It is often divided into type 1 and type 2. It is a degenerative eye condition and is often hereditary, *see also* RETINAL ATROPHY.

precipitate Solid particles that settle out to the bottom of a solution.

preclipping Clipping a conscious patient several hours prior to surgery; this allows more efficient use of theatre time, and allows loose hairs to be shed outside the theatre; it may need more staff, however, and can be impossible with uncooperative patients or painful surgical sites.

prednisolone Synthetic steroid with similar action to cortisone; it has analgesic and anti-inflammatory properties; at high doses it is immunosuppressive. Treatment should not be withdrawn suddenly as adrenal insufficiency can occur; dogs should be given the medication in the morning, and cats in the evening, so that the dose pattern follows the normal cortisol peak. The common side-effects include polyphagia, polyuria and polydipsia; prednisolone should not be given to pregnant animals.

pregnancy diagnosis Confirmation that an animal is carrying one or more offspring; a variety of tests are available, depending on the species and the stage of gestation; tests include abdominal palpation, ultrasound, hormone assays, vaginal mucus smears and radiography. Other signs corroborate: failure to return to oestrus, prominent teats, enlargement of the mammary glands, behaviour changes and significant weight gain.

pregnancy toxaemia Metabolic disorder occurring in late pregnancy, due to the high demands of the fetus or inadequate nutrition of the mother; rare in small animals but common in sheep.

pregnant mare serum gonadotrophin (PMSG) Hormone produced by mares to help sustain pregnancy; purified PMSG can be used in other species to stimulate the formation of ovarian follicles and spermatogenesis.

prehensile Used for grasping.

premedication Drug given prior to another agent, usually to counter side-effects; examples include use of an anti-emetic prior to chemotherapy, and the widespread use of sedatives, analgesics and antisialogogues prior to anaesthesia.

premolars The teeth in the upper and lower jaws between the canine teeth and the molars, *see also* CARNASSIAL TOOTH.

preparation room The room where animals are prepared for theatre; anaesthesia may be induced here, the patient clipped, the surgical site given an initial scrub, intravenous catheters inserted, etc.

prepatent period The time between infection of a host with a parasite and the excretion of infective forms, e.g. eggs, larvae, by that host.

prepuce The sheath that covers the penis.

prescapular lymph node The palpable lymph node located just cranial to the scapula.

prescription A written legal instruction to a pharmacist to supply a certain drug to an owner, for treatment of an animal under the signing veterinary surgeon's care.

presentation (1) The clinical signs and symptoms shown by an animal. (2) The relationship between the long axis of the fetus and the birth canal; presentations may be longitudinal, transverse or (rarely) vertical, *see also* POSITION, POSTURE.

pressure bandage Pad of absorptive material applied firmly with a bandage to control haemorrhage; usually used on the distal limb; should not be left on for more than 24 hours.

pressure sore *see* DECUBITAL, ULCERS.

prevalence The number of cases of a disease within a specified population at any point in time, *see also* INCIDENCE.

preventive medicine Branch of veterinary medicine dealing with the prevention of disease in individual animals or groups; preventive medicine includes the use of vaccines, control of environmental factors, hygiene, etc.

priapism Prolonged erection of the penis.

primary haemorrhage Blood loss immediately following rupture of a vessel.

primidone An anticonvulsant used for the control of epilepsy, *see also* EPILEPSY.

primigravida Describes an animal that is pregnant for the first time.

prions Minute particles smaller than viruses of a protein-like nature that are considered to be the infective agent for BSE, scrapie and the new form of CJD of humans.

probe A blunt-ended instrument used for assessing the depth of a tract or recess.

proctitis Inflammation of the rectum.

proctoscopy Endoscopic examination of the rectum.

prodromal Preceding, occurring before, e.g. a prodromal phase may be recognised before an epileptic seizure.

pro-oestrus The phase of the reproductive cycle occurring immediately before oestrus; during pro-oestrus, there is follicular growth and maturation, the uterus enlarges and the endometrium hypertrophies; in the bitch there is vulval oedema and bleeding, *see also* ANOESTRUS, DIOESTRUS, METOESTRUS, OESTRUS.

progeny All the offspring of a single animal.

progeny testing Assessing the usefulness of a breeding animal by looking at the quality of their offspring.

progestagen A drug with progesterone-like activity, e.g. megestrol acetate.

progesterone Hormone produced by the corpus luteum that develops after a follicle has released its ovum; the hormone sustains pregnancy and inhibits return to oestrus.

proglottid The mature, gravid segment of a tapeworm that is released into the faeces; these sac-like structures typically appear like rice grains and contain the eggs.

prognathism Having the lower jaw longer than the upper jaw; undershot.

prognosis The likely outcome of a disease.

progressive axonopathy (PA) A rare giant axonal neuropathy reported in German shepherd dogs and inherited as an autosomal recessive trait; affected dogs show paresis and pelvic limb ataxia, typically at 1 year of age; the disease worsens and there is no cure.

progressive retinal atrophy (PRA) *see* RETINAL ATROPHY.

projectile vomiting Propulsive vomiting; may be associated with mechanical abnormalities such as pyloric stenosis.

prolactin Hormone secreted by the anterior pituitary, stimulating lactation.

prolapse The displacement of a structure or organ from its usual location, e.g. prolapsed rectum, uterus, etc.

prolapsed third eyelid Swelling of the free border of the nictitating membrane or third eyelid; may require surgical correction.

pronation Rotation of the paw so that the palmar or plantar surface faces ventrally; the opposite of supination.

prone Position where an animal is lying on its ventral surface, with its back uppermost.

prophylactic A treatment used to prevent a disease.

proprioception The sense of spatial awareness and limb positioning.

proptosis Protrusion of the eyeball.

prostaglandins Group of diverse molecules formed from fatty acids; they can have hormone-like effects in the body, and can be potent inflammatory mediators; synthetic prostaglandin analogues are used to regress the corpus luteum, leading to abortion or induction of parturition.

prostate The male accessory sex gland situated at the neck of the bladder, surrounding the urethra; it secretes fluid into the urethra for sperm transport.

prostatitis Inflammation of the prostate. **Benign, hypertrophic prostatitis** A common consequence of ageing; enlargement may be associated with a degree of prostatitis, and is often subclinical; in some cases the hypertrophy may cause dysuria or constipation, often with tenesmus; steroid hormones may be used to cause the gland to regress, or castration can be performed.

prosthesis An artificial replacement, e.g. a hip prosthesis.

protamine zinc insulin An insoluble insulin preparation with a duration of action of approximately 24 hours.

protein Large molecule made from amino acids; proteins function as enzymes and hormones; they are used as structural building blocks for body tissues; there is constant turnover of protein in the body; when fat and carbohydrate reserves are used up, protein can also be catabolised to release energy.

proteinuria Presence of protein in the urine; causes include renal disease, inflammation elsewhere in the urogenital tract, haematuria and natural secretions such as semen.

***Proteus* spp.** Genus of Gram-negative bacteria that are commensals of the gastrointestinal tract, and common pathogens.

prothrombin Precursor of thrombin, formed by the liver, *see also* THROMBIN.

protoplasm The cytoplasm or ground substance of a cell.

proton An elemental particle carrying one positive charge; it is the equivalent of the nucleus of a hydrogen atom, and is commonly represented as H^+, *see also* ELECTRON.

protozoa Unicellular parasitic organisms such as *Coccidia.*

proud flesh Exuberant granulation tissue that may be produced during second intention wound healing; the tissue is vascular but aneural; if the tissue rises above the level of the epithelium, the epithelial cells cannot migrate across to cover the defect; proud flesh can be reduced with astringents such as copper sulphate, or may require surgical cutting back.

proximal Towards the centre or origin.

pruritis Itchiness, irritation of the skin; a common sign in many skin diseases.

pseudoarthrosis A fibrous articulation that develops between two bone ends when the usual articular surfaces are no longer in apposition, e.g. the fibrous joint that allows functional movement of the hip after femoral head excision.

pseudocyesis False pregnancy, *see also* OESTROUS CYCLE.

***Pseudomonas* spp.** Gram-negative motile rod-shaped bacteria; found commonly in stagnant water and decaying matter; some species are pathogenic and are associated with urinary, ear, gastrointestinal and wound infections.

pseudopodia Cytoplasmic projections from unicellular organisms that help them to move.

pseudopregnancy False pregnancy, *see also* OESTROUS CYCLE.

pseudorabies Aujeszky's disease, infectious bulbar paralysis or mad itch; acute disease caused by a herpes virus; the natural host for the virus is the pig, although many other species may be affected; after a 2–10 day incubation period, affected animals become pyrexic, agitated and increasingly pruritic; signs progress rapidly and death usually occurs within 24–48 hours.

pseudotuberculosis Granulomatous disease or enteritis caused by *Yersinia* spp.; the organism is zoonotic, so suspected cases should be handled with extreme care.

psittacine Term used to describe climbing birds, e.g. parrots and budgerigars.

psittacosis Ornithosis, chlamydiosis; disease of psittacine birds caused by the intracellular organism *Chlamydia psittaci*; signs include ruffled feathers, green/grey diarrhoea and conjunctivitis; the disease is zoonotic, causing a 'flu-like syndrome in man that may occasionally be fatal; treatment of affected birds may be attempted, but due to the zoonotic risk, euthanasia is usually performed.

psoriasis An erythematous, scaling skin disease in man with secondary bacterial infection. No equivalent disease in dogs.

Psoroptes ovis Surface-living mite of sheep, that causes intense irritation with scratching and wool loss; sheep scab is no longer a notifiable disease.

psychology The study of an animal's behaviour in its normal environment.

ptosis Drooping of the upper eyelid so that the palpebral fissure is narrowed; occurs with lesions of the oculomotor (III) cranial nerve, e.g. Horner's syndrome.

ptyalin The enzyme in saliva that breaks starch down into sugar; salivary amylase.

puberty Sexual maturity.

pubic symphysis The joint between the left and right pubic bones of the pelvis; the cartilaginous joint weakens in late pregnancy to aid expulsion of the fetus.

pubis The most ventral bone in the hemipelvis, contributing to the acetabulum and the obturator foramen.

pudendal Relating to the region around the external genitalia.

puerperium The time from birth to the end of uterine involution.

pulmonary Relating to the lungs.

pulmonary embolus A small blood clot that lodges within a vessel in the lungs; some may be subclinical, while others may cause sudden onset dyspnoea.

pulmonary oedema Inflammation of lung tissue, with build-up of oedema fluid within the alveoli; the most common cause is left-sided heart failure, although other causes include paraquat poisoning, hypoproteinaemia and smoke inhalation. There is usually dyspnoea and wet respiratory noises; diuretics and oxygen should be administered, and stress minimised; the primary cause should be treated, and antibiotics may be given to prevent secondary infection.

pulmonary valve The valve of the heart that opens when the right ventricle pumps blood towards the lungs, and then closes off the base of the pulmonary artery preventing backflow or regurgitation. Three cusps close together as a tight seal.

pulmonic stenosis Congenital malformation of the cusps of the pulmonic heart valve, with narrowing of the artery; affected animals are stunted and have poor exercise tolerance. Signs of right-sided heart failure may develop and there is a harsh systolic murmur; ECG, radiography and ultrasound confirm the diagnosis; dilation of the narrowing (balloon valvuloplasty) or patch grafting may be attempted.

pulpitis Inflammation of the pulp cavity within a tooth.

pulsate Throb.

pulse The palpable thrill that can be felt in a superficial artery where it passes over bone; in the normal animal there is a palpable thrill for each beat of the heart; pulse is usually referred to in terms of the rate (number of beats per minute), rhythm (regular, irregular, galloping, etc.) and character (weak, full, bounding, etc.).

pulse deficit Term used when the number of pulses felt is less than the number of beats of the heart; if there is an arrhythmia, some heart beats will be premature, and will occur before the ventricles have filled correctly – the peripheral pulse associated with this beat may be weak, or not able to be felt at all; the greater the pulse deficit, the more serious the cardiac abnormality.

punch biopsy An instrument for taking small skin biopsy samples.

punctate Dotted or pitted.

puncture Make a small hole with a sharp, pointed instrument, stab.

pupa Part of the life cycle of an insect.

pupil The gap in the centre of the iris, through which light passes to the retina; the size of the pupil is regulated by the iris.

pupillary light reflex (PLR) When a bright light is shone into the eye, the pupil should constrict (direct response); there is also a consensual response, with the other pupil constricting too. When the stimulus is removed the pupils should rapidly dilate; the PLR tests the function of the optic (II) and oculomotor (III) cranial nerves.

purgative Agents that decrease gastrointestinal transit time; strong purgatives should be avoided as they may irritate the mucosa, cause pain and can lead to potassium depletion, *see also* LAXATIVE.

purine One of the component bases of DNA and RNA.

Purkinje cell Inhibitory neuron found in the cerebellum; plays an important role in regulating muscle tone.

Purkinje fibres The network of fibres that conduct the waves of depolarisation over the heart.

purpura Haemorrhagic condition, thought to be immune-mediated and usually following another illness; ecchymoses, petechiae or areas of haemorrhage and oedema arise spontaneously.

purulent Pus-like; containing pus.

pus Thick liquid composed of bacteria, leukocytes (predominantly dead neutrophils) and necrotic tissue debris.

pustule A small swelling containing pus, often a skin blister.

putrefaction The process of tissue decomposition brought about by bacteria.

pyaemia Severe septicaemia, with the presence of pus in the blood.

pyelitis Pus in the renal pelvis and urine; usually due to an ascending urinary tract infection.

pyelogram Radiographic contrast study of the kidney.

pyelonephritis Inflammation of the renal pelvis and cortex; due to infection from the bloodstream, or ascending from the ureters.

pyknosis Shrinking and condensing of the nucleus of a cell; often a sign of impending cell death.

pyloric stenosis Congenital or acquired narrowing of the pylorus, so that gastric emptying is delayed; affected animals vomit frequently, and may bring up food that they have eaten several days earlier. Vomiting may be projectile; surgical correction is usually required, *see also* PYLOROMYOTOMY, PYLOROPLASTY.

pyloromyotomy The muscle layer of the pyloric sphincter is cut surgically to increase the size of the opening from the stomach into the duodenum; care is required to ensure that the incision does not penetrate the mucosa; the effectiveness of the technique may be limited in the long term due to the development of fibrous scar tissue.

pyloroplasty Permanent surgical correction of pyloric stenosis, where a longitudinal incision is made across the pylorus, through all tissue layers; the incision is then closed transversely.

pylorus The canal between the stomach and duodenum; bound by a muscular collar – the pyloric sphincter.

pyoderma Bacterial infection of the skin; may be surface, e.g. moist dermatitis, superficial or deep; a wide range of bacteria have been implicated, but the most common is *Staphylococcus intermedius.*

pyogenic Capable of forming pus.

pyometra Presence of pus in the uterus; a common problem in nulliparous bitches and prevented by spaying. Pyometra may be open or closed, depending on the state of the cervix; affected animals are depressed, polydipsic and may vomit; with open pyometra there is a vulval discharge; the animal has usually been in oestrus within the previous 8–12 weeks; treatment is ovariohysterectomy.

pyonephritis Pus in the renal cortex.

pyothorax Pus within the thoracic cavity.

pyrethrum Insecticide based on plant extracts.

pyretic Having a raised body temperature, fevered.

pyrexia Fever; elevated temperature.

pyrexia of unknown origin (PUO) *see* PYREXIA.

pyrogen An agent that produces pyrexia in an infected animal.

pyuria Pus in the urine.

Q

Q fever Zoonotic disease caused by the rickettsial organism *Coxiella burneti*; affects mainly sheep and cattle and is characterised by pyrexia, abortion or pneumonia.

q.i.d. L. abbreviation, 'four times daily'.

QRS complex Part of the electrical trace on an ECG representing depolarisation of the ventricles of the heart.

Q wave The downward phase of the QRS complex on an ECG trace; indicates early contraction of the ventricles.

quadriceps femoris Muscle mass lying cranial to the femur; consists of four separate muscles which arise from the pelvis and proximal femur and insert on the patella; they act to extend the stifle and flex the hip.

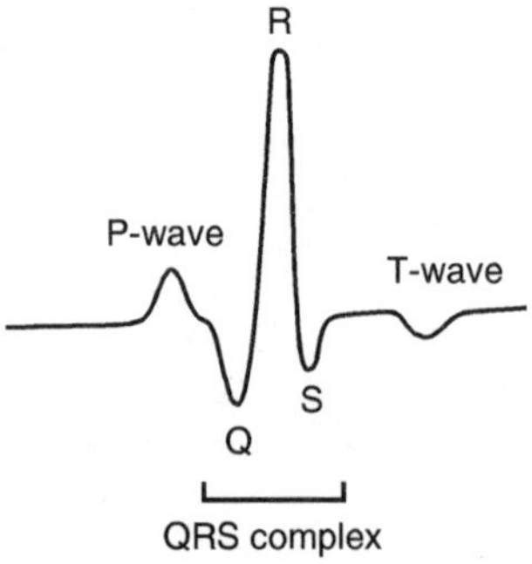

QRS complex

quadriparesis Weakness affecting all four limbs, with neurological deficits but the animal is still able to make stepping movements.

quadriplegia Paralysis of all four limbs, *see also* TETRAPLEGIA.

quadruped A four-footed animal.

quality control A method of evaluating the accuracy or efficiency of a procedure; should routinely be applied to all practice laboratory tests.

quarantine Statutory isolation period, usually longer than the incubation period of a disease, for animals being brought into a country or region, *see also* RABIES.

quaternary ammonia compound Group of disinfectant compounds based on ammonium hydroxide; suitable for skin preparation, non-toxic but inactivated by soap or organic matter.

queen Female cat of breeding age.

quinalone Antibiotic drug occasionally used in cases of resistant infections as nalidixic acid. Fluorinated quinalones are derivatives used as antibacterial agents, *see also* CIPROFLOXACIN.

R

rabbit Small mammal now the third most popular domestic pet. An efficient digester of cellulose by its almost unique process of caecotrophy. Pet rabbits are prone to dental disease as nutritional needs are still not fully understood.

rabies Disease of the central nervous system of mammals, caused by a rhabdovirus; transmitted mainly via bites; incubation may be as long as 4 months; signs include bouts of hyperexcitability, weakness and difficulty swallowing; not present in the UK, and imported mammals have to go through a period of quarantine; elsewhere, the disease is controlled by vaccination.

Rabies (Importation of Cats, Dogs and Other Mammals) Order 1974 (amended 1977) Act of parliament controlling the importation of mammals into the UK, setting down standard periods of quarantine. Currently under review.

rachitic Suffering from rickets.

radiation The electromagnetic spectrum of rays such as radio waves, light, X-rays and gamma rays; the radiation of a short wavelength and high energy can penetrate tissue and ionise molecules.

radiation protection adviser Qualified person (e.g. holder of Diploma in Veterinary Radiography) who advises a practice on radiation procedures and safety, in line with the Code of Practice.

radiation protection supervisor Employee of the practice who is responsible for radiation safety on a daily basis.

radiculitis Inflammation of a spinal nerve root, the main presenting sign being pain.

radiculomyelopathy Pathological condition of the spinal nerve roots and white matter of the spinal cord, *see also* CHRONIC DEGENERATIVE RADICULOMYELOPATHY.

radioactive Able to spontaneously emit X-radiation.

radiocarpal joint The joint between the distal radius and radiocarpal bone.

radiodense Unable to be penetrated by radiation, e.g. lead; radio-opaque; the more radiodense a material, the whiter it will appear on the finished radiograph.

radiograph The developed and fixed X-ray film, showing the negative image of the object that has been radiographed.

radiographer A technician trained to take radiographs.

radiography Diagnostic imaging of a part of the body using X-radiation.

radio-isotope A molecule that spontaneously emits radiation, losing energy and changing to a more stable form.

radiologist Specialist trained in the interpretation of radiographs and other diagnostic imaging techniques.

radiology The science of the use of radiation for diagnosing and treating disease.

radiolucent Able to be penetrated by X-radiation; the more radiolucent a material is, the darker it will appear on the finished radiograph; gases are the most radiolucent substances.

radio-opaque *see* RADIODENSE.

radiotherapy The use of radiation for the treatment of disease, especially neoplasia.

radius Main bone of the forearm, running from elbow to carpus.

rale A respiratory noise heard on auscultation; may be moist, gurgling, dry, crackling, etc.

ramify Divide into branches.

ramus Anatomical term meaning a branch.

ranula A fluid-filled swelling (mucocoele) under the tongue, often due to obstruction of the duct of the sublingual salivary gland; may be drained surgically or treated conservatively.

raphe A line of join, e.g. the linea alba.

raptor A bird of prey.

rarefaction Becoming less dense.

rate The speed at which something happens.

rationale The scientific reasoning behind the management of a patient.

react Respond to a stimulus.

reactionary A fairly rapid response to a situation, such as reactionary haemorrhage, that occurs after an animal's blood pressure has risen again following surgery or shock.

reactionary haemorrhage Leakage of blood from vessels within 24 hours of an injury or post-operatively; primary haemorrhage occurs immediately after injury, while secondary haemorrhage may develop 7–10 days later.

rebreathing circuit Type of anaesthetic circuit that includes a soda lime canister to absorb carbon dioxide from the exhaled gases; thus, the remaining gases can be inhaled again by the patient, as long as sufficient oxygen remains. Rebreathing circuits include the to-and-fro (for animals under 20 kg) and the circle (for animals over 20 kg). Rebreathing circuits are generally more economic to run but the level of anaesthesia is more difficult to control accurately compared with non-rebreathing circuits.

recessive Genetic term used to describe a trait that is only apparent in the homozygous animal; the trait will not be apparent if other dominant alleles are present.

recipient The patient who receives donated blood, tissues, etc.

reconstitute Return to the original state; term used to describe the addition of diluent to a vaccine or sterile water to a powder to make a solution that can be injected.

recovery Return to consciousness after general anaesthesia; recuperation from a disease.

recrudescence Recurrence of a disease after a period of remission.

rectal prolapse Protrusion of part of the rectal wall through the anal sphincter; results from prolonged tenesmus, e.g. severe diarrhoea, perineal hernia, prostatic hypertrophy. A prolapse may be replaced manually, although a purse-string suture may be required for 24–48 hours to prevent recurrence; if the rectal tissue is not viable, resection and anastomosis is performed.

rectal pull through Surgical technique for the removal of rectal lesions that could not be removed via the abdomen; a circumanal incision is deepened, and the rectum freed and exteriorised by applying traction to stay sutures.

rectifier Part of the electrical circuit of an X-ray machine that converts the alternating current to a direct current.

rectovaginal fistula Connection between the rectum and vagina, usually due to tearing of tissues during parturition.

rectum The terminal portion of the gastrointestinal tract, extending from the colon to the anus.

recumbent Lying down, unable to stand.

reduce Put back in its normal anatomical position; term used to describe the realignment of fracture fragments.

reducing valve Valve on an anaesthetic machine between the cylinder and the flow meter, which reduces the pressure of the gas and allows small adjustments in flow rate to be made.

referral The seeking of a second opinion from another veterinary surgeon or specialist. Referral may be suggested by the first veterinary surgeon, or may be requested by the owner; it is the ethical duty of the referring veterinary surgeon to provide a case history, and the second vet should not examine the animal without this document or the permission of the referring vet.

reflex An involuntary response to a stimulus, e.g. pupil constriction when a light is shone into the eye, the knee jerk response when the patellar tendon is tapped.

reflux Backward flow; commonly used to describe the movement of gastric contents back into the oesophagus.

refractometer An instrument that measures the deflection of light passing through a material; hand-held refractometers are used to measure the specific gravity and total protein levels of liquids such as urine and CSF.

regional anaesthesia Local anaesthetic technique where conduction in a specific nerve is blocked, providing anaesthesia of the region innervated by that nerve.

regurgitate (1) Backward flow of blood through incompetent valves. (2) A passive movement of food from the oesophagus back to the mouth; usually occurs soon after feeding, but may occur up to 24 hours later; associated with mega-oesophagus, persistent right aortic arch, oesophageal stricture, etc; may also be normal in nursing animals, snakes, birds, etc.

rehydration The supply of fluids to a dehydrated patient, *see also* FLUID THERAPY.

relapse The return of a disease.

relaxant A drug that reduces muscle tone; may be used during an anaesthetic protocol to provide good relaxation of skeletal muscle, but as the respiratory muscles will also be affected the patient will need to be ventilated, *see also* VENTILATOR.

relaxin A hormone secreted by the corpus luteum during pregnancy; relaxin causes a softening of the cervix and loosening of pelvic ligaments prior to parturition.

remission Reduction in symptoms; period during which the disease disappears.

renin The enzyme that converts angiotensinogen to angiotensin I.

renin–angiotensin system The homeostatic mechanism controlling sodium excretion and water loss from the kidneys; if extracellular fluid and sodium are lost, the kidney produces more renin, which increases levels of angiotensin I; this is converted to active angiotensin II in the lungs and other tissues, and stimulates aldosterone production, thirst and vasoconstriction.

reproduction The process by which animals produce offspring.

resection Surgical removal of tissue.

resistance The force opposing the movement of air through the respiratory system.

resorption Removal of tissue by absorption, e.g. bone resorption during disuse; resorption of fetuses during early pregnancy.

respiration The cellular process where molecules are oxidised to release energy and form carbon dioxide and water; on a gross scale, the process also involves breathing, and carriage of oxygen to the tissues via the red blood cells.

respiratory acidosis Increased amount of carbon dioxide carried in the blood stream, resulting in lowering of the pH of the blood; causes include hypoventilation due to painful chest trauma, suffocation, etc.

respiratory alkylosis Increase in the pH of the blood, due to hyperventilation, e.g. panting.

restraint Manual or chemical means of handling an animal.

resuscitation Reviving a patient when respiration has ceased (heart may also have stopped beating); the measures include establishing a patent airway, administering oxygen, external cardiac massage or internal cardiac massage and drug therapy, *see also* INTERMITTENT POSITIVE PRESSURE VENTILATION.

retained afterbirth Failure to expel the fetal membranes soon after whelping/kittening, etc; symptoms include pyrexia and an unpleasant vulval discharge.

retained cartilage cores Localised delay or failure of endochondral ossification, so that columns of cartilage remain in some growth plate areas; the distal radius is most commonly affected; the significance of these cartilage cores, which are eventually replaced by bone, remains unclear.

retained meconium Failure of the neonate to pass the meconium soon after birth, resulting in abdominal cramps and increased chance of infection; neonates should be observed carefully to ensure that they receive adequate colostrum and pass the meconium.

retch Gagging response, often immediately prior to vomiting.

rete A fibrous network.

reticulocyte An immature red blood cell.

reticulo-endothelial system A system comprising cells from the bone marrow, spleen, liver and lymphoid tissue; the cells share a common embryonic ancestry, and are involved in fighting infection, antibody and blood cell production.

retina The light-sensitive membrane lining the back of the eye.

retinal atrophy Degeneration of the retina, broadly divided into forms affecting the photoreceptors (generalised progressive retinal atrophy, or PRA) and those affecting the pigment epithelium (RPED). The conditions are inherited, generalised PRA occurring in many breeds, including setters, poodles and retrievers. The first clinical sign is often night blindness, and the condition worsens until the animal is totally blind; a control scheme operates in the UK, run by the Kennel Club and British Veterinary Association and annual ophthalmological examinations are required, *see also* RETINAL PIGMENT EPITHELIUM DYSTROPHY.

retinal dysplasia A congenital condition, where the retina is thrown into folds or rosettes; breeds affected include the beagle, Rottweiler, Yorkshire and Bedlington terriers, labrador, cocker and English springer spaniel.

retinal haemorrhage Bleeding between the retina and the choroid, or sometimes into the vitreous humour. It may be the result of trauma or some hereditary defect such as collie eye anomaly, retinal dysplasia etc. Detachment of the retina also occurs.

retinal pigment epithelium Part of the retina; the single cell layer between the photoreceptors (rods and cones) and the choroid.

retinal pigment epithelium dystrophy (RPED) Disease of the RPE, where deposits of brown lipopigment build up, leading to destruction of photoreceptors and retinal atrophy; the peripheral retina remains intact and so sight is poor, particularly in bright light, but total blindness is rare; affected breeds include the retrievers, spaniels, briard, sheepdogs and collies.

retinaculum A fibrous band of tissue that acts as a retaining strap to hold a tendon or ligament in the correct place.

retractor A surgical instrument used for holding tissues away from the operating site; may be self-retaining or hand-held.

retrobulbar Lying behind the globe of the eye but within the orbit, e.g. retrobulbar abscess.

retroflexion bending back upon itself, e.g. the bladder may be exteriorized and retroflexed during a cystotomy, so that the incision can be made into the dorsal bladder wall.

retrognathia Having the lower jaw shorter than the upper jaw; overshot.

retrograde In the reverse direction.

retrograde urethrography Positive contrast agent is injected into the urethra and fills towards the bladder, in the opposite direction to normal urine flow.

retrovirus A family of viruses including HIV, maedivirus and visna.

rhabdomyoma Benign tumour of striated (skeletal and cardiac) muscle.

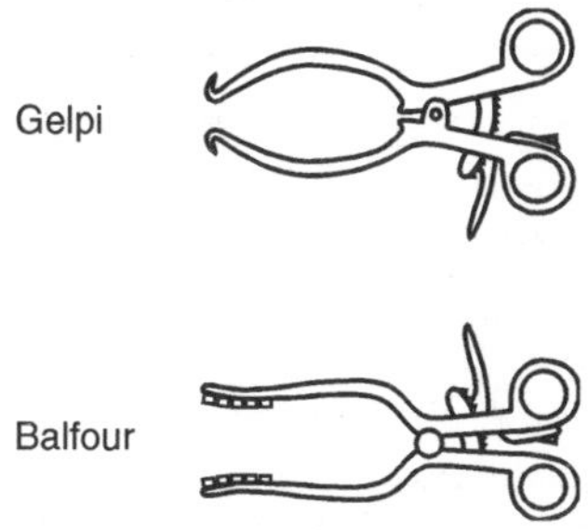

Retractors, two types: Gelpi and Balfour

rhabdomyosarcoma Malignant tumour of striated (skeletal and cardiac) muscle.

rhabdovirus Group of bullet-shaped viruses that includes rabies virus.

rheumatoid arthritis An immune-mediated, erosive, inflammatory polyarthropathy; cartilage and bone are eroded within affected joints, the condition progressing towards an ankylosed end stage. Treatment options include analgesics, immunosuppressive therapy, cytotoxic drugs and gold injections.

rhexis Rupture of a blood vessel, resulting in frank haemorrhage.

rhinarium The hairless area of the nose around the nares.

rhinitis Inflammation of the nasal mucous membranes within the nasal chambers and sinuses.

rhinotomy Surgical opening of the nasal passages.

rhodopsin The pigment in the rods of the retina; visual purple; the pigment is bleached by the action of sunlight but is restored in the dark.

rhonchus A musical sound heard during inspiration or expiration, when air is passing through constricted bronchi and bronchioles.

rib Curved bones forming the thoracic wall.

ribonucleic acid (RNA) A single-strand, helical molecule consisting of ribose sugars, linked by the purines adenine and guanine, and the pyrimidines cytosine and urasil; messenger RNA carries the genetic code from DNA in the nucleus out to the cytoplasm of a cell; ribosomal RNA controls protein synthesis within the cell and transfer RNA brings specific amino acids to the ribosomes for protein synthesis.

ribosome An intracellular granule of ribonucleic protein that is the site of protein synthesis.

rickets Skeletal disease occurring in puppies fed a diet lacking vitamin D and phosphorus; rare nowadays; leads to failure of endochondral ossification, with painful enlargement of the growth plates. **Renal rickets** Also occur if the conversion of vitamin D to its active metabolites by the kidney is impaired and phosphate excretion is blocked, as in some congenital renal disorders; in these cases mineral is absorbed from the skeleton, to a degree where the mandibles become soft and malleable (rubber jaw).

***Rickettsia* spp.** Pleimorphic Gram-negative bacteria causing diseases such as Rocky Mountain spotted fever.

RIDDOR Legislation governing the recording of accidents in the workplace, making it the responsibility of the injured person to ensure that the accident book is filled in, although anyone can fill in the book on behalf of the injured person.

Rideal–Walker test Measure of the effectiveness of a disinfectant at killing micro-organisms.

rigor mortis Stiffening of a cadaver that occurs 1–6 hours after death; rigor mortis then wears off after approximately 24 hours, depending on the ambient temperature.

RIM test A rapid immunological test for FeLV, where the p27 antigen is bound by antibody conjugated to colloidal gold.

rima glottidis The space between the two vocal cords at the entrance to the larynx.

Ringer's solution Isotonic solution, a physiological aqueous solution for fluid therapy; contains sodium chloride, potassium chloride and calcium chloride; used to replace water loss and as a topical physiological salt solution, *see also* HARTMANN'S SOLUTION.

ringing The fitting of a numbered metal band around a bird's leg for identification.

ringworm Fungal skin disease, *see also* DERMATOPHYTOSIS, *MICROSPORUM CANIS, TRICHOPHYTON.*

road traffic accident (RTA) Common type of accident suffered by dogs, cats and other animals; any animal that has been in an RTA should be examined as soon as possible to assess the extent of the injuries, and treated for shock.

Robert Jones bandage A useful first aid and orthopaedic support bandage for the distal limbs; the dressing includes several thick layers of cotton wool or padding, that are then firmly compressed by bandage; the central toes are left uncovered.

rodent ulcer Eosinophilic granuloma; an erosive lesion most commonly affecting the upper lip in cats; possibly has an immune mechanism and generally responds to steroids, although antibiotics may also be indicated if there is secondary infection.

rod Light-receptive cell forming part of the neuroretina; contain rhodopsin and provide night/dusk vision.

Romanovsky's stain A compound stain containing eosin and methylene blue, used for differential white cell counts and examination of blood smears.

rongeurs Surgical instrument with jaws for cutting and removing bone.

rose bengal A red/pink stain used occasionally in bacteriology.

Rose–Waaler test An immune-based test carried out on a blood sample to help confirm a diagnosis of rheumatoid arthritis.

rostellum The cranial part of the scolex (mouthpart) of a tapeworm, often carrying a ring of hooks to anchor the parasite to the intestinal wall.

rostral Term used to describe structures on the head that are towards the nose.

rotavirus Group of RNA viruses with a wheel-like structure; a common cause of diarrhoea in neonates.

Rothera's test A test for the presence of ketone bodies, where urine is mixed with reagent and develops a purple colour if ketones are present.

roughage The indigestible fibre in the diet.

rouleau formation Aggregation of erythrocytes in a blood smear to form long columns; a normal finding in the horse when it looks like a pile of coins.

round ligament The distinct band of fibrous tissue running in the lateral edge of the broad ligament of the uterus.

roundworm Group of fleshy endoparasitic worms that occur mainly in immature animals, *see also* ASCARID, *TOXOCARA CANIS.*

Royal Army Veterinary Corps (RAVC) The part of the army in the UK that provides veterinary care for horses, dogs, etc. used in the armed forces.

Royal College of Veterinary Surgeons (RCVS) The governing body of the veterinary profession. Individuals must be registered with the RCVS to practice in the UK; the RCVS draws up professional codes of conduct, advises government on legislative issues and oversees veterinary and veterinary nurse training and examination. The RCVS has to maintain a register of veterinary surgeons and veterinary nurses.

Royal Veterinary College (RVC) Founded in London in 1792 and presently has the largest UK intake of veterinary students and is also involved with veterinary nurse training.

rub, pericardial Sound heard on auscultation when the two layers of the pericardium rub over each other.

rub, pleural Sound heard on auscultation when the visceral and parietal layers of the pleura rub against each other.

rubber jaw *see* RICKETS.

rubor Redness; one of the classical signs of inflammation.

ruga, pl. rugae A fold, particularly in the lining of the stomach.

rumination Regurgitation of food from the rumen back up to the mouth for further chewing, before being swallowed again; an important part of the digestive process in ruminants.

ruminant Herbivorous animal with a four-chambered stomach, consisting of the rumen, reticulum, omasum and abomasum.

rupture A traumatic tear in the wall of an organ.

ruptured bladder Tearing of the bladder wall due to trauma or overdistension, e.g. blocked urethra.

ruptured spleen Traumatic tearing of the capsule of the spleen that may result in significant and life-threatening internal haemorrhage, neoplasia is another cause.

rush pin A metal pin, used as a pair for internal fracture fixation.

S

S–A node The sino-atrial node is situated in the right atrium muscle; it initiates the heart beat by the discharge of rhythmic electric impulses, *see also* A–V NODE.

S–T segment The part of the electrocardiogram trace at the end of each cycle that represents the repolarisation of the ventricles.

Sabouraud Culture medium used in mycotic disease diagnosis; has a low pH of 5.6 and additional glucose content, *see also* RINGWORM.

sabulous Sandy-like, usually used when referring to calculi material in the cat with urethral obstruction, *see also* CALCIUM OXALATE, FELINE UROLOGICAL SYNDROME, STRUVITE.

sac Term for a purse-like structure, the respiratory system of birds depends on such air-filled cavities.

saccule Indicates a smaller purse or bag: the small cavity at the base of the semicircular canals of the ear is the saccule connecting to the utricle.

sacculitis, anal Inflammation of the lining of the anal sacs; causes the production of foul smelling liquid; irritation to the perineal area may make the dog slide or 'scoot' or bite at the hind quarters, *see also* ANAL SAC DISEASE.

sacral Relates to the area of the back known as the sacrum.

sacral artery The final part of the dorsal aorta continues to the tail as the median sacral artery.

sacral dysgenesis Disease where there is a failure of bone development, sometimes associated with urinary incontinence.

sacrococcygeal The area posterior to the sacrum running to the coccygeal vertebrae.

sacrococcygeal agenesis A failure of development of the vertebrae of the area; seen in old English sheep dogs or 'bob tails'.

sacrococcygeal fusion An extension of the fused vertebrae that make up the sacrum into the first coccygeal veterbrae; a condition sometimes seen on X-ray.

sacrococcygeal luxation The result of accidents to the pelvic region; nerve damage is the main complication.

sacroiliac The cranial end of the sacrum articulates with the wing of the ilium on either side; the joint is usually fibrous and may be easily damaged in road traffic accidents; especially liable to such injury is the cat dragged under a vehicle.

sacrolumbar The articulation of the sacrum with the last lumbar vertebrae, often the site of pain on palpation in older dogs, *see also* DEEP PAIN SENSATION.

sacrosciatic ligament The fibrous band that connects the sciatic tuberosity of the ilium to the sacrum.

sacrum The three fused vertebrae at the base of the spine with a narrow triangular shape have this special name, from the Greek word for 'sacred bone'.

Saddler's list PML legislation in the UK allows certain retail outlets for equine goods to sell anthelminthics which would otherwise be on a pharmacy prescription basis.

safe light Method of illumination in photographic dark room that allows the operator to view negatives without harming the image; the colour of filter used must be suitable for each type of X-ray film.

sagittal Like an arrow cutting an object into two; the sagittal plane is therefore parallel to the median plane.

SAIDS Simian acquired immunodeficiency syndrome; virus infection of primates similar to 'AIDS'.

salicylate Salt used medicinally in many products such as aspirin; it has antipyretic and anti-inflammatory properties; the first pharmaceutical discovery made was that willow tree bark was of benefit in rheumatic disorders.

saline (normal saline) Common salt or sodium chloride is widely used in nursing as a solution for flushing wounds and for fluid therapy; normal saline is isotonic at 0.9% solution.

saliva Secretion in the mouth that lubricates the food, maintains a protective coat on the mucous membranes, has some digestive enzyme content and, especially in cats, is a valuable substance for washing and grooming the rest of the body.

salivary Relates to the production of saliva.

salivary ducts The tubular connection of one of four pairs of salivary glands with the mouth.

salivary glands The four paired glands found in the dog and cat are zygomatic, sublingual, mandibular and parotid.

salivary mucocele Leakage of saliva from a damaged duct results in a subcutaneous swelling. The first injury or obstruction of a duct may be unnoticed but often an enormous non painful swelling appears at the angle of the jaws, *see also* MULTILOCULAR RANULA.

Salmonella Group of Gram-negative bacteria associated with enteric diseases. Distinguished on culture as non-lactose-fermenting organisms, *see also* MACCONKEY, ZOONOSIS.

salping- Relates to the uterine tubes, salpingitis may be a cause of infertility.

salpinx (1) The uterine tube. (2) The auditory tube.

salt Chemical definition is a combination of a base and an acid. Sodium bicarbonate is an example of a salt. **Bile salt** Substances found in the liver secretion that help in the digestion of fats. **Common salt** Sodium chloride. **Epsom salts** Magnesium sulphate, formerly used for wound lavage, poulticing and for its laxative properties.

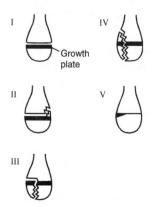

Salter–Harris fracture classification

Salter–Harris fracture classification Classification system for fractures in skeletally immature animals which involve the growth plate region of long bones.

sample (1) Specimen usually collected for laboratory tests. (2) Statistically the number that needs to be analysed to produce an accurate picture of the whole population.

sand Gritty material with a silica base. May be the cause of irritation to dogs running on sand surfaces – especially racing greyhounds.

sanguineous Prefix word relating to blood; pus with a pinkish blood tinge is sanguino-purulent.

saphenous vein Superficial vein on the lateral aspect of the hind leg above the tarsus. Site of venepuncture as an alternative to the forelimb or the neck.

saprophyte Free-living group of bacteria usually feeding on dead or decaying matter.

Sarcocystis Genus of parasitic protozoa that are closely related to *Coccidia*. Dogs are the final hosts for some species and oocysts appear in the faeces; they are not associated with canine disease. The intermediate host such as sheep or humans may have the disease sarcocystosis.

sarcoid A small tumour on the skin surface, not usually malignant.

sarcolemma The plasma membrane covering the striated muscle fibres.

sarcoma Malignant tumour, *see also* LYMPHPOSARCOMA, OSTEOSARCOMA.

Sarcoptes External parasite species, cause of pruritus and mange. The mites are usually detected by skin scrapings which may have to be taken from several sites or sometimes it is necessary to use blood tests to confirm a suspected problem.

sarcoptic mange A type of mange that is characterised by intense itchiness, caused by *Sarcoptes scabiei* that may be very difficult to find in skin scrapings. An antibody test is available to examine the blood for exposure to a previous infection with the mite.

sartorius muscle Muscle on the inner surface of the hind limb, the so-called 'tailor's muscle' from the time when such workers sat cross-legged on the floor and the muscle hypertrophied.

SAT Serum agglutination test.

saws Used orthopaedically, may be oscillating or wire, *see also* GIGLI SAW.

SC Subcutaneous route, sc or sq are alternatives.

scab A crust on the skin surface, *see* SARCOPTIC MANGE.

scabies Human disease caused by *Sarcoptes scabiei*.

scala tympani Part of the cochlea of the ear.

scald Moist heat necrosis of the superficial skin layers, but sometimes deep penetration if the hot fluid unavoidably remains in contact with the skin, *see also* BURN.

scaler Instrument to remove dental calculus, *see also* ULTRASONIC.

scalpel Instrument for cutting; detachable blades of various shapes are available, *see also* BARD–PARKER.

scan A method of producing an image used diagnostically as in ultrasound or computed tomography.

scaphoid bone Skeletal bone found in the carpus.

scapula Triangular skeletal bone forming the top of the shoulder and the joint with the humerus, *see also* GLENOID CAVITY.

scar Fibrous contracted tissue, the result of healing after an incision, burn, scald, abscess, etc.

scatter (1) Implies a wide distribution. (2) Incident photons in radiography that may interact with solid tissues. **Back scatter** The type of diversified ionising radiation in X-ray work; cassettes are designed to absorb and reduce this effect, tables must be covered with lead rubber.

scattered or secondary radiation The amount is small in cats, thin patients and whenever a lower kV is used; it causes blackening of X-ray plates thus reducing image quality. Always a hazard to personnel and precautions are necessary.

scavenging of anaesthetics Safety measures should be used to remove toxic and hazardous gases from the operating room. Active and passive systems are available.

Schirmer tear test Method of measuring tear secretion and flow by the use of prepared strips of absorbent paper suspended from the lower eyelid.

schisto- Prefix for a split, as in schistosomus for a fetus with an open or split abdomen.

Schroeder–Thomas A type of external fixation splint that was used in the treatment of injury to the proximal limb of cats.

Schwann cells Cells that wrap around the nerve axons to form a myelin sheath which increases the speed of conduction, *see also* MYELIN.

scissor Instrument with apposed two blade action used frequently in surgical procedures. May be curved or straight, blunt or sharp tipped, *see also* MAYO SCISSORS.

scissor bite Description used for the closure of the incisor teeth favoured by most dog breeds; a slight overlap of the upper jaw over the lower jaw front teeth, *see also* OVERSHOT JAW.

sclera The tough outer casing of the sensitive structures of the eye; it is a continuous globe structure except for the optic nerve exit and the transparent cornea in front.

scleritis Inflammation of the sclera; may be a localised raised patch or a general reddening of the 'white' of the eye, *see also* GLAUCOMA.

scolex The head of the tapeworm that attaches to the host's intestine wall either using suckers or a series of hooks, *see also* ROSTELLUM.

scoliosis Condition of curvature of the spine, usually a lateral displacement of the neck and back. It may be congenital or acquired, *see also* KYPHOSIS.

-scopy Word used to describe the examination of a part.

scours Popular descriptive term for diarrhoea.

scraping Implies taking superficial or deep samples of skin to detect ectoparasites.

screening (1) Term in general use for any series of tests to look for diseases. The Guthrie test was the first such test used on human babies to look for phenylketonuria by one drop of urine. (2) Used to include fluoroscopy or dynamic image intensification.

screw Metal fixation device for attaching bone plates or holding fracture fragments in place.

screwtail Inherited condition in the bulldog where the short tail is distorted and presses into the perineum.

scrotal Relating to the sac that contains the male organs for sperm production and the accessory epididymis.

scurf Popular description of skin scales seen more easily in black and dark coated breeds, *see also* *CHEYLETIELLA*, ZINC.

scurvy Disease of humans associated with vitamin C deficiency. Only guinea-pigs can be affected by a similar deficiency as other animals synthesise vitamin C.

scybalum A lump or mass of hard faeces.

seasonally polyoestrus The reproductive cycle pattern seen in the cat, *see also* OESTRUS.

sebaceous Relates to the production of the greasy skin substance sebum. The sebaceous glands are the main sites for finding the parasite *Demodex*.

seborrhoea Skin disorder characterised by excess scaling or sometimes a greasy form is associated with overactive sebaceous glands masking the keratinisation defect.

sebum The oily substance that helps seal the skin against water loss and at the same time acts as a bacteria barrier.

second intention healing Where the incision, if sutured, has failed to heal or an open wound where there has to be granulation tissue formed before the epithelium can cover it over.

secondary Indicates something that develops later.

secondary generation Such anticoagulant rodenticides were developed as a safer way of killing rats and mice without harming pets.

secondary haemorrhage The type of bleeding that occurs at least some 24 hours after an injury, may be due to infection of the blood clot or a delayed clotting problem.

secondary radiation *see also* SCATTER.

secondary sexual characters Those that develop on maturation, or in the bitch and queen the mammary glands only grow in pseudopregnancy or in pregnancy.

secretin Hormone associated with the production of pancreatic and intestinal juice.

section The act of cutting or dividing up. **Caesarean section** The delivery of one or more fetuses by cutting into the abdominal wall and the uterus, *see also* HYSTERECTOMY.

sedation Method of preparing an animal for surgery or helping it to relax during a time of excitement by the use of medication.

sedimentation The settling out of the solid parts of a suspension.

sedimentation rate The rate at which erythrocytes settle in a standing blood sample; observed under standard conditions it was used as a test for many chronic conditions.

seeing practice Traditional term for veterinary students attending the workplace to learn the art as well as the science of their veterinary duties.

seizure General term used for an epileptic fit or in humans for a heart attack.

self-trauma Damage done to an animal by its own actions of biting, scratching or rubbing at a painful or irritating part, *see also* PRURITUS.

selenite broth An enriched culture medium used in the identification of *Salmonella*.

selenium Chemical element, used in the treatment of conditions such as muscular dystrophy, often combined with vitamin E.

semen White fluid ejaculated from the penis during reproductive activity, rich in spermatozoa. **Frozen semen** Method of preserving genetic material in liquid nitrogen at −197°C.

semen diluent Buffered solution used during the preservation of collected semen.

semicircular canals The balance centre of the inner ear, contained in the bony labyrinth.

semilunar Either of the two heart valves shaped like half moons that allow the forward flow of blood from the ventricles, *see also* AORTIC VALVE, PULMONARY VALVE.

semimembranosus muscle A muscle of the group that occupies the caudal aspect of the thigh known as the 'hamstring group'.

semi-permeable membrane A separating layer that only allows water and small molecule-sized particles to pass through. Diffusion across the SPM is the basis of osmotic pressure, a process with many examples in physiology.

semitendinosus muscle Muscle of the hind leg group that occupies the caudal aspect of the thigh known as the 'hamstring group'.

senile The state of physical and mental deterioration that is part of the ageing process.

sensitisation An alteration in the reaction of the body to the introduction of a foreign substance.

sensory Relating to the part of the nervous system that carries the receptors and the transfer of this received information to the spinal cord and the brain.

sensory nerve An afferent nerve conveying information of stimuli received.

sentient An animal that is able to feel and in some people's minds is also able to be sensitive with emotions.

sentinel dog Guard dog.

sepsis The presence of infection in tissues or the blood causing inflammation and tissue destruction, *see also* BACTERAEMIA, TOXAEMIA.

septal A division or dividing membrane.

septal defect Usually a congenital fault, as in a hole between the two ventricles or the atria.

septicaemia Condition where bacteria are multiplying in the blood stream; toxins add to the problem, *see also* TOXAEMIA.

septum A dividing wall as in the nose or heart.

sequelae The after-effects; any disorder or pathological condition that follows a disease.

sequestration Forming a dead or separate part especially after bone injury.

sequestration, feline corneal Seen as a black raised spot in the cornea, it is an avascular response to injury.

seroconversion Part of the production of the immune state, measured by the formation of circulating antibodies.

serology Study of components of blood serum, e.g. for antibody and antigen presence; may be used diagnostically, *see also* ANTIBODY.

seroma An accumulation of fluid usually under the skin following surgery or an injury; may appear on the outside as a tumour-like mass, *see also* HAEMATOMA.

seropurulent A discharge that is thinner in constituency than normal pus and may indicate a foreign body or a recovery stage after infection.

serosa The name for any serous membrane.

serotonin Hormone and neurotransmitter, found in many tissues and may be associated with sleep.

serotype The characteristic of a bacterial group recognised by its antigens, *see also* MOLECULAR.

Sertoli cell A specialised cell in the testicular tissue that helps the spermatids to mature; may become neoplastic in the older dog with the production of oestrogens, *see also* CRYPTORCHID.

Sertoli cell tumour Neoplastic growth within the testis that may produce oestrogens causing feminisation. This is a particular risk with the intra-abdominal retained testes of the cryptorchid.

serum Biological fluid noted for its antibody content but contains all the liquid elements of plasma once fibrinogen and the blood cells have been removed in the clot. Usually obtained by taking a blood sample in a plain (preferably glass) container and allowing it to stand long enough to clot. The cool part of a room or a 5°C refrigerator may help the clot to retract and free the serum.

serumal Relating to the production of serum.

serum alkaline phosphatase (SAP) A labile enzyme used in estimation of liver damage and bone activity.

service (1) Relates to the physical act of mating; term most used in large animals but occasionally used by dog breeders. (2) Any provision of supplies or procedures, e.g. a laboratory service.

sesamoid Small bone that lies within a tendon, often at a joint flexure point.

sesqui- Infrequently used word for one and a half.

sessile Flat or adherent, close to the surface.

sex (1) The basic difference in the gametes produced by an organism used in reproduction of the species. (2) Word used to find out in birds, kittens and puppies, etc. future development into male or female and whether suitable for breeding as pairs.

sexarche The age at which an individual first becomes involved in breeding.

sex-linked A gene located on a sex chromosome that will always pass a characteristic to the next generation, usually on the X-chromosome.

sex pili Gram-negative bacteria have cell-wall structures that allow them to stick to the lining of the host's intestine, respiratory or urinary system. Sex pili are also the manner in which bacteria reproduce by conjugation, passing DNA from donor to recipient cell.

sexual Relating to breeding or secondary sexual characteristics and behaviour.

sexual behaviour Any usual or unusual activity associated with reproduction.

sexual cycle Oestrous cycle or in some male animals such as deer in the rutting season.

sexual maturity The time when breeding is possible; may be delayed in some male animals when there are no external signs of maturation.

SGOT Serum glutamic–oxaloacetic transaminase – used as a liver damage test.

SGPT Serum glutamic–pyruvic transaminase – used as a test for degree of liver cell damage.

shaft The portion of a long bone between the two epiphyses, *see also* DIAPHYSIS. May also be used to describe the hair's main length.

shampoo A suspension of detergent and medication used in grooming and for the medical treatment of skin diseases.

sharps Term used for needles and blades that have to be disposed of in rigid containers under the *Disposal of Clinical Waste Regulations.*

sheath (1) The outer covering, as used in the microscopic structure of the hair; nerves have myelin sheaths and synovial sheaths cover tendons. (2) Popular word used to describe the male's prepuce.

Sherman bone plate Traditional form of implant used in fracture repair by internal fixation; the weakness is the narrow part between each screw hole.

shock Profound physiological change in the body with circulatory collapse as the result of trauma, bacterial toxins or allergic response, *see also* FLUID THERAPY.

short chain fatty acid (SCFA) Important in the production of the watery faeces associated with many diarrhoea conditions.

shoulder The first joint of the proximal limb, between the scapula and the humerus.

shunt A passage connecting two anatomical channels or a diversion. **Left-to-right shunt** Diversion of the blood from the left side to the right side of the heart, usually due to a defect in the septum. **Porto-systemic shunt** Congenital disease seen in growing puppies where blood from the intestines passes direct to the right atrium without being processed in the liver.

SI units A standard of 'system international' units all relating to the litre; it replaced many of the traditional words used in measurement.

sialagogue A drug that promotes the secretion of saliva.

silent heat An unobserved breeding period; accounts for presumed anoestrus in bitches, etc.

silk suture Traditional fine permanent material used for suturing eyelids, etc.

silver Metallic element, also used to describe the coat colour of some breeds.

silver halide Part of the photographic developing process; involves the conversion of exposed particles of silver bromide into black particles of metallic silver which remain on the final plate.

silver nitrate Prepared in sticks, it may be used as a chemical cautery to control bleeding or treat superficial warts.

simian Describes a member of the ape and the monkey family.

sinoatrial node The microscopic area of the heart muscle that sets the pace of the beat.

sinus (1) A blind ended infected tract or drainage channel. (2) Term used anatomically for any air- or fluid-filled cavity.

sinus arrhythmia During the pulse measurement of the normal patient, the pulse rate increases on inspiration and decreases on expiration; considered to be a sign of a functioning heart and a normal variation of the heart beat rhythm.

sinusitis Inflammation of one of the sinus cavities of the skull, often the result of an upper respiratory tract infection.

skatole A protein breakdown product that causes one of the characteristic odours of fresh faeces.

skeleton The bony framework that supports the body and largely determines its shape.

skeletal muscle The voluntary muscles under control of the nervous system, *see also* STRIATED.

skin The outer covering and therefore the largest organ of the body. Variously covered with hair, feathers and scales and carrying pigment, *see also* CUTIS, DERMIS, EPIDERMIS.

ski slope Term used in radiological diagnosis to describe the anconeal process shape when affected by osteophytes, *see also* OSTEOCHONDROSIS.

skull The skeletal structure of the head made up of many fused bones; the mandible is the only articulating structure.

skyline view One used radiographically to get an angled or silhouetted view of a structure.

sleep A natural state of unconsciousness in which brain activity is not apparent. **Put to sleep** A term for euthanasia, difficult to be certain about; a signed authority is best obtained to avoid confusion with the owner thinking it is a form of anaesthesia that is being described. **Rapid eye movement (REM) sleep** Describes a stage of sleep where the muscles of the eye are in constant motion, equated with dreaming.

slide A piece of glass used in examination under the microscope. **Acetate tape slide** Used in obtaining superficial parasites of the skin for transfer to the laboratory.

sling A support for an injured part of the body, helps to promote rest, *see also* EHMER SLING, VELPEAU SLING.

slough A piece of dead tissue, often peals away from the living tissue underneath. **Anaesthetic slough** A necrotic area of skin and underlying vein due to perivascular injection of an irritant such as thiopentone.

slow Not rapidly developing; some infections are due to a slow virus, *see also* LEUKAEMIA, PRIONS.

small A dimunitive term as used in small bowel or in small pox.

small intestine Includes the duodenum, jejunum and ileum.

smear A method of examining a specimen under the microscope by spreading a film across a glass slide.

smell Odour or fragrance detected by the receptor cells of the mucous membrane covering the ethmoturbinate bones of the nose.

smoke injury Animals involved in fires may cough only slightly at first but then develop pneumonia and pulmonary oedema due to the inhaled smoke particles becoming attached to the lower bronchial airway, even into the alveoli.

smothering One cause of neonatal death due to overcrowding of puppies and kittens.

snake Reptiles are often kept as pets; the nurse should ask the attendant of any poisonous propensity before handling the patient.

snoring Reverberating noise from the soft palate and pharynx on inspiration or exhalation; adjusting the head position may reduce the noise produced.

snuffles Nasal sound produced by cats after sinusitis; small mammals with upper respiratory tract infections also breathe like this.

social Relates to animals living in a community.

social behaviour Behaviour of a domestic animal that is not harmful to its fellow members, especially those in the same group or locality.

social distance The spacing out of animals such as birds on a telephone line or cats in suburban gardens.

social order The hierarchy that allows animals to coexist without constant fighting; depends on dominant and submissive behaviour patterns.

socialisation Process of adapting to living with other animals or humans; one of the necessary duties of a 'puppy walker' is to introduce the recently weaned animal to human carers and other external experiences.

soda A salt containing sodium, often associated with the release of carbon dioxide. Old (flat) soda water is a first-aid drink for dogs that have vomited frequently. **Baking soda** Sodium bicarbonate, used for teeth cleaning or in dilute solution as a skin wash. **Washing soda** Sodium carbonate; a large crystal makes an effective emetic for a dog.

Soda lime Used in anaesthetic circuits to absorb carbon dioxide; consists of a colour indicator for the combination of sodium hydroxide and calcium hydroxide, together with silicates to reduce dust.

sodium Chemical element; symbol Na for natrium, hence hyponatraemia for low serum level.

sodium bicarbonate A salt used in first aid and as an antacid.

sodium carbonate Used as an emetic, *see also* VOMIT.

sodium chlorate Cause of severe poisoning in dogs accidentally ingesting weedkiller.

sodium chloride Common salt, used in emergency oral fluid therapy.

sodium cyanide Poisonous substance used in certain chemical plants, sometimes causing fish to die in contaminated watercourses.

sodium hydroxide Caustic soda used in degreasing and is strongly alkaline.

sodium hypochlorite Mild antiseptic used for sterilising feeding bottles, etc.

sodium lactate Compound included in Hartmann's solution to provide bicarbonate.

sodium pump Cell regulating mechanism to maintain the isotonic state.

soft palate The caudal part of the pharynx that can be used to seal off the nasopharynx, oesophagus and the larynx.

solanine Toxic compound found in green potatoes.

solar Relating to the sun. **Nasal solar dermatitis** Crusty dermatosis known as 'collie nose'.

solar burns Dermal necrosis, especially due to ultraviolet radiation.

solution A mixture in which a solid is evenly distributed in the liquid solvent.

solvent The liquid in which another substance is dissolved to form a solution; some propellant and volatile liquids have been used for their stimulatory effects on humans, *see also* POISON.

soma The entire body excluding the germ cells.

somatic Cells that relate to the animal's body, *see also* NERVE.

somatostatin Hormone secreted by the pituitary and the islets of Langerhans cells in the pancreas; inhibits the production of insulin and glucagon.

somatotrophin The growth hormone.

soporific Sleep-inducing substance.

sore A name for any abrasion or ulcerating area. **Bed sore** Pressure sore usually on the elbow or bony prominences, *see also* DECUBITUS. **Pressure sores** General term for any skin damage in a recumbant animal, most often on the elbows but can occur on the shoulders or hind legs of greyhounds.

sour crop Fermenting condition of the bird's alimentary tract; the dilated oesophagus may cause a distension of the neck.

space Any unfilled area. **Dead space** A surgical term for a cavity left after an excision; is liable to fill with serum or blood. **Epidural space** Space outside the spinal cord membranes usually containing fat; used for filling with an anaesthetic substance, *see also* REGIONAL ANAESTHESIA. **Intercostal space** The space occupied by muscles between two ribs and provides an access point to the chest. **Subarachnoid space** The space between the arachnoid mater and the pia mater, the membranes around the brain and spinal cord; contains the cerebrospinal fluid.

spasm A sustained involuntary muscle contraction, most serious when it restricts a channel such as the airway, *see also* BRONCHOSPASM, LARYNGOSPASM.

spasmolytic Medication that relieves spasms of smooth muscle.

spastic (1) Characterised by spasms. (2) An individual suffering from spastic paralysis.

spay From an early English word meaning to neuter the female, *see also* GELD.

specialist In the veterinary context, a person recognised by the Royal College of Veterinary Surgeons as having a named RCVS Diploma or a person who has been recognised as having specialist skills such as a Fellowship Diploma by examination or meritorious contributions to learning. A more general definition in the medical or dental world is one who by special studies concentrates on one particular branch of that profession.

specific Particular, one that is clearly distinguishable from others.

specific drug A medicine that has particular properties to cure a disease.

specific gravity The relative density of a liquid.

specimen (1) A sample usually obtained from the animal patient. (2) May mean an unusual or unique sample.

spectinomycin Broad-spectrum antibiotic used mainly against Gram-negative bacterial infections.

spectrum, broad Medication with a wide band of activity against micro-organisms.

speculum An instrument, usually trumpet-shaped, for examining or dilating a body orifice to see inside.

sperm The male animal's output for reproductive purposes, *see also* SPERMATOZOA.

spermatic cord Suspensory ligament structure of the testis that contains an artery, a vein, a nerve and a muscle as well as the vas deferens.

spermatid A juvenile or developing spermatozoa produced by meiotic division, one development stage before the functioning spermatozoa.

spermatocyte The germ cells produced by the spermatogonium.

spermatogenesis The process of maturation of spermatozoa that takes place within the testis; the cells lie in the seminiferous tubules eventually passing into the epididymis. Reduction division or meiosis is an important stage in the development so that only half the genetic information is available for the fertilisation of the ova, *see also* MEIOSIS.

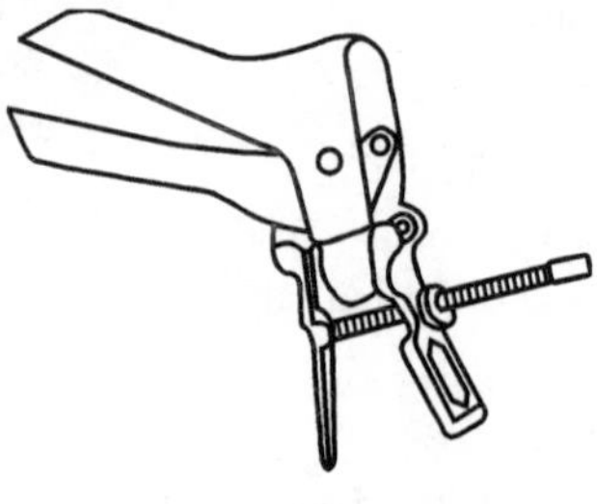

Cusco vaginal speculum

spermatozoa The mature male sex cells. The tail allows for movement by swimming in a fluid medium and the head (acrosome) allows for penetration of the ova when fertilisation may take place. In the dog spermatozoa can survive for 5 days in the fallopian tube of the bitch after mating.

spermaturia Reflux into the bladder of spermatozoa remaining in the prostate area of the vas deferens.

spermiogenesis The second stage of maturation where the spermatids are developed to form spermatozoa.

spewing Popular term for vomiting, *see also* EMESIS.

sphenoid bone The bone at the base of the skull behind the eyes, so called because of its wedge shape.

spheroma Any tumour shaped like a sphere or ball.

sphincter A circular muscle whose function is to keep an orifice closed until such time as the contents need to be discharged from within or, in the case of the pupil, the iris dilates to allow more light to reach the retina.

sphincterotomy An incision into a sphincter to allow easier passage of contents.

sphygmo- Prefix relating to the pulse in the animal's circulation.

spica bandage A cloth wound around repeatedly in a figure-of-eight pattern, so a series of V-marks appear on the outside surface of the bandage.

spicule A small fragment, often spike-shaped.

spider Member of the *Arachnida*, an invertebrate: some are terrestrial, some aquatic, some aerial.

spider monkey Small monkey from the New World group, with long legs and long tails as they are active tree climbers.

spike A sharp point; used to describe the trace on an encephalogram of brain cell activity, *see also* EPILEPSY.

Spilopsylla cuniculi The most common rabbit flea; acts to spread the myxomatosis virus, *see* VECTOR.

spina bifida Developmental fault of the neural tube where the newborn has part of the spinal cord unprotected by vertebrae.

spinal Relates to part of the central nervous system and bony vertebral column.

spinal anaesthesia Regional anaesthesia for certain segments of the spine, *see also* EPIDURAL.

spinal column The vertebrae that make up successive parts of the spine.

spinal cord The nerve tissue that occupies the spinal column, *see also* CENTRAL NERVOUS SYSYTEM.

spinal muscular atrophy Rare inherited disease affecting movement, with eventual paralysis.

spinal nerve Paired nerves run from the spinal cord to various structures, exiting between the vertebrae.

spinal reflex A reflex action that involves the nerve impulses passing through localised segments of the spinal cord.

spinal shock Paralysis that develops above and below an injury to the spinal cord accompanied by many of the other circulatory signs of shock.

spindle cell tumour Neoplasm of skin structures, may be malignant in the vertebrae.

spine (1) A sharp prominence; in reptiles a modification of the skin. (2) Anatomical feature of the skeleton such as the ridge down the scapula or the whole length of the backbone.

spinous process Bony prominence, well developed in the thoracic vertebrae and less strongly developed in the cervical and lumbar regions.

spirit An alcohol-based liquid; industrial methylated spirit has been used as a disinfectant and for topical application to the unbroken skin.

spirolactone A diuretic substance used when other agents such as frusemide are not removing fluid adequately.

spironolactone An oral preparation for inducing diuresis, anatogonises the hormone aldosterone.

splanchnic Relates to the abdomen contents or viscera. The splanchnic nerves are part of the sympathetic nervous system, *see also* AUTONOMIC NERVOUS SYSTEM.

spleen One of the abdominal viscera, lies adjacent to the stomach. Its main function is to act as a reservoir for erythrocytes.

splenectomy Surgical removal of the spleen. The removal of the spleen may be necessary for such gross enlargement; often associated with anorexia and abdominal discomfort.

splenomegaly Enlargement of the spleen, causes include neoplasia, gastric torsion or the action of some drugs e.g. barbiturates.

splint A supporting structure, was used in first aid for fixing displaced or fractured bones.

spondylo- Prefix relating to the spine or vertebrae.

spondylosis The production of bony spurs along the ventral borders of the vertebrae, resulting from chronic instability.

spongiform encephalopathy A degenerative condition of the brain characterised on post mortem by softened or spongy areas, *see also* BSE, CREUTZFELDT–JAKOB DISEASE, KURU.

spontaneous abortion Loss of the fetus(es) without apparent external or infectious cause; indicates a hormonal or auto-immune problem.

sporadic Indicates an irregular or once-only event; sometimes meaning at distantly placed locations.

spore Resistant stage of a bacterium such as *Clostridia* or a fungal infection.

sprain Injury to a ligament caused by sudden over-stretching, *see also* STRAIN.

spray freezing Type of cryosurgery when liquid nitrogen is jetted on to a surface until an ice ball forms.

spraying Undesirable behaviour in cats when urine is used to mark territory including the living areas of the house, *see also* PHEROMONES.

spur veins Veins on the lateral surface of the thorax that lie subcutaneously and can inadvertently be punctured when giving vaccines or other injections by the subcutaneous route. The name comes from similar veins on the horse damaged by the rider's spurs.

sputum Expectorated mucus from the bronchial tubes and lungs, rarely produced in dogs as there is a tendency for such material to be swallowed.

SQ (sub q) tunnel An abbreviation for the subcutaneous route for giving drugs or an entry point for a drain or feeding tube.

squab An immature pigeon often poorly feathered.

squamous A thin, plate-like layer.

squint Anglulation of the eyes. Seen in some cats; may be divergent or convergent.

Stader splint Method of bone fixation using half pins, no longer used.

stain Substance used to delineate a structure; may be used in microscopy or for a corneal ulcer.

standard Regular or normal level.

standard deviation Statistical measurement of the normal variation allowed in a healthy population of animals for biochemical and other parameters.

standard operating procedures Health and Safety Regulations in the UK require these to be written and followed for anything involving a hazard to humans, *see also* COSHH.

stapes One of the three small bones that form a chain across the middle ear, this one being stirrup-shaped.

staphylo- Prefix relating to the bunch of grapes appearance of the causal organism.

Staphylococcus Important group of Gram-positive bacteria, often the cause of severe skin infection and food toxin illnesses.

staphyloma The exception to bacterial infection, as it is the swelling of the eye sclera or cornea due to injury or raised intra-ocular pressure.

staples Method of closure of skin incisions also used in gastrointestinal surgery.

stapling Method of tissue repair, *see also* STAPLES.

starch Carbohydrate compound used in storage; enzyme action (ptyalin and amylase) is needed to release sugars.

starvation Either enforced or voluntary deprivation of food; may have irreversible long-term consequences.

stasis Lack of flow as with an intestine obstruction, *see also* ILEUS.

static A form of electrical discharge that can mark undeveloped film, caused by the films in storage being agitated.

stationary anode The part of the X-ray tube that produces the ionising radiations.

stationary grid Device used in radiography to reduce scatter when X-raying thicker parts of the body, more than 10 cm thick.

status epilepticus A severe form of epileptic attack where the body remains in a constant spasm rather than the usual tonic–clonic convulsions of fits, *see also* EPILEPSY.

steatitis Indicates the inflammation of fatty tissue, often followed by softening with necrosis, *see also* PANSTEATITIS.

steatorrhoea Excessive fat in the faeces, making them pale coloured and greasy.

Steinmann pin An intramedullary pin used for fracture fixation.

stem cell Bone marrow haematopoietic cell that allows either for red or white cells to be formed.

stenosis Narrowing or contraction of an opening, mainly used in describing blood vessel narrowing, e.g. pulmonary stenosis.

Stenson's duct Anatomical name for the parotid gland's drainage of saliva to the mouth.

stercus Another word for faeces. Often the adjective is used as stercorous.

stereotypic Behaviour pattern with constant repetition of what may be a quite complicated action. Seen in animals confined in cages for a long time.

sterile (1) Aseptic, incapable of producing micro-organism growth. (2) Infertile or barren, may apply more common in males than females.

sterilisation The process of destroying all micro-organisms and spores.

sternal Relates to the lower surface area of the thorax over the sternum.

sternal recumbency When the animal lies on its chest with limbs equally placed on either side.

sternebrae The chain of sternal cartilages that makes the lower side of the thoracic cavity.

sternocostal The area where the ribs join the sternum.

sternum Flat structure in mammals made of eight cartilaginous structures (sternebrae) that receive the ribs to support the thorax but allow for flexibility whilst breathing.

steroid An organic four-ring compound produced naturally by the adrenal cortex and as hormones have potent effects. Steroids are also synthesised and used medically and one form is used as a cat anaesthetic, *see also* ALPHAXALONE.

stertor Difficult respiration with a characteristic snoring.

steth(o)- Prefix relating to the chest area.

stifle The complex joint between the femur and the tibia and fibula and the associated sesmoid bones and cartilages; also known as the knee.

stilboestrol Synthetic oestrogen formerly used as a milk suppressant and for mesalliance. Has benefits in some forms of urinary incontinence.

stillborn When a fetus is born but there is no evidence of life.

Stille shears A pattern of shears for cutting plaster casts.

stimulant Any medication that stimulates reflex activity, appetite or demeanour.

sting Injury by the proboscis of an insect or a silicone tipped plant, usually followed by intense irritation.

stippling Body colour pattern; also appears in the haematological examination of red cells as an indicator of anaemia.

stirrup Popular name for the stapes bone found in the middle ear, *see also* ANVIL, STAPES.

stitch Knotted fibre or suture used in repairs.

stitch abscess A reaction to slow dissolving soluble suture material, sometimes associated with wound infections.

stoma An orifice, may be natural like the mouth or surgically produced, *see also* URETHROSTOMY.

stomach Storage organ of the alimentary tract; can distend in carnivores; acidification and digestion of swallowed food should occur in it, *see also* GASTRIC TYMPANY.

stomatitis Inflammation of the mucous membranes of the buccal cavity.

-stomy Surgically to produce a permanent hole, often for drainage of contents.

stone It was the hardness of phosphate calculi that gave this name, *see also* CALCULUS.

stool Word used in human nursing for faeces outside the anus; originally from a 'close stool' or wooden seat used by persons in the production of the product.

strabismus Squint, deviation of the pupil direction.

strain (1) To over-stretch, especially a muscle injury. (2) Also used to indicate a particular subtype of an organism. (3) The popular use is to filter or press hard to make something pass through, *see also* TENESMUS.

strangulated Restriction of the blood flow, as in partial torsion of a hernial sac.

stratum A layer or anatomical structure, as in the outer layer of the cornea.

strepto- Implies a twisted chain of bodies.

Streptococcus Bacterial group whose Gram-positive organisms always appear in pairs or in short chains.

streptomycin An aminoglycoside antibiotic to be used with caution because of ototoxicity especially in cats.

stress Physiological state as a result of injury, disease and worry such as a caged animal in a trap. Stress can be measured by blood pressure changes and cortisol secretion levels apart from behavioural observations.

striated Stripe marked; in histology the marking on voluntary or skeletal muscle fibres.

stricture A narrowing of an orifice such as a blood vessel or the oesophagus after a foreign body injury.

stridor Louder and harsher than a wheeze; difficult breathing noise from the larynx or trachea, *see also* LARYNGEAL PARALYSIS.

strip, mammary A technique used in the treatment of mammary neoplasia, less popular now that individual gland removal and histological sampling is preferred as a less radical alternative to a total excision of all the tissues.

strobila Tapeworm structure arrangement where a chain of proglottids grow away from the head end; a method used for dispersing the tapeworm ova in the host's faeces.

stroke General term for a sudden weakness developing in humans; the result of a reduction in the blood supply to a part of the brain, often from a thrombus, embolism or intracranial haemorrhage. Owners describe a similar sequence in dogs but they may confuse such attacks with those of vestibular disease. **Heat stroke** Examples of hyperthermia and sudden collapse in animals may be due to water deprivation and confinement in a closed space such as a walled yard or a car left in the sun.

struvite Otherwise known as triple phosphate, it is the commonest calculus found in dogs and is also found in cats.

stud tail Bare area on the dorsum of the tail seen in breeding animals and short-haired breeds as they grow older; sebaceous gland activity may be detrimental to hair follicle function.

stump amputation Description of a limb or tail that has had its distal part removed for surgical reasons.

stupor A state of near unconsciousness with poor response to external stimuli such as noise or light.

Stuttgart disease Historical term in England for advanced nephritis with mouth ulceration; term unknown by veterinary students from Germany, *see also* LEPTOSPIROSIS.

styloid As in stylo-hyoid, pen-shaped or pointed structure; used in anatomy.

styptic Something to stop bleeding; assisting blood to clot chemically.

sub- Prefix for beneath, below.

subarachnoid The space between the arachnoid membrane and the pia mater; provides a channel for cerebrospinal fluid.

subclavian The area of the axilla or 'under the armpit' or clavicle.

subclinical Describing a disease that is suspected but has not developed with positive symptoms.

subconjunctival The potential space below the conjunctiva of the eyelid or the sclera that can be used for injecting medication into.

subcutaneous The most frequently used route for injections in pet practice; the layers beneath the skin are almost painless to approach and have an adequate blood supply.

subcutis Term for the area below the dermis or skin layer, composed of adipose and loose connective tissue, *see also* CELLULITIS.

subfertility State of poor reproductive function so that apparently normal matings produce less than the expected results.

subjective Indicates it is something experienced by an individual; there may be symptoms not apparent to others.

sublingual artery One of the available pulse points, and the adjacent vein may be used as a site for injecting an anaethetised patient.

sublingual glands Paired salivary glands that are found under the tongue, *see also* RANULA.

subluxation Partial dislocation of a joint where there is still some contact between the bones' articular ends, *see also* LUXATION.

submandibular The area below the mandibles subject to swelling after injury or infection.

submandibular lymph nodes Soft nodules that usually can be palpated in the angle of the jaw.

submaxillary Below the eyes, adjacent to the maxilla bone.

submental organ Area of sebaceous glands on the chin of the cat; concerned with scent marking but cats may develop a sebaceous folliculitis in this area.

subnormal temperature Body temperature below normal; varies with the species. Temperatures should always be checked a second time before reporting or charting as it can be a sign of a failing metabolism, *see also* TOXAEMIA.

substantia propria The structure that makes up the main thickness of the cornea; it has no blood supply but has sensory nerves.

substrate The substance on which an enzyme reacts. The enzyme increases the speed of the reaction (catalysis) to change the substrate.

sucking Vacuum-assisted means of moving air or liquids into the mouth.

sucking lice One of the two main groups of lice that feed on animals. *Linognathus* is the most common species in the dog.

sucralfate Preparation used in the treatment of gastric irritation; the aluminium sulphate helps to protect the gastric mucosa.

sucrose Cane sugar used medicinally in water to reduce thirst of vomiting dogs; it requires the enzyme sucrase to make the carbohydrate available as a nutrient, *see also* SUGARS.

suction Vacuum apparatus required during surgery to remove fluids and to re-inflate the thoracic cavity contents after pneumothorax.

sudoriferous Smelling of sweat.

suffocation Cessation of breathing as a result of drowning or smothering in puppies or other new-born animals.

sulcus (1) One of the clefts or inward folds of the brain surface. (2) May also be used to describe a groove or furrow in other anatomical structures such as the heart or the penis. **Gingival sulcus** Groove in the gum where it meets the tooth.

sulpha drugs (USA sulfa) Describes those in the suphonamide group.

sulphonamide One of the first chemotherapeutic groups of drugs used against bacteria, developed before penicillin; the clinical use of this group has decreased in recent years.

sulphosalicylic acid test Original test for protein in the urine; largely superseded by dipstick tests. Positive test is turbidity in the urine sample.

sunburn Inflammation of the skin by ultra-violet rays; severe cases cause skin necrosis but unlikely in breeds that have some amount of natural pigmentation.

sunstroke Heat accumulation is more the result of fluid loss and an inability to replenish by drinking rather than damage to the brain.

super- Prefix for better than, excessive or above the normal.

supra- Prefix for above, higher than the rest.

supravital stains Stains used in the laboratory on living cells, to detect inclusions and other cellular material including *Haemobartonella* and *Babesia* species.

surfactant Substance similar to a detergent that is important in the functioning of the lungs so that the alveoli can open at birth and reduces surface tension in pulmonary fluid.

surgery (1) The branch of medical work that deals with injuries, growths, deformities and the removal of unwanted parts by operation or manipulation. (2) Also used to denote a place – veterinary surgery.

surgical Adjective for anything treated by cutting, freezing, burning, etc. or relating to the work performed by the veterinary surgeon.

surgical anaesthesia Describes a level of anaesthesia sufficient to undertake an act of surgery.

surgical shock Physiological state that develops as a result of trauma during surgery; to some extent should be preventable, *see also* FLUID THERAPY.

suture (1) Method of assisting the closure of a wound; also can be used to describe the type of material used in stitching. (2) Anatomically the junction between flat bones.

suxamethonium Drug used to relax voluntary muscles; respiration may then have to be assisted.

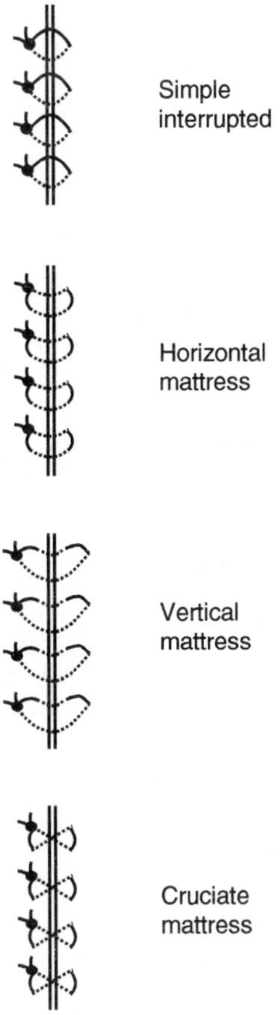

Suture patterns: simple interrupted, horizontal mattress, vertical mattress and cruciate mattress

swab Pad of absorbent material, may be attached to a stick when used to collect laboratory specimens.

swaged needle The type of needle where the suture material is 'welded into' the metal so causing no drag when the needle passes through delicate tissues.

sweat glands Known as sudiferous glands that are only active on the nose and the pads of dogs and cats.

swimmer Popular term for a puppy that fails to stand on its front legs whilst still in the nest; may be the result of an overweight puppy with too rapid growth or one of the obscure muscular dystrophy conditions.

sylvatic rabies The type found in wildlife including foxes; woodland animals are no more susceptible than urban living creatures to the virus infection.

symbiosis A relationship of peaceful co-existence in which there should be mutual aid and benefit.

symblepharon Eyelids adhering to each other and to the eyeball as a result of sticky discharge. Normal state of the new-born puppy or kitten.

sympathetic The part of the autonomic nervous system that works closest to the effects of adrenaline. The 'fright, flight, frolic' response is initiated by the sympathetic nervous system and followed up by the secretion of adrenaline (epinephrine) for a sustained response, *see also* ADRENALINE.

sympathomimetic Producing the results similar to stimulation of the post-ganglionic part of the sympathetic nervous system, *see also* ADRENERGIC, ISOPRENALINE.

symphysis A junction or place where two bones join each as in the pelvis.

synapse Junction of two nerves; production of acetylcholine or noradrenaline as a neurotransmitter allows the chemical transmission of an electrical impulse in the nerve, *see also* NEURON.

synarthrosis Cartilaginous junctions allowing little or no joint movement.

synchondrosis Type of cartilaginous joint which is converted to bone in adult life but remains a point of weakness, *see also* MANDIBULAR SYMPHYSIS.

synchysis scintillans Small particles seen in the posterior chamber of the eye in older animals; may contribute to a bluish reflective haze from the vitreous but not considered a cause of blindness, *see also* ASTEROID HYALOSIS.

syncope Sudden collapse similar to human fainting. May be cardiac in origin with a temporary cerebral anaemia or the result of hypotensive drugs such as acetylpromazine.

syndrome, physiological A group of symptoms that give a clinical picture but not necessarily a disease that can be named, *see also* CUSHING'S SYNDROME, KEY–GASKELL SYNDROME.

synechia An adhesion from the iris to the lens or the cornea; potentially dangerous as a cause of cataract. Classified as anterior or posterior depending on the attachment place.

synergism The state of working together; often applied to medication such as the use of two antibiotics simultaneously to enhance the effects of both.

synorchism An adhesion between the two testes so that they are fused into one mass.

synovial fluid Fluid closely related to plasma but with extra lubrication that occurs in joint spaces; it provides nutrients for the cartilage and has become the subject of research in the prevention of arthritis.

synovitis Inflammation of a synovial membrane; usually the sac becomes filled with serous fluid but there may be infection with pus present.

synovium Synovial membrane lining joints and the fluid it produces.

synthesis Production of a substance in the body or the manufacture of a compound that may be the replica of a natural product.

syringe Surgical tool for introducing a substance into the body, or sometimes for withdrawing a fluid such as blood from a vein or other internal site, *see also* HYPODERMIC, BIOPSY.

syrinx An adaptation of the bird's trachea to produce a voice box.

systemic circulation The part of the blood flow that takes oxygenated blood to all parts of the body and then returns deoxygenated blood to the heart, *see also* PULMONARY CIRCULATION.

systemic lupus erythematosus (SLE) An auto-immune disease characterised by chronic skin changes, *see also* LUPUS.

systemic vascular resistance (SVR) The systemic vascular resistance maintains the blood pressure after blood is pumped into the elastic arteries. SVR is largely controlled by a precapillary sphincter mechanism under the control of the sympathetic nervous system.

systole The contracting phase of the heart, especially when the ventricles force the blood out through the arteries.

systolic murmur Noise produced during the ejection phase of the heart's cycle usually associated with aortic valve incompetence and regurgitation of blood. Always potentially dangerous as a cause of dilation of the ventricles and heart failure.

T

tablet Solid drug formulation. Tablets with enteric coatings should not be broken; the enteric coating either protects the stomach from contact with an irritant drug or prevents degradation of an acid-labile agent.

tachycardia Elevated heart rate; common causes include pain, stress (adrenaline), hypotension and drugs such as atropine; exercise and excitement are non-medical causes.

tachypnoea Elevated respiratory rate; common causes include pain, shock, airway obstructions, effusions and pneumonia; panting, exercise and excitement are non-medical causes.

***Taenia* spp.** A genus of cestodes (tapeworms); endoparasitic worms that infect carnivores. All have an intermediate host, such as mice, where the cysticercus stage develops; adult worms are long and ribbon-like, and eggs are shed in the faeces in packets (proglottids) resembling rice grains; proglottids have a single genital pore. Species include *T. hydatigena, T. pisiformis, T. ovis, T. multiceps, T. serialis* and *T. taeniformis*, *see also* *DIPYLIDIUM CANINUM, ECHINOCOCCUS GRANULOSUS, TAENIA TAENIFORMIS.*

Taenia taeniformis A cat tapeworm.

tail biting A habit developed by some dogs; may be difficult to control as the tail is awkward to bandage; an Elizabethan collar may be required, or a plastic tail guard; severe self-mutilation can necessitate amputation of the tail in persistent cases.

tail-fold pyoderma Infection of the skin fold that is located at the base of the tail in breeds with a corkscrew tail, such as the bulldog and pug.

tail gland Region towards the base of the tail on the dorsal surface, where there are numerous sebaceous glands and the skin tends to be thickened, *see also* CIRCUM-ANAL GLANDS.

tail-gland hyperplasia Hyperplasia of the sebaceous glands of the tail, with the formation of an oval patch of alopecia; associated with generalised seborrhoea and testicular tumours, *see also* SEBORRHOEA, STUD TAIL.

tail shedding Many species of lizard can voluntarily shed their tail as an escape mechanism and thus, the tail should not be used as a means of restraint.

talocrural joint The articulation between the tibia/fibula and the talus; tibiotarsal joint; inaccurately called the hock.

talus One of the bones in the proximal row of tarsal bones; articulates with the tibia and fibula proximally and with the calcaneus laterally (there is little movement at this latter joint).

tamponade Compression of the heart due to an increased volume of fluid within the pericardium, e.g. haemopericardium due to haemangiosarcoma; signs include dyspnoea, tachycardia and muffled heart sounds; may require emergency pericardiocentesis.

tapetal Relating to the tapetum.

tapetum Reflective, non-pigmented part of the retina, just above the optic disc.

tapeworm *see* *TAENIA* SPP., *DIPYLIDIUM CANINUM*, *ECHINOCOCCUS GRANULOSUS*.

target Part of the anode (within the X-ray tube head) that is bombarded by the focused, high-energy electron beam to produce X-rays; the target is usually made from a hard-wearing metal such as tungsten and rotates at high speed.

target cell Type of red blood cell seen in some anaemic patients, having pigment around the periphery and centrally.

tarsal Relating to the tarsus or hock.

tarsal glands Meibomian glands located within the tarsal plate, along the borders of the eyelids.

tarsal plate The thin fibrous layer that gives shape to the eyelid margins.

tarsometatarsal joint Articulation between the distal row of tarsal bone and the metatarsal bones in the hind leg; there is little movement at this level.

tarsorrhaphy Suturing together of the eyelids to protect the cornea, e.g. during ulcer healing.

tarsus The collection of seven bones between the tibia and the metatarsal bones; the talus, calcaneus, central tarsal and first to fourth tarsal bones; the hock.

taste Sensation produced by molecules put in the mouth; taste is relayed via the facial (VII) and glossopharyngeal (IX) cranial nerves.

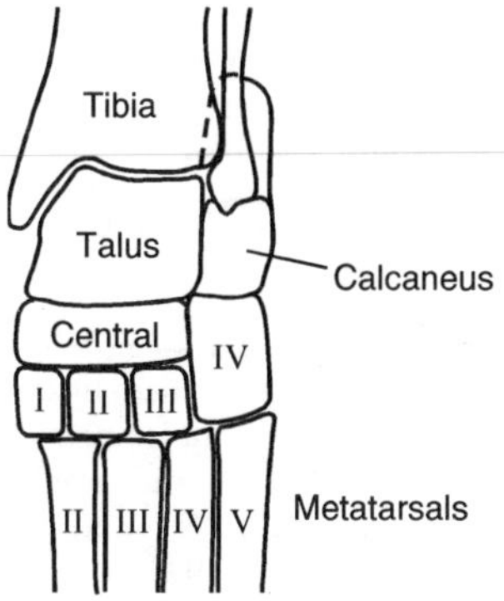

Tarsus: cranial view, left hind

tartar The hard deposit that builds up on teeth; dental calculus, *see also* CALCULUS.

tattooing Permanent means of identifying animals; used in greyhound racing, with a tattoo being placed inside the ear flap.

taurine Amino acid essential in the diet of cats as they cannot synthesise it themselves; signs of taurine deficiency include infertility and central retinal degeneration. The condition is rare now as cat foods have adequate levels of taurine, but deficiency can arise if cats are fed on dog food long term.

taxonomy The scientific and systematic classification of living organisms into groups.

T cell Thymus-derived lymphocytes that confer cell-mediated immunity.

tears Fluid secreted by the lacrimal gland ventromedial to the eye, which bathes the cornea and conjunctiva; tears then drain via the nasolacrimal duct into the nasal chambers where they evaporate.

tear staining Discolouration of the coat at the medial canthus of the eye due to the chronic overflow of tears, *see also* EPIPHORA.

teat Nipple; usually arranged in pairs along the thorax and abdomen.

technetium A radioisotope that emits gamma rays; it can be linked to several different molecules which are taken up by specific organs; in the veterinary field it is used mainly for bone scans.

tectum A roof-like covering.

teeth Dentition; teeth have one or more roots, a pulp cavity, dentine and a covering of tough enamel. Full dentition composes incisors, canines, premolars and molars; carnassial teeth are the large crushing first molar on the mandible and fourth upper premolar.

teeth clipping The teeth of rats, mice, gerbils, hamsters and rabbits are open-rooted and so the teeth grow continuously. If there is malocclusion, where the upper and lower teeth fail to meet correctly, the teeth will require periodic clipping; hard foods should be provided to minimise the problem; signs that clipping is necessary include drooling saliva, inappetence and pawing at the mouth; incisors are most commonly affected but it should be remembered that the cheek teeth may also be overgrown.

telangiectasis Dilation of capillaries or end blood vessels.

telencephalon The olfactory bulbs, cerebral cortices and basal nuclei constitute the telencephalic part of the brain.

telogen The resting phase in the hair growth cycle, *see also* ANAGEN.

telogen effluvium Shortening of the anagen (growth phase) of the hair cycle, so that many hairs enter the telogen (resting) phase at the same time; these hairs are then shed a few weeks later; this moulting may be part of the normal hair growth cycle, or can follow an illness, pregnancy, lactation or drug therapy.

temperament The demeanour of an animal; its character and psychology.

temperature A measure of the degree of heat; measured in °C: room temperature is taken to be 20–24°C, the incubation of bacterial culture plates is usually performed at 37°C. Refrigerators operate at 4°C and freezers at –20°C, *see also* HYPERTHERMIA, HYPOTHERMIA, PYREXIA, APPENDIX 1.

temporomandibular joint The joint of the lower jaw, with articulation between the condylar process of the vertical ramus of the mandible and the temporal bone of the skull; the jaw is closed by the action of the temporal, masseter and pterygoid muscles, and opened by the digastricus.

temporal The region overlying the temporal bone, forming the caudodorsal portion of the skull.

tendinitis (tendonitis) Inflammation of a tendon, usually a result of a strain injury; may be chronic or acute; treated with rest and anti-inflammatories, followed by controlled exercise.

tendon Tough, fibrous band connecting a muscle to a bone.

tenesmus Excessive straining to urinate or defecate; associated with constipation, colitis, urinary calculi and other obstructions.

Tenon's capsule The dense fibrous connective tissue of the periorbita, surrounding the rectus and retractor muscles.

tenorrhaphy The sutured repair of severed tendons; appropriate suture patterns include Bunnell, Bunnell–Mayer, horizontal mattress and Kessler locking loop.

tenosynovitis Inflammation of a tendon and its tendon sheath.

tenotomy Surgical sectioning of a tendon to correct a defect caused by shortening of the tendon.

tension band wire Orthopaedic technique used to internally secure fragments that tend to distract under the pull of muscles and tendons, *see also* WIRING.

tensor Any muscle that acts to create tension in a body area, e.g. tensor fascia lata muscle contracts to increase the tension in the fascial planes over the thigh.

teratogen A substance that causes abnormal development and malformation of a fetus.

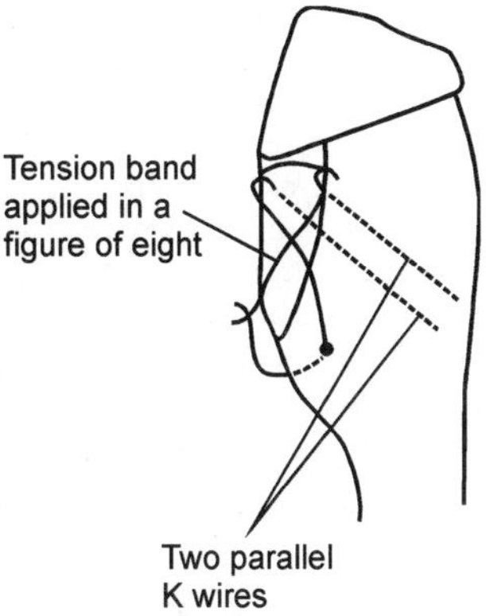

Tension band wiring for fixation of avulsed tibial crest

teratoma A tumour of embryonic origin consisting of cells that would not normally be found at the tumour location; most commonly affect the ovaries and testes.

testicle *see* TESTIS.

testis, pl. testes The male reproductive gland, located within the scrotal sac; sometimes known as the testicle, *see also* GONAD.

testosterone An androgenic, steroid-type hormone formed by the Leydig (interstitial) cells of the testes, but also in small amounts by the ovaries; causes the development of male characteristics, libido and secondary sexual organs.

test tube Basic laboratory apparatus; a glass vial in which chemical reactions can be carried out.

tetanus Disease affecting many species, caused by *Clostridium tetani*; characterised by progressive tetanic (sustained) muscle contractions, due to the effect of bacterial neurotoxin on the CNS; the organism enters via accidental wounds, bites, surgical sites, etc; treatment is with antitoxin and antibiotics, but the prognosis is guarded, with death due to respiratory or cardiac failure. Vaccine is used routinely in man, and staff working with animals should ensure that they have in-date cover. Symptoms are due to the exotoxin tetanospasmin, cats are more resistant than dogs to the effects.

tetany Protracted muscle spasm, *see also* ECLAMPSIA.

tetra- Four.

tetracycline Broad spectrum, bacteriostatic antibiotic; may sometimes cause yellowing of the teeth if given to immature animals.

tetralogy of Fallot A serious congenital cardiac abnormality comprising pulmonic stenosis, ventricular septal defect, displaced aorta and right ventricular hypertrophy, resulting in a right-to-left shunt; affected animals are often stunted and have poor exercise tolerance; there is a systolic murmur and ECG changes. The condition is confirmed by ultrasound or angiography; surgical correction may be attempted but the outlook is guarded.

tetraparesis Weakness affecting all four legs; however, if the weight of the animal is supported it is still able to make coordinated stepping movements.

tetraplegia Paralysis of all four legs, with no stepping movements, *see also* QUADRIPLEGIA.

tetraploid Having four times the haploid number of chromosomes, *see also* DIPLOID, HAPLOID.

thalamus Part of the diencephalon, deep within the brain, surrounding the third ventricle; it acts as the major sensory relay centre for information passing up to the cerebral cortex.

theatre Room set aside for performing aseptic surgical procedures.

theobromine A methylxanthine derivative; a myocardial stimulant and diuretic; also dilates the coronary arteries and relaxes smooth muscle; occurs naturally in chocolate, and overdose has been reported in dogs, the signs being vomiting, diarrhoea, diuresis and collapse; treatment is symptomatic, *see also* CHOCOLATE POISONING.

theophylline A widely used methylxanthine; a bronchodilator, with positive inotropic and chronotropic effects on the heart; used in the management of congestive heart failure and other cardiogenic pulmonary disease.

therapeutics The science of the use of drugs to treat disease.

thermocautery Electrocautery; use of an electric current to generate heat that controls haemorrhage, or can be used to cut through tissue.

thermometer Instrument for measuring temperature; consists of a mercury column sealed under vacuum, which contracts or expands depending on the temperature. The clinical thermometer has a glass neck in the mercury tube just above the reservoir that stops the column falling back down after the temperature has been read, and thus needs to be shaken down before use.

thermophile A bacterium that thrives at temperatures above 50°C.

thermoplastic Material that softens when heated and hardens again as it cools; used as splinting and casting materials.

thermoregulation Control of body temperature; body temperature is regulated by the hypothalamus. When body temperature drops, skin blood vessels constrict, the coat stands on end and shivering is used to generate heat; conversely, when body temperature rises, peripheral blood vessels dilate to increase heat loss, sweating occurs and animals start to pant, *see also* HEAT STROKE, HYPERTHERMIA, HYPOTHERMIA.

thiamin *see* VITAMIN B_1.

thiaminase An enzyme present in raw fish that breaks down thiamin; thus, animals fed exclusively on raw fish are likely to develop thiamin deficiency.

thiazide diuretics Group of diuretics, e.g. hydrochlorothiazide, which increase urine production and sodium ion excretion.

thiopentone sodium The agent most widely used for the induction of general anaesthesia; provided as a powder, which is made up into a 2.5% solution using a sterile technique. Administered intravenously; it rapidly crosses the blood–brain barrier, inducing narcosis; there is a period of apnoea; stored in body fat; accidental perivascular injection is irritant due to the high pH, *see also* BARBITURATES.

third eyelid *see also* NICTITATING MEMBRANE.

thirst The desire to drink and the primary regulator of water intake; the thirst centre is located in the hypothalamus.

Thomas–Schroeder splint A frame used as a means of external fracture support; time-consuming to apply, it has been largely superseded by other casting and splinting materials.

thoracic Relating to the thorax and chest area.

thoracic duct The main route for the return of lymph to the circulation; lymph draining from the viscera and pelvic limbs runs into the cysterna chyli, which in turn becomes the thoracic duct, running alongside the aorta and azygous vein; the duct opens into the left brachiocephalic vein within the thorax.

thoracolumbar Relating to the loin region over the last few thoracic and first few lumbar vertebrae.

thoracocentesis Insertion of a needle or catheter into the thoracic cavity to drain off free fluid or air.

thoracotomy Surgical opening of the thorax; once the thorax is opened the negative pressure is lost and lung tissue will collapse; thus, some form of ventilation is required, e.g. IPPV, use of a ventilator.

thorax The chest cavity; bounded by the ribs, intercostal muscles and the diaphragm, it contains the heart, lungs, great vessels, pleura, thymus and mediastinum.

thrill A palpable vibration accompanying a cardiac murmur.

thrombin The enzyme that converts fibrinogen to fibrin, to assist in blood clotting; the liver synthesises the precursor, prothrombin, which circulates as a plasma protein, and is activated to thrombin at sites of blood vessel damage.

thrombocyte Blood platelet.

thrombocytopenia Reduction in the number of circulating platelets; may be due to bone-marrow suppression, immune-mediated disease, chronic haemorrhage, DIC, etc.

thromboembolus An embolism arising from a thrombus, *see also* EMBOLISM.

thrombolytic An agent that dissolves a thrombus.

thrombosis The process of thrombus formation.

thrombus A blood clot.

thrush (1) Term used for an infection with the yeast *Candida albicans*. (2) Used to describe a chronic infection of a horse's foot.

thymol A phenolic compound that may be used to preserve urine samples that cannot be examined immediately.

thymoma Benign neoplasm of the thymus, located within the anterior mediastinum; clinical signs may arise because the neoplasm puts pressure on vital structures such as the trachea or cranial cava.

thymus A gland lying within the anterior mediastinum; it is part of the lymphatic system, and is most active in the late fetal stages and in neonates; the gland processes T lymphocytes, priming them for their role in cell-mediated immunity.

thyroglobulin The form which thyroid hormones are stored in by the thyroid gland; consists of thyroid hormone linked to a colloid.

thyroid The bi-lobed endocrine gland in the neck that secretes thyroid hormone to control metabolic rate (from follicular cells), and calcitonin (from the parafollicular C cells), *see also* CALCITONIN, GOITRE, HYPOTHYROIDISM, HYPERTHYROIDISM, THYROXINE.

thyroid cartilage One of the main cartilages of the larynx.

thyroidectomy Surgical removal of the thyroid gland, used to treat hyperthyroidism.

thyroid hormones Thyroxine (T_4) and tri-iodothyronine (T_3); the hormones produced by the thyroid gland; these hormones stimulate cell metabolism, increase heart rate and blood pressure and stimulate gut motility; they are also necessary for growth and reproduction.

thyroid stimulating hormone (TSH) Hormone produced by the anterior pituitary gland, stimulating the release of thyroid hormones from the thyroid.

thyroxine T_4; the main thyroid hormone.

tibia The main bone of the distal hind leg, running from stifle to tarsus.

tibial tuberosity The bony prominence at the cranioproximal end of the tibia in the midline; it is the insertion point for the patellar ligament.

tibiotarsal joint The articulation between the distal tibia and the talus.

tick Arthropod, blood-sucking ectoparasite. Those of veterinary importance are mainly of the genus *Ixodes*; oval body, four pairs of legs and a well-developed beak (capitulum); go through larval and nymph stages and are not generally host specific. Ticks themselves may cause local irritation and pruritis, but they also act as vectors for many diseases, e.g. *Babesia*; ticks can be removed manually but care must be taken to ensure the mouthparts are totally removed (swabbing with ether first may help).

tick fever Febrile disease caused by biting ticks that carry *Rickettsia* or *Babesia canis*.

tick paralysis Flaccid weakness and paralysis reported in the USA and Australia, due to neurotoxins injected by some species of tick.

tidal volume The volume of air that passes in and out of the airways during one normal respiratory cycle.

tie Part of the mating process in dogs, when the muscles in the vagina of the bitch contract around the penis of the stud dog so that it cannot be withdrawn. The dog may step over the bitch's back during this stage, so that they stand back-to-back; the tie can last from a few seconds up to an hour, but the animals should not be separated during this time. Device unique to canines to promote fertility, not seen in other animals that live in packs or groups.

Tieman catheter Bitch urinary catheter.

titre The amount or levels of a substance.

to-and-fro circuit Type of anaesthetic circuit incorporating a soda lime canister so that gases can be rebreathed. Exhaled air passes through the soda lime into a reservoir bag, and is then rebreathed back through the soda lime; the circuit is economical to run, but can only be used on animals over 7–10 kg due to the resistance.

tocopherol Vitamin E.

toe The distal digit, comprising the first, second and third phalanges.

toggle Surgical technique for repair of hip luxations, where a synthetic round ligament is passed through a tunnel drilled in the femoral head, and anchored on the medial side of the acetabulum using a metal toggle-pin.

tongue The muscle mass occupying the oral cavity; used for chewing and swallowing; carries taste buds and caudally directed papillae.

tonic (1) Having tone; used to describe a muscle that is under tension. (2) Medicine said to increase appetite and sense of well-being.

tonicity The osmotic pressure of a solution.

tonometry Measurement of pressure; a tonometer may be used to measure intraocular pressure in suspected cases of glaucoma.

tonsil The collection of lymphoid tissue located in the pharynx, caudal to the palatoglossal arch; they are partially covered by the tonsillar fold of the soft palate.

tonsillectomy Surgical removal of the tonsils.

tonsillitis Inflammation of the tonsils.

tophus A urate plaque deposited in soft tissues, most commonly in periarticular fibrous tissue.

topical Applied locally.

torpor Lethargy.

torsion Twisting, *see also* GASTRIC TORSION, VOLVULUS.

torticollis Spasm of cervical muscles so that the head is twisted to one side.

total ear canal ablation (TECA) Surgical removal of both the horizontal and vertical parts of the external ear canal; used to treat severe otitis externa.

total lung capacity The total amount of air within the respiratory system; equal to the vital capacity plus the residual volume.

total plasma protein The amount of protein carried in the blood stream (predominantly albumin, globulins and fibrinogen); as these molecules do not diffuse out of the circulation, plasma proteins are used to assess an animal's state of hydration.

tourniquet A constricting band or bandage applied to control haemorrhage; they must be released every 10–15 minutes to prevent excessive tissue ischaemia and subsequent necrosis, *see also* ESMARCH BANDAGE.

towel clip Self-retaining clamp with two points, used to anchor surgical drapes.

toxaemia Presence of toxins from infectious agents within the blood stream.

Toxascaris leonina A nematode (roundworm) of the dog and cat;

may cause visceral larval migrans in humans, *see also* ASCARID.

toxic Harmful, poisonous.

toxic epidermal necrolysis (TEN) Rare, immune-mediated disorder characterised by the acute onset of severe ulceration of the skin and mucous membranes; most commonly an allergic response to drugs, but may also be associated with infections and neoplastic conditions; guarded prognosis.

toxin A poisonous substance, biological in origin.

Toxocara canis Common nematode (ascarid) of the dog, also affects cats; the L2 stage causes ocular larval migrans and visceral larval migrans in humans. Adult worms are round, fleshy and 10–20 cm long; large worm burdens in puppies can cause clinical signs; controlled by regular worming, especially of pregnant bitches and puppies, and hygiene.

Toxocara cati Ascarid worm specific to the cat.

toxocariasis Infection with *Toxocara* nematodes.

toxoid A toxin that has been processed so that is no longer harmful to the body, but retains its antigenicity; used to produce active immunity, e.g. tetanus toxoid.

Toxoplasma gondii A coccidial parasite of the cat, that can use many mammals and birds as intermediate hosts; most cats are asymptomatic and may periodically excrete the protozoa; the oocysts take at least 24 hours to become infective and so daily cleaning of litter trays is a useful control measure; in intermediate hosts, the parasite has a predilection for the CNS and muscle, causing diverse neurological signs and cysts; the zoonotic form of the disease can lead to fetal abnormalities, fever and myalgia; diagnosis is confirmed by muscle biopsy (cysts) or demonstrating a rising antibody titre to the organism.

T plate Bone plate in the shape of a letter 'T', which is used for some distal radial fractures and carpal arthrodesis.

trabeculum, pl. trabeculae A network of tissue, e.g. bone.

trace element Mineral required in the diet in small amounts, e.g. iron, copper, zinc, manganese. Cobalt is necessary for vitamin B_{12}.

trachea The wind-pipe, running from the larynx, down the neck and into the thorax, bifurcating at the level of the base of the heart into the right and left main bronchi. The tube is composed of C-shaped rings of cartilage linked by a tough membrane; lined with mucosa.

tracheal Relating to the trachea.

tracheal collapse Congenital dorsoventral flattening of the tracheal rings, seen most commonly in toy breeds; affected sections of the trachea collapse on inspiration, creating an upper airway obstruction and generating a classic hard, dry cough; if mild, the condition may be managed using bronchodilators, corticosteroids and antitussives; surgery involves supporting the trachea by using prosthetic rings.

tracheal hypoplasia A rare congenital disorder, associated with laryngeal hypoplasia; the prognosis is guarded.

tracheal rupture Trauma to the trachea can lead to rupture of the tracheal membrane; a large tear will cause marked respiratory distress necessitating immediate action; small tears can lead to gradual subcutaneous emphysema and pneumothorax or pneumomediastinum.

tracheal stenosis Rare condition, with narrowing of the tracheal lumen; possibly secondary to rough intubation.

tracheal worm *see* FILAROIDES OSLERI.

tracheitis Inflammation of the mucous membrane lining the trachea, *see also* KENNEL COUGH.

tracheostomy Creation of a permanent opening in the neck into the trachea.

tracheotomy Creation of a temporary opening in the neck into the trachea; may be elective, e.g. tracheotomy may facilitate the reduction and repair of jaw fractures, or may be an emergency measure, e.g. laryngeal foreign body.

tract A pathway or route.

traction Application of a drawing force, e.g. to overcome the pull of contracted muscles to allow fracture reduction or correction of a luxation.

trait A characteristic.

tranquilliser An ataractic; a drug that calms a patient without sedating; in practice, most tranquillisers have some degree of sedative effect.

trans- Prefix, across or through.

transcription The conversion of the genetic code from a length of DNA into mRNA.

transcutaneous electrical nerve stimulator (TENS) Analgesic device that delivers small electric pulses via pads placed over a painful focus; the current blocks the pain message from the area before it is perceived by the brain.

transformer Part of the X-ray machine that converts the alternating mains current into a direct current.

transfusion Transfer of blood from a donor animal to a recipient.

transfusion reaction Response to an incompatible blood transfusion; signs include salivation, restlessness, vomiting, abdominal cramps, jaundice, DIC, pyrexia and collapse.

transitional cell carcinoma Malignant tumour of transitional epithelial cells.

transitional epithelium A region of epithelium bridging two different types, e.g. changing from squamous to columnar epithelium.

transitional vertebra Rare abnormality where a vertebra has some of the characteristics of vertebrae from an adjacent region, e.g. L7 having transverse processes that are fused to the pelvis (a characteristic of sacral vertebrae).

transit time The time taken from ingestion to the appearance in the faeces.

transmissible Able to be passed from one individual to another.

transmissible venereal tumour (TVT) A sexually transmitted granulomatous tumour of the penis, prepuce, vulva or vagina in the dog; extremely rare in the UK.

transplacental Able to pass across the placenta.

transudate Fluid that has passed through cells or across a membrane into a body cavity or onto the skin, the direction of transfer depending on the osmotic pressure on either side.

transverse At right angles to the long axis.

trauma Physical or mental injury.

travel sickness Motion sickness; common in animals transported by car, etc.; acepromazine has a central effect to reduce travel sickness.

trematode Flatworm endoparasites, e.g. fluke.

tremor Repetitive, involuntary movement.

trephine A surgical instrument used to remove a circle of bone to allow access to the brain, nasal sinuses, etc.

triceps Muscle mass caudal to the humerus, the main action of which is to extend the elbow.

trichiasis The presence of aberrant hairs around the eye, e.g. on prominent skin folds, which irritate the corneal surface; require surgical removal.

Trichodectes canis The common biting louse of the dog; an intermediate host for *Dipylidium caninum.*

trichobezoar A hairball.

trichomoniasis Disease caused by infection with a *Trichomonas* spp. protozoal parasite; a common disease in pigeons, with inappetence, diarrhoea and respiratory signs; antiprotozoal agents can be given in the drinking water, but poor hygiene and overcrowding should also be addressed.

***Trichophyton* spp.** Fungi causing ringworm; may affect dogs, cats, man, etc.; do not generally fluoresce under UV light, *see also* *MICROSPORUM.*

Trichuris vulpis The dog whipworm.

tricuspid Having three cusps; the heart valve between the right atrium and ventricle.

trigeminal neuralgia Pain due to irritation of the trigeminal (fifth cranial) nerve.

triglyceride Glycerol molecule with three attached fatty acid chains.

trigone The triangular region at the neck of the bladder.

Tripsin-like immunoreactivity (TLI) Test commonly used to assess exocrine pancreatic insufficiency, *see also* PANCREAS.

trismus An early sign of tetanus; inability to open the mouth due to spasm of the masseter muscles, *see also* TETANUS.

trocar A sharp metal probe that fits into a sleeve.

trochanter A bony prominence; there are greater, lesser and third trochanters on the proximal femur.

trochlea A smooth, articular surface of bone.

Trombicula autumnalis Harvest mites; only the larval stage is parasitic and affects dogs, cats and man; can cause seasonal pruritis in the summer and autumn.

trypsin Digestive enzyme that breaks down protein; secreted as trypsinogen by the exocrine pancreas.

tube feeding Method of force-feeding anorexic patients or animals that cannot eat and swallow normally; techniques include nasogastric, pharyngostomy, gastrostomy and PEG tubes.

tuber calcis The proximal prominence of the calcaneus; the point of the hock.

tubercle (1) A small bony eminence. (2) A granulomatous nodule.

tuberculosis Disease caused by *Mycobacterium tuberculosis*; typical lesions are granulomatous nodules with a necrotic centre, that can occur in any tissues; rare – cats are more frequently infected by the oral route than dogs.

tubule A small tube.

tulle A wound dressing; a gauze mesh impregnated with paraffin wax.

tumify Swell.

tumour Means swelling, usually is a neoplasm or 'growth'; may be benign or malignant; due to the unchecked, abnormal proliferation of cells, *see also* NEOPLASM.

tunica A coat or covering.

turbinate Scroll-shaped bones within the nasal chambers.

tympanic bulla Bony ventral extension of the petrous temporal bone; may become involved in middle ear disease.

tympanic membrane The membrane at the end of the horizontal ear canal, separating the external ear from the middle ear.

tympany Bloat.

Tyzzer's disease Disease of rats, mice, gerbils, etc. caused by *Bacillus piliformis*; causes sudden death, diarrhoea and lethargy; highly contagious; antibiotics and supportive treatment can limit the disease in contacts; attention to hygiene is also important.

U

Uberreiter's syndrome Traditional name for the eye disease that has a breed specificity in German shepherds; seen as a chronic superficial keratitis or pannus, *see also* PANNUS.

ulcer A full-thickness crater or erosion defect in the surface of the skin or mucous membrane, often surrounded by a zone of inflammation. **Corneal ulcer** Defect in the corneal epithelium; stains with fluorescein. **Decubitus ulcer** Pressure sore ulcer on the point of the elbow, *see also* BED SORE. **Gastric ulcer** Seen after endoscopy or radiography; may be treated with ranitidine or cimetidine to protect the mucosa. **Indolent ulcer** A non-healing ulcer, particularly a corneal ulcer. **Rodent ulcer** Specific condition of the cat's nasal area, *see also* EOSINOPHILIC, RODENT ULCER.

ulcerative colitis Medical condition, usually in the larger breeds of dog, *see also* COLITIS.

ulcerative glossitis Painful condition of the cat's mouth with ulcers on the tongue surface, usually caused by the herpes virus FCV. It is associated with the feline lymphocytic gingivitis stomatitis complex, *see also* GINGIVITIS.

ule- (ulo-) (1) Scars, scar tissue. (2) The gums.

ulnar Relates to the smaller of the two bones of the forearm or the medial aspect.

ultra- Prefix meaning beyond, in excess of or on top of.

ultracentrifuge Method of removing particles using a high centrifugal force perhaps assisted by a vacuum.

ultrafiltration The type of filtration in the nephron to remove waste material.

ultramicroscopic Particles too small to be visualised with the highest power light microscope, *see also* VIRUS.

ultrasonic Sound waves too high for the human ear to be aware of, that are increasingly used for diagnostic imaging, cleaning teeth, cleaning surgical instruments, etc.

ultrasound Sound waves of extremely high frequency, over 20 000 Hz; real-time is used to record these images in a scanning device.

ultraviolet High-frequency but short wavelength invisible rays beyond the normal spectrum of light seen; cause skin damage but may be used for bacterial sterilisation, *see also* VITAMIN D, WOOD'S LAMP.

umbilical cord The connection of the fetus to its placenta and then to the mother.

umbilical hernia Point of weakness in the midline where fat or other viscera may bulge outwardly from inside the abdomen with a skin 'lump'; may have a hereditary basis due to incomplete fusion in the midline.

umbilical infection The patent umbilicus of the new-born can easily become infected; peritonitis and septicaemia may result.

umbilicus The area of connection of the fetus to its placenta and the mother.

unciform Shaped like a sickle or a hook.

Uncinaria The name of one of the two genuses of hookworm found in the UK.

Uncinaria stenocephala Nematode infection of dogs, unusual in that it may cause skin lesions on the feet through larval migration. Sometimes known as the northern hookworm.

unconscious A state of deep sleep-like unawareness of surroundings with reduced responses to external stimuli; often the result of a head injury or administration of anaesthetic agents, *see also* COMA.

underdevelopment (1) In X-ray developing, it is a fault recognised by the greyish flat background in place of the normal black of exposed parts of the film. (2) May mean poor growth, as found in the ovaries or testes of late maturing animals.

undershot Condition of the mandible where the incisor teeth of the lower jaw are placed in front of those in the upper jaw.

undescended testis The visible defect may be bilateral or unilateral, where the normal migration of the testis into the scrotum soon after birth fails for a genetic or hormonal reason, *see also* CRYPTORCHIDISM.

undifferentiated Error of development when a primitive feature still remains; is important in biopsy cell diagnosis of malignancy.

ungual Relates to the hooves, nails or the claws.

uni- Single or one of a kind.

unicellular A one cell structure, typical of bacteria and of protozoa.

unilateral One side of the body.

union Coming together or forming a junction, *see also* FRACTURE.

uniparous Giving birth to a single offspring; more typical of human reproduction than of pet animals; sometimes called primiparous as in a pregnancy that produces one young capable of survival.

unmyelinated Description of nerve axons that have no myelin sheath.

unsaturated Fats that have a structure with one or two double bonds in their carbon chain structure; they are considered beneficial in some skin and circulatory disorders.

ununited Refers to the non-healing fracture or when an epiphysis does not join with a diaphysis. Common in osteochondrosis of the elbow where part of the anconeal process fails to fuse with the main head of the ulna, *see also* OSTEOCHONDROSIS.

unstriated The type of muscle that moves involuntarily, as in smooth muscle of the viscera or the more specialised cardiac muscle.

upper Above, but sometimes words such as cranial, rostral or oral may have a similar usage.

upper motor neurons Efferent neurons with cell bodies in the brain, whose axons run down the spinal cord to synapse with the lower motor neurons. They initiate and control muscle movements.

upper respiratory tract Refers to the nose, paranasal sinuses, nasopharynx and the larynx.

upsaliensis A type of *Campylobacter* infection that has become recognised as a not uncommon cause of dog diarrhoea. Named from the Swedish veterinary centre at Uppsala.

urachus The part of the umbilical cord that connects to the bladder; usually a solid fibrous cord at birth but sometimes it will remain open and dribble urine, when it is known as a 'pervious urachus'.

uraemia Elevated levels of urea in the blood, usually associated with kidney disease; the harmful effects of urea are not as great as some of the other products retained, *see also* AZOTAEMIA.

uraemic fits Convulsions may be due to many causes but in advanced renal failure, often accompanied by hepatic failure, toxic products such as ammonia have deleterious effects on brain function.

uranoschisis An alternative name for a cleft palate.

urate Dalmatians normally excrete high levels of urate as part of their metabolism; a salt with ammonia sometimes forms in acid urine and may be one of the types of calculus found.

urea Nitrogenous compound, produced in the liver as a less toxic substance than the ammonia that results from protein metabolism. Commonly measured in the laboratory as a simple indicator of renal function.

urease Enzyme that will break down urea; a constituent of one of the stick tests for measuring blood urea. Many bacteria produce a urease. A test for *Helicobacter* that colonise the stomach is the urease test.

ureter A tube that connects the pelvis of the kidney to the neck of the bladder. **Ectopic ureter** A misplaced tube that drains directly into the vagina and is a possible cause of incontinence in the 'difficult to house train' puppy.

ureteral Relates to the ureter.

ureteral calculus One of the concretions causing dysuria, *see also* CALCULI.

ureteral obstruction Caused by a combination of an obstructing body and a spasm of the smooth muscle.

ureterocolostomy Surgical method of connecting the ureter to the colon to bypass the bladder; the operation is a ureteroenterostomy.

ureteropyelography Method of radiographic examination of the kidneys and ureters using an intravenous contrast medium.

ureterovaginal fistula Abnormality said to be produced by incautious spaying surgery.

urethra Tube from the bladder to the exterior – short in the female and longer and narrower in the male.

urethral Relating to the urethra.

urethral calculus Small stone or concretion causing a total or partial obstruction to the flow of urine; most frequently found at the point where the urethra is restricted by the shape of the os penis and less frequently where the urethra curves round from the floor of the pelvis.

urethral obstruction A calculus is the most common obstruction but trauma or scar tissue may have a similar effect.

urethral plug More typical of feline urolithiasis syndrome when small calculi form an obstruction with mucilagenous protein.

urethral stricture A narrowing, often a sequel to calculus damage or a previous urethrotomy.

urethritis Inflammatory condition of the urethra, may be associated with calculi.

urethrorectal fistula Result of a developmental defect in producing a cloaca or sometimes after a birth canal trauma by a tear of the vagina roof, *see also* FISTULA.

urethrostomy A hole after a surgical incision into the lumen of the urethra, usually to relieve an obstruction and help in the passage of calculi out of the bladder. A permanent opening may be needed, *see also* STOMA. **Perineal urethrostomy** Incision made between the anus and the scrotum. **Scrotal urethrostomy** Incision made at the level of the scrotum, sometimes accompanied by castration.

urethrotomy The surgical incision into the urethra when an opening is created.

-uria Word ending relating to a condition of urine, *see also* POLYURIA.

uric acid Naturally produced end product of purine breakdown, found especially in bird excrement. May be one cause of calculi in the urinary tract.

urinalysis The testing of urine for diseases such as diabetes, nephrosis, etc.

urinary Relates to the urine production and excretion mechanisms.

urinary calculus 'Stones' in the tract anywhere between the kidney and the tip of the penis.

urinary energy (UE) Urinary energy is the loss of energy in urine from food and the breakdown of endogenous metabolised proteins.

urinary incontinence Some failure of the mechanism that allows urine to be stored in the bladder until the appropriate time for bladder emptying.

urinary territory marking Behaviour mechanism that allows urine to be emptied from the bladder in any appropriate place to show an individual animal has visited the spot.

urination The controlled and periodic emptying of the bladder through the urethra; applies equally to males and females, *see also* MICTURATE.

urine Complex solution of excreted products produced by the kidneys and the major route of nitrogen excretion.

urinogenital Relates to the tracts involved in reproduction as well as the excretory system for urine.

urinometer Laboratory instrument formerly used for estimating the specific gravity of urine.

urobilin Pigment substance formed by the oxidation of urobilinogen.

urobilinogen Product of the breakdown of bilirubin when bacteria act in the intestine; some may be absorbed back into the blood stream then excreted by the kidneys.

urochrome One of the colouring agents of urine produced from bile pigments.

urogenital Relates to both systems, *see also* URINOGENITAL.

urography Radiographic examination of the urinary tract, *see also* PNEUMOCYSTOGRAM.

urolith A stone in the bladder or urethra; common causes are struvite, ammonium urate, calcium oxalate, silicate and cystine.

urolithiasis The state of producing calculi in the urinary tract.

URT Upper respiratory tract.

urticaria Allergic response; involves oedema and a vascular response to mast cell degradation, *see also* NETTLE RASH.

uterine Relates to the breeding organ of the female.

uterine adenocarcinoma One of the commonest causes of death in un-neutered female rabbits.

uterine horn The part of the uterus leading to the ovary as two tubes running cranial to the main body; especially important in multiple birth animals. Birds have two but only the left one is functional.

uterine milk Used for the internal secretion of mucoid milk-like fluid that surrounds the fertilised egg before implantation.

uterine prolapse Eversion of the uterus so it reaches the exterior through the vulva; often a sequel to a difficult birth and the expulsion of fetal membranes.

uterine stump granuloma Chronic inflammation and discharge as a result of leaving part of the cervix in place as a focus of infection; often associated with unabsorbed ligature material.

uterine tube The connection between the fimbriae and the uterine horn; the site of fertilisation of the ova, *see also* FALLOPIAN TUBE, OVIDUCT.

uterus Found in the female as an important hollow organ; during pregnancy functions first for the development of the fetus and later the surrounding smooth muscle of the uterus wall is used to propel the developed offspring to the outside world, *see also* DELIVERY.

UTI Urinary tract infection

utricle A little sac-like cavity, found in the ear where the macula responds to the position of the head with respect to the pull of gravity. The name is also used for the cavity in the prostate gland used for fluid storage that connects with the urethra.

uvea Term used for those vascular and pigmented structures occupying the middle part of the eyeball within the outer sclera: ciliary body, lens suspension, iris and the choroid.

uveal tract Name for the vascular area of the eye choroid, ciliary body and iris.

uveitis Inflammation of the uvea; may be an important cause of blindness, *see also* IRIDOCYCLITIS.

uvula Pendulous structure at the back of the soft palate, not evident in domestic animals.

V

V-plasty Surgical technique for the repair of full-thickness eyelid defects; a V-shaped section, encompassing the defect, is removed and the conjunctiva and skin are then closed in two separate layers.

vaccinate Administer a vaccine.

vaccination Inoculation of an individual with antigenic material to stimulate artificial active immunity, *see* APPENDIX 8; vaccination protocols usually consist of two primary injections (although only one may be required with live vaccines), followed by regular boosters.

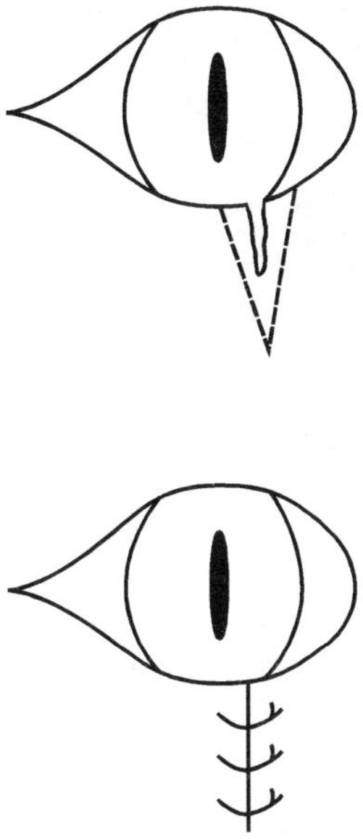

V-plasty (eyelid)

vaccination reaction Anaphylactic reaction following the administration of a vaccine; rare, *see also* ANAPHYLACTIC SHOCK.

vaccine Any preparation of antigenic material that will stimulate an immune response, e.g. bacterial wall proteins, killed bacteria, attenuated virus, toxoid.

vacuole Fluid-filled cavity within the cytoplasm of a cell; surrounds material that is being digested by the cell.

vacutainer Blood collection system consisting of a tube sealed under a vacuum, a holder and a needle; the apparatus allows blood sampling without the operator coming into contact with the blood; tubes are available containing a range of anticoagulants.

vacuum A space containing no gas or gas at a very low pressure.

vagina Part of the female reproductive tract; a muscular tube extending from the cervix to the vulva, *see also* TIE.

vaginal smear A smear made from the cells lining the vagina, which may be used to determine the stage of oestrus cycle in the bitch. Red blood cells appear in the smear during pro-oestrus, while keratinised epithelial cells predominate during oestrus; vaginal mucus may also be sampled for pregnancy diagnosis in the bitch, the ferning pattern of the mucus having a characteristic formation during pregnancy.

vaginitis Inflammation of the vagina.

vaginoscope Speculum for dilating the vulva and vagina to facilitate examination and urinary catheterisation.

vaginate Enclosed in a sheath.

vaginovesical Relating to the vagina and the urinary bladder.

vagolytic A drug inhibiting the effects of the vagus nerve.

vagomimetic A drug whose effects mimic the actions of the vagus nerve.

vagus The tenth cranial nerve; it is motor and sensory to the pharynx, larynx, lungs and digestive tract, controlling important autonomic functions such as swallowing and digestion.

valgus Angular limb deformity with outward rotation of the foot away from the midline.

valve A flap-like structure or fold of a membrane within a vessel to limit the flow to one direction only, e.g. the mitral (bicuspid) valve which prevents blood flowing back from the left ventricle to the atrium, vein valves.

vane Structure of the bird's wing composed of the barbs and barbules. Separated into inner and outer webs by the central shaft.

vaporiser The part of an anaesthetic circuit where the liquid volatile agent is converted to a vapour; older types include the Boyle's bottle; the more modern vaporisers are temperature and pressure compensated to provide a controlled and accurate percentage of anaesthetic agent in the gaseous mix, irrespective of changes in flow rate and cooling.

varicosis Dilation of a vein.

varus Angular limb deformity with inward rotation of the foot towards the midline.

vas deferens, pl. vasa deferentia Part of the male reproductive tract; paired vessels that carry spermatozoa from the epididymis to the urethra.

vascular Having a blood supply; tissues that become avascular, e.g. as a result of trauma, are non-viable.

vascular ring anomaly Developmental abnormality where a ring of intrathoracic blood vessels constricts the oesophagus, leading to difficulty swallowing, regurgitation and megaoesophagus cranial to the constriction, *see also* PERSISTENT RIGHT AORTIC ARCH.

vasculogenic shock Imbalance between circulating blood volume and tissue oxygen requirements due to excessive vasoconstriction.

vasectomy Surgical transection of the vasa deferentia, rendering the male sterile, *see also* VAS DEFERENS.

vasoactive Having an effect on the tone and diameter of a blood vessel.

vasoconstriction Narrowing of blood vessels due to the contraction of smooth muscle in the vessel wall.

vasodilatation Widening of the lumen of a blood vessel; due to relaxation of smooth muscle in the vessel wall.

vasomotor Able to constrict and dilate, thus changing diameter; term is applied to blood vessels.

vasopressin Antidiuretic hormone (ADH); produced by the posterior pituitary gland; increases water resorption by the kidneys.

vector An invertebrate animal such as a tick or a mite, that carries a parasite from one vertebrate host to another.

vecuronium bromide A non-depolarising neuromuscular blocking agent.

vein A thin-walled blood vessel, carrying deoxygenated blood towards the heart (NB the pulmonary vein carries *oxygenated* blood to the heart from the lungs).

Velpeau sling A foreleg bandage that may be used to prevent weight-bearing, e.g. after reduction of an elbow luxation.

velvet disease Parasitic disease of tropical fish, caused by *Oodinium* spp.

Venables plate Metal bone plate with circular screw holes, used for internal fixation of fractures.

venae cavae The great veins; the cranial vena cava is formed by the union of the right and left brachiocephalic veins and carries deoxygenated blood back to the heart from the head, neck, forelimbs and cranial thorax; the caudal vena cava is formed by the union of the common iliac veins and brings blood to the right atrium of the heart from the caudal thorax, abdomen and hind limbs.

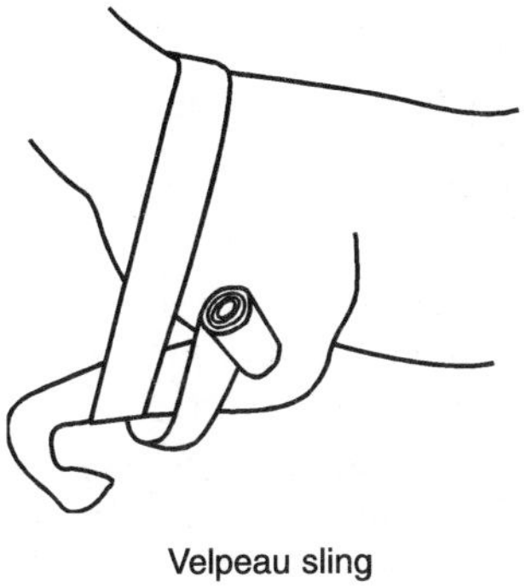
Velpeau sling

venepuncture *see* VENIPUNCTURE.

venereal disease A disease that is transmitted at mating, *see also* TRANSMISSIBLE VENEREAL TUMOUR.

venipuncture Puncture of a vein with a needle to obtain a blood sample or inject a solution.

venography Radiographic study where positive contrast media are injected into a vein; for example, ionic contrast media may be injected into the hepatic portal vein to demonstrate a portosystemic shunt.

venom Poisonous substance produced by many snakes, scorpions, etc.; antisera to specific venoms may be available.

venous sinus Normal dilations and enlargements of veins, e.g. the venous sinuses around the spinal cord beneath the dura mater.

vent *see* CLOACA.

ventilate Provide with oxygen during anaesthesia; anaesthetised patients may be ventilated if necessary by squeezing the reservoir bag, or by using mechanical ventilators, *see also* INTERMEDIATE POSITIVE PRESSURE VENTILATION, VENTILATOR.

ventilation–perfusion mismatch Any imbalance between alveolar ventilation and the pulmonary blood flow, resulting in hypoxia.

ventilator Mechanical apparatus to automatically supply oxygen to a patient, e.g. Bird, Manley, minivent; the respiratory rate and tidal volume are set so that ventilation is adequate; useful when muscle relaxants have been given as part of the anaesthetic protocol.

ventral Towards or near the lower body surface or belly; includes the undersurface of the neck and tail.

ventral slot Surgical technique that involves a ventral approach to the cervical spine and the removal of a rectangular area of bone and intervertebral disc material from two adjacent vertebrae, thus relieving pressure on the spinal cord; a surgical option for some cases of cervical disc prolapse and wobbler syndrome.

ventricle A chamber, e.g. ventricles of the heart, ventricles of the brain, laryngeal ventricles.

ventricular arrhythmia Any irregularity in the pattern of cardiac ventricular contractions.

ventricular fibrillation Life-threatening cardiac arrhythmia where the ventricles fail to contract in a coordinated fashion, but quiver instead; inadequate blood volume is supplied to the brain, resulting in rapid loss of consciousness and death if the normal rhythm is not restored rapidly.

ventricular septal defect (VSD) Any defect (usually congenital) in the muscular wall between the right and left ventricles. A VSD allows blood to move from the left (high pressure) side of the heart into the right (low pressure) ventricle, leading to right ventricular overload and pulmonary congestion. A murmur is often audible and the defect is found in association with other cardiac abnormalities such as tetralogy of Fallot and pulmonic stenosis.

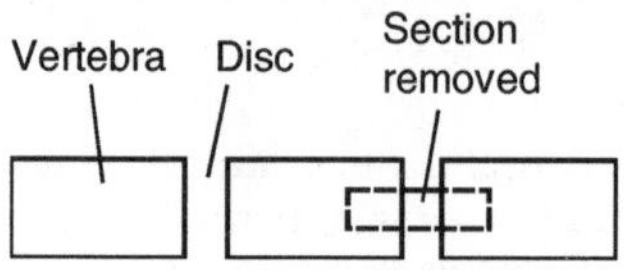

Ventral slot

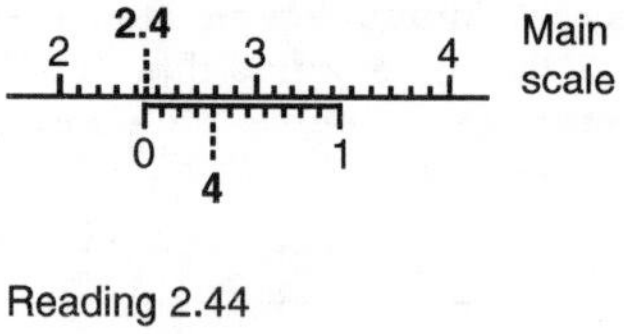

Vernier scale

ventrodorsal In a direction from the ventral surface towards the spine.

venule Small vessel receiving deoxygenated blood from a capillary.

vernier scale A scale that accurately measures small distances; the vernier scale on the stage of a microscope is used to pinpoint the exact position of an object so that it can be relocated; a reading is obtained by seeing which mark on the main scale is closest to the zero on the short scale and the next decimal place is obtained by seeing where the marks on the two scales align.

vertebra, pl. vertebrae Bone of the spinal column; cervical, thoracic, lumbar, sacral and caudal (coccygeal).

vertebrate An animal having a spine, made up of vertebrae.

vertical transmission Transmission of a disease from one generation to the next, usually passed from mother to offspring.

vesical Relating to a bladder, usually the urinary bladder.

vesicle A fluid-filled blister.

vesicovaginal Relating to the bladder and vagina.

vestibule A space leading to the entrance to a canal.

vestibular disease Disease of the vestibular apparatus of the inner ear, leading to head tilt, circling and ataxia.

vestibulocochlear nerve The VIIIth cranial nerve, the vestibular component providing information concerning the orientation of the head, and the cochlear division mediating hearing; lesions along the nerve give rise to symptoms such as head tilt, ataxia, nystagmus and deafness.

Veterinary Surgeons Act 1966 Parliamentary act which governs the veterinary profession and restricts the right to practise to members of the Royal College of Veterinary Surgeons.

vibrissa Stiff, sensory hairs located on the muzzle of many species.

villus, pl. villi Finger-like projection of tissue; found in the small intestine and the placenta; the projections greatly increase the surface area over which diffusion and absorption of molecules can occur.

vincristine An anti-neoplastic alkaloid used in the treatment of lymphosarcoma and leukaemia, *see also* CYTOTOXIC.

viraemia Having virus particles in the blood stream.

virile Possessing male characteristics and able to reproduce.

virulence A measure of the power of a pathogen to cause disease.

virulent Highly pathogenic and able to cause disease.

virus Infectious agents that are smaller than bacteria and are incapable of growth or reproduction outside a living host cell; viruses contain either RNA or DNA but not both.

visceral larval migrans (VLM) A syndrome in humans due to the migration of *Toxocara canis* larvae through the tissues; symptoms depend on the location of the larvae, but include fever, jaundice and ocular disturbances.

viscous Sticky, thick, glutinous.

viscus, pl. viscera Any organ within the pleural, pericardial and peritoneal cavities.

vision The ability to see.

vital capacity The volume of air that can be expelled after taking a maximally deep breath.

vitamin A dietary component other than fat, protein, carbohydrate and inorganic salts; present in small amounts in the food but essential for growth, reproduction and good health.

vitamin A Retinol; a fat-soluble vitamin used in the synthesis of rhodopsin and in cell division and differentiation. Foods with high vitamin A content include liver and fish; deficiency leads to reproductive failure, night-blindness and xerophthalmia, and is rare in all species other than terrapins; hypervitaminosis A, e.g. in cats fed solely on fish or liver, accelerates bone remodelling and leads to the formation of exostoses; widespread exostoses may limit movement in the spine so animals may have difficulty grooming themselves, and exostoses around the optic nerves may impair vision.

vitamin B A water-soluble complex of substances (thiamine, riboflavin, niacin, pyridoxine, pantothenic acid, folic acid and biotin) that are important coenzymes in many cell metabolic processes; toxicities are rare as any excess is readily excreted; deficiency causes anaemia, etc.

vitamin C Ascorbic acid; water-soluble vitamin found predominantly in fresh fruit and vegetables; adequate vitamin C is manufactured in the liver of most animals other than primates and guinea-pigs, and thus is not required in the diet.

vitamin D A steroidal calciferol complex formed by the action of sunlight on precursor molecules; fat-soluble; important for bone and teeth formation; excess vitamin D leads to elevated blood calcium levels resulting in calcification of soft tissue, anorexia and weight loss; deficiency causes rickets and osteomalacia.

vitamin E α-tocopherol; fat-soluble vitamin important as an antioxidant; deficiency causes muscular dystrophy and pansteatitis.

vitamin K A fat-soluble factor necessary for the biosynthesis of prothrombin, and thus important in clotting; deficiency results in clotting disorders; used as part of the treatment for warfarin poisoning.

vitiligo A skin condition characterised by the appearance of depigmented patches; thought to have an underlying auto-immune mechanism.

vitreous The jelly-like material filling the posterior chamber of the eye.

viviparous Giving birth to live young.

vivisection Scientific experimentation using animal models.

vocal fold Membranes covering the vocal chords; the folds project into the larynx and are used to produce sound.

vocational Practical training for a profession or occupation, *see also* NATIONAL COUNCIL FOR VOCATIONAL QUALIFICATION.

volar On the undersurface of a fore or hind foot, *see also* PALMAR, PLANTAR.

volatile A substance that evaporates readily.

Volkmann canal The network of canals within bone that carry blood vessels from the surface to the Haversian systems.

Volkmann curette A small spoon-shaped curette used for obtaining cancellous bone graft material.

voltage The electrical potential difference between two points.

voluntary Under conscious control of an individual.

volvulus Obstruction of a hollow organ due to twisting, e.g. gastric volvulus.

vomeronasal organ A structure at the base of the nasal septum; thought to play a role in olfaction.

vomit Expulsion of stomach contents through the mouth.

vomiting Autonomic reflex where stomach contents is ejected via the mouth; sometimes confused with regurgitation, *see also* REGURGITATION.

vomitus The material expelled during vomition.

von Willebrand disease An inherited bleeding disorder due to lack of clotting factor VIII. Spontaneous haemorrhage may occur, e.g. epistaxis, or it may follow routine surgery such as spaying; an autosomal dominant characteristic; has been reported in several canine breeds, but particularly the Dobermann pinscher and German shepherd dog.

von Willebrand factor A clotting factor essential for platelet adhesion and aggregation.

vulva The female external genitalia.

W

Wallerian degeneration The degeneration that occurs to the portion of a nerve fibre distal to the point of injury; characterised by demyelination and resorption of the axon.

warfarin Potent anticoagulant used as a rodenticide; also used therapeutically in some prothrombotic disorders, such as DIC. The accidental consumption of warfarin by pets should be treated with vitamin K and emetics, *see also* COAGULATION DISORDERS.

warm-blooded Able to thermoregulate and maintain a body temperature higher than that of the external environment.

wart Verrucose benign growth, often due to papilloma virus infection.

washing soda Sodium carbonate; may be used as an emergency measure to induce vomiting if an animal has recently ingested a non-irritant poison, *see also* EMETIC.

waste, clinical All waste materials generated by a business, such as a veterinary practice, that may be contaminated with animal matter, e.g. bedding, bandages, swabs; also includes drug packaging; has to be disposed of in labelled yellow bags.

waste, pathological Animal tissue such as excised tumours, uteri, etc., generated by a business; disposed of in labelled red bags.

water Chemically H_2O; liquid consisting of hydrogen and oxygen; a major constituent of all animal and vegetable tissues; vital to sustain life. Animals require access to water at all times unless specifically contraindicated for short periods, e.g. prior to general anaesthesia, during water deprivation tests.

Waters' canister Part of a rebreathing anaesthetic circuit; a canister packed with soda lime where exhaled carbon dioxide is reabsorbed, *see also* SODA LIME.

wean Put onto solid food and remove access to maternal milk (gradual is best).

web The sheet of tissue bridging the space between each of the toes.

wedge ostectomy Surgical technique used to correct an angular limb deformity; a wedge of bone is removed from the region of greatest curvature and the fracture reduced using a bone plate or external fixation device; the technique results in some shortening of the limb, although this is not usually of functional significance.

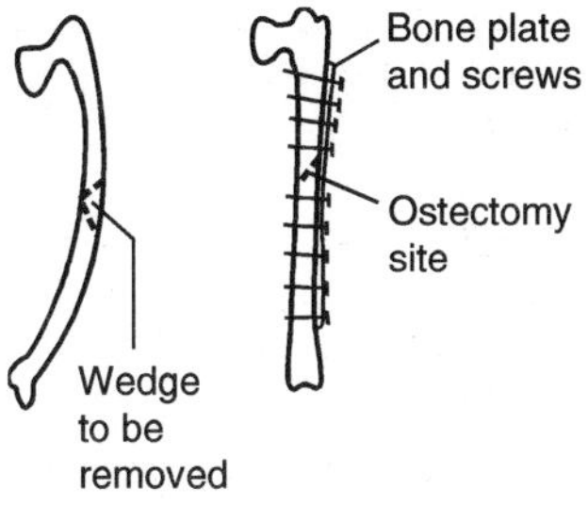

Wedge ostectomy

weight The force exerted on a body by the gravity of the earth. Body weight or heaviness is usually measured in kilograms (kg). **Atomic weight** The mass (in grams) of 1 mole (6×10^{23}) of atoms of an element. **Molecular weight** The sum of the atomic weights of the atoms in a molecule.

weight loss Reduction in body weight; may be desirable in obese animals or may be associated with many disease states; body weight will reduce if calorific intake is below the metabolic requirement, or if metabolic needs increase, e.g. burns, post-surgery.

Weil's disease Disease caused by *Leptospira icterohaemorrhagiae*; characterised by pyrexia and jaundice, *see also* ICTERIC, JAUNDICE.

welfare Well-being of the animal; an important responsibility of all people caring for animals.

West's retractors Self-retaining retractors with curved teeth; used for holding soft tissues out of the surgical field.

wet tail A common condition in recently weaned hamsters, characterised by profuse diarrhoea; possibly due to stress and *Escherichia coli* infection.

wheal An area of reddened, oedematous skin; part of the classic inflammatory response (pain, redness, heat, swelling and loss of function).

wheat-sensitive enteropathy Allergy to the gluten in ingested wheat products, resulting in malabsorption, weight loss and chronic diarrhoea; mainly reported in Irish setters and West Highland white terriers; treatment involves feeding a gluten-free diet.

wheeze Audible whistling sound made during dyspnoeic breathing.

whelp (1) Give birth to puppies. (2) Refers to unweaned puppies – whelps.

whipworm *Trichuris* spp., nematodes; endoparasite that may occasionally cause diarrhoea in dogs, but is of more clinical significance in warmer climates; adult worm is about 7 cm long with a slender anterior portion; eggs are barrel-shaped with a plug at each end.

white blood cell (WBC) Leukocyte; any cell formed by the reticuloendothelial system; neutrophils, eosinophils, basophils, small and large lymphocytes and monocytes all belong to this group.

white blood cell count Laboratory technique for counting the number of WBCs per unit volume of blood; process may be mechanised, or can be carried out using a counting chamber; having ascertained a total WBC count, a differential count can then be done by counting 100 WBCs in a smear.

white muscle disease Muscular dystrophy resulting from a lack of vitamin E; rare, but used to be seen in calves and lambs.

white spot External disease of fish due to the parasite *Ichthyophthirius mutifiliis*; white areas appear, especially around the gills, but may break out over much of the fish; proprietary treatments are available based on malachite green solution.

whorl Circular patch of hair.

withdrawal reflex Normal protective response with flexion of the limb joints away from a painful stimulus; may be elicited by pinching the toes or the webbing between the toes; as the stimulus is increased the more proximal limb joints should also be flexed; used to assess neurological function and responses during anaesthesia.

Willis, circle of Ring of arterial blood vessels within the cranium at the base of the brain; formed by the paired internal carotid arteries and vertebral arteries; supplies blood to the mid- and forebrain.

Winslow, foramen of *see* EPIPLOIC FORAMEN.

wiring A technique for fracture fixation; may be used as a modified means of stabilisation in birds. **Cerclage wiring** Internal fixation technique where wire is wrapped tightly around two bone fragments to hold them together; cannot be used as the sole method of fixation but is a useful adjunct for long spiral fractures that are inherently stable. **Hemicerclage wiring** A wire suture is anchored through a drill hole in one bone fragment and wrapped around the external circumference of the second fragment. **K wire** A thin metal pin that may be used to anchor fracture fragments; may be used as cross pins, or used to hold fragments temporarily while other fixation devices are applied; useful fixation technique for some epiphyseal fractures in young animals where the fracture line may cross a growth plate; also used in tension band wiring to hold the figure-of-eight wire in position. **Tension band wiring** Internal fixation technique for bony fragments that are likely to avulse or distract, such as the tibial crest; the fragment is secured with two parallel K wires and wire is then wrapped around the pins and through a hole drilled in the bone in a figure-of-eight.

wobbler syndrome Cervical spondylopathy; a neurological condition characterised by progressive ataxia and neck pain; particularly common in young Great Danes and older Dobermann pinschers; due to pressure on the cervical spinal cord from unstable discs, deformed vertebrae or hypertrophied spinal ligaments; may be managed conservatively but many affected dogs require surgery such as ventral slotting or cervical fusion.

Wolff's law The law describing the normal response of bone to the stresses placed upon it; bone remodels constantly such that it is deposited in areas that are subjected to stress and is removed from regions that do not experience stress; thus, bone is resorbed when a limb is immobilised.

womb Uterus.

Wood's lamp Ultraviolet lamp used to detect fluorescent hairs in the coat infected with *Microsporum* spp. of ringworm; fluorescence is typically an apple green or yellow and is most commonly seen on the ears, around the face and on the paws.

wool eating Behavioural disorder of dogs and cats that can rapidly become a habit; may be associated with early weaning and sucking reflexes. Similar behaviour may be seen in rabbits that make nests with their own and other rabbits' fur.

work up Term used to describe the logical and thorough diagnostic approach to a case, including the rational use of tests such as radiography, laboratory tests and electrodiagnostic testing.

worm Common endoparasite of all animals and man; various roundworm and tapeworm species inhabit the gastrointestinal tract. The stages of the life cycle may involve migration through body tissues; some worms target lung tissue, e.g. *Aelurostrongylus abstrusus,* urinary tract, e.g. *Capillaria putorii* or blood vessels, e.g. *Dirofilaria immitis.* Although generally controlled by routine worming and good hygiene measures, a number of worms cause serious zoonotic diseases, *see* APPENDIX 4; appropriate worming preparations should be used for the specific worms in question.

wound Trauma to the body resulting in tissue damage and a break in continuity; includes surgical wounds, incised wounds (made by sharp objects) and puncture wounds (opening is small compared with the depth of the wound).

wrist Lay term for the carpus.

wrymouth Lateral displacement of the mandible and teeth – a show fault in dogs.

wryneck Torticollis.

X

xanthochromic Yellow-coloured; deposition of yellow pigments is commonly associated with jaundice, *see also* JAUNDICE.

xanthoma Benign, granulomatous lesion of the skin; due to deposition of cholesterol to form fatty, yellow plaques and nodules.

X-chromosome The sex chromosome present in both the sexes, males being heterozygous (XY) and females being homozygous (XX).

xenograft Tissue/organ grafting technique where the donor and recipient are from different species, *see also* HETEROGRAFT.

xerophthalmia Dryness of the conjunctiva and cornea, resulting from vitamin A deficiency; can predispose to corneal ulceration.

xiphisternum *see* XIPHOID PROCESS.

xiphoid cartilage Cartilaginous (distal) portion of the xiphoid process, where the linea alba and rectus abdominis muscle insert.

xiphoid process Xiphisternum; the most caudal sternebra; continues as a cartilaginous projection and is the insertion for the abdominal muscles.

X-linked A trait carried by a gene on the X (female) chromosome; if the gene results in disease, all males will be affected as they have one X and one Y chromosome, while females may be affected or carriers, depending on whether they have one or both X chromosomes with the gene.

X-radiation Invisible ionising radiation that is part of the electromagnetic spectrum; it has a shorter wavelength than visible light, penetrates tissue and affects photographic film; produced in the X-ray tube head by bombarding a metal target (usually tungsten) with high speed electrons. The absorption of X-radiation by tissue depends on the density and atomic weight of the material; chronic exposure to radiation is damaging to tissues, *see also* RADIATION.

xylazine A sedative/hypnotic that is used as a premedicant, or in combination with ketamine to provide anaesthesia; may also be used to induce vomiting in cats.

xylocaine Proprietary name for the local anaesthetic agent lignocaine hydrochloride.

xylose A five-carbon sugar; poorly absorbed from the small intestine and so is used in some specialised tests for intestinal function.

Y

Y-chromosome Sex chromosome only present in males.

Y-fracture A combination of an intercondylar and a supracondylar fracture of the distal humerus or femur, resulting in three fracture fragments; more commonly seen affecting the humerus, where there is separation of the two sides of the condyle through the articular surface and the supratrochlear foramen; also known as a T-fracture; requires prompt internal fixation to ensure joint mobility and function are restored.

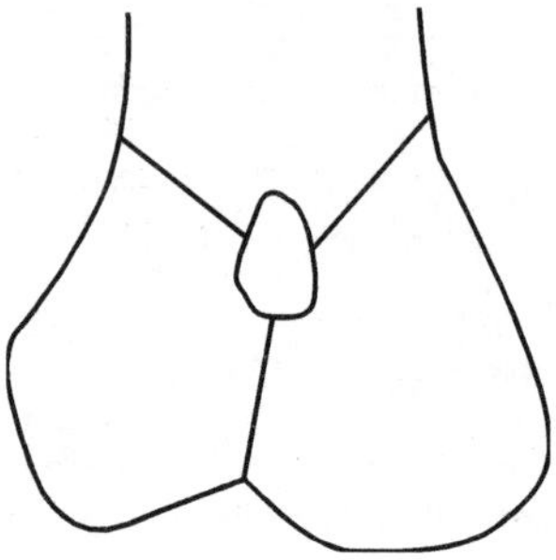

Y-fracture in distal humerus

yeast Unicellular fungus; in the diet it can be a source of B vitamins; a commensal of the skin and oral cavity, but is also associated with ear infections, stomatitis, dermatitis and enteritis if present in high numbers, e.g. in immunocompromised patients, *see also* *MALASEZZIA*.

yellow fat disease *see* PANSTEATITIS.

Yersinia enterocolitica Organism causing pseudotuberculosis, a rare disease characterised by lethargy, weight loss and chronic diarrhoea.

***Yersinia* spp.** Enteropathogenic Gram-negative rods that cause enteritis, colitis and diarrhoea; possibly zoonotic; affect dogs, cats, chickens, horses and cattle.

yolk sac Structure within the embryo that contains yolk, the nutritive material for the developing fetus.

Z

Z-plasty Surgical technique for relieving tension on a skin incision by making two parallel incisions and joining them to create two triangular skin flaps which are then rotated and sutured.

Ziehl–Neelsen stain Bacteriological staining method where the fixed smear is flooded with red Ziehl stain and heated for 1 minute, followed by decoloration in acid-alcohol and counter-staining with methylene blue; acid-fast organisms, such as *Mycobacteria* spp., stain red, *see also* ACID FAST.

zinc A metallic dietary mineral and trace element necessary as a cofactor for a number of metalloproteases and other enzymes; deficiency is rare as dietary sources are generally adequate, but some animals may have poor uptake, and thus respond to supplementation.

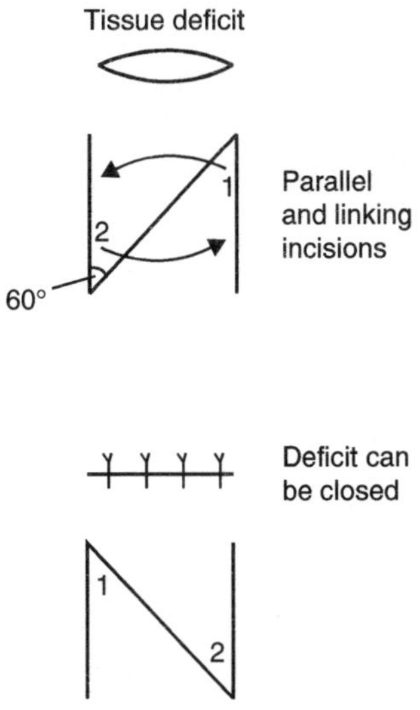

Z-plasty

zinc-responsive dermatosis Hyperkeratotic skin disorder, characterised by crusty lesions around the eyes and mouth, thought to be due to a defect in zinc uptake; treatment is to provide a zinc supplement in the diet.

Zimmer splint A light finger splint made for humans, consisting of a thin aluminium strip lined with a layer of foam padding; available in several widths and can easily be cut to length, although sharp metal ends should be rounded off. Useful as a first-aid splinting material or can be included within the layers of a support bandage to provide additional external support; only suitable for cats and small dogs.

zona pellucida The membrane initially surrounding the fertilised ovum.

zonary placentation Type of placentation found in the dog and cat, where the villi from the atlantochorion form a discrete broad band across the placenta – this is in contrast to other species where the villi are diffuse (mare, sow) or concentrated at sites known as cotyledons (ruminants).

zonule of Zinn Small zone on the anterior face of the vitreous body of the eye, consisting of fine ligamentous strands that run from the ciliary processes to the equator of the lens and hold the latter structure in place.

zonulysis A technique in cataract surgery to free the lens, to make it easier to remove.

zoogamy Reproduction using the fusion of two gametes.

Zoo Licensing Act 1981 Parliamentary act governing all zoos and open collections of non-domestic animals.

zoology The study of the biology of animals.

zoonosis A disease that can be communicated between animals and man, *see also* APPENDIX 4.

zygapophysis Alternative name for the articular process on a vertebra.

zygomatic arch Cheekbone.

zygote The fertilised ovum, formed by the fusion of two haploid gametes thus restoring the usual diploid number of chromosomes.

Appendix 1:
Temperature, pulse and respiratory rates for various species

Species	*Temperature in °C (°F)*	*Pulse rate/min*	*Resp. rate/min*
Dog	38.3–38.7 (100.9–101.7)	60–120	15–30
Cat	38.0–38.5 (100.4–101.6)	100–140	20–30
Rabbit	37.0–39.4 (99.0–103.0)	220	38–65
Guinea-pig	39.0–40.0 (102.2–104.2)	130–190	90–150
Hamster	36.0–38.0 (98.0–101.0)	300–600	33–127
Gerbil	38.0–39.0 (100.4–102.2)	100–150	40–80
Rat	37.5–38.0 (99.8–100.5)	260–340	70–150

Appendix 2:
Biochemistry parameters for cats and dogs

		Normal range	
Test	*Units*	*Canine*	*Feline*
Albumin	g/l	25–37	21–39
Alkaline phosphatase (ALP)	U/l @ 30°C	<80	<60
Alanine aminotransferase (ALT)	U/l @ 30°C	<25	<20
Aspartate aminotransferase (AST)	U/l @ 30°C	<25	<35
Bilirubin (total)	μmol/l	<16	<10
Calcium	mmol/l	2.3–3.0	1.6–2.4
Cholesterol	mmol/l	3.8–7.0	1.9–3.9
Creatinine	μmol/l	<106	80–180
Creatine kinase (CK)	U/l @ 30°C	<100	<80
Globulin (total)	g/l	23–52	15–57
Glucose	mmol/l	2.0–2.5	4.3–6.6
Phosphorus	mmol/l	0.8–1.6	1.4–2.6
Potassium	mmol/l	3.5–5.6	3.5–5.6
Sodium	mmol/l	135–154	147–155
Total protein	g/l	54–77	54–78
Urea (BUN)	mmol/l	1.7–7.4	6.0–10.0

Normal parameters for urine for dogs and cats

Species	*pH*	*Specific gravity*
Canine	5.2–6.8	1.018–1.045
Feline	6.0–7.0	1.020–1.040

Appendix 3:
Haematology parameters for dogs and cats

Test	*Units*	*Normal range* Canine	*Normal range* Feline
Red blood cells	$\times 10^{12}/l$	5.0–8.5	5.5–10.0
Haemoglobin (Hb)	g/100 ml (g%)	12.0–18.0	9.0–17.0
Packed cell volume (PCV or haematocrit)	%	37–57	27–50
MCV	fl	60–77	40–55
MCH	pg	19–23	13–17
MCHC	g/100 ml (g%)	31–34	31–34
White blood cells	$\times 10^9/l$	6.0–15.0	4.0–15.0
Mature neutrophils	$\times 10^9/l$	3.6–10.5	2.5–12.5
	%	60–70	45–75
Band neutrophils	$\times 10^9/l$	0–0.3	0–0.45
	%	0–2	0–3
Lymphocytes	$\times 10^9/l$	1–4.8	1.5–6.5
	%	12.0–30.0	25–33
Eosinophils	$\times 10^9/l$	0.1–1.5	0.1 -1.8
	%	2.0–10.0	4.0–12.0
Monocytes	$\times 10^9/l$	0.18–1.5	0–0.6
	%	3.0–10.0	0–4
Basophils	$\times 10^9/l$	rare	rare
	%	rare	rare
Platelets	$\times 10^9/l$	200–500	200–600

Appendix 4: Zoonotic diseases

Disease	*Causative agent*	*Symptoms*
Brucellosis	*Brucella abortus*, from infected cattle	Undulent fever
Campylobacter	*Campylobacter* spp	Diarrhoea
Cat scratch fever	Various organisms	Cellutitis at site of scratch or bite, fever, septicaemia
Cheyletiella	Surface-living mite	Skin irritation
Chlamydia psittaci	Intracellular parasite causing psittacosis and feline pneumonitis. Passes to humans by inhaling chlamydia in air-borne dust or cage contents of infected birds	Psittacosis. Fever, dry cough, muscle pain and headaches. Pneumonia can be fatal. Condition responds to tetracycline or erythromycin
Echinococcus granulosus	Cestode found in intestines of dogs and sheep	Hydatid cyst can develop in liver, lungs or brain. Treated by anthelminthics, drainage of cyst and surgical removal of cyst wall which is a hazardous procedure. In the worst case malignant cyst tumours can develop in people
Fleas	*Ctenophalides felis* and *C. canis* from cats and dogs	Rarely live on humans but can cause severe irritation from bites
Leptospirosis	Gram-negative spirochaetal bacteria *L. canicola* and *L. icterohaemorraghiae* found in dog and rodents	Weil's disease. Fever which can affect liver causing jaundice, meninges causing meningitis and often the kidneys are affected
Listeriosis	*Listeria monocytogenes*	Meningitis
Orf	Orf virus, mainly from sheep and cattle	Fever and skin granulations

Appendix 4: (*continued*)

Disease	*Causative agent*	*Symptoms*
Rabies	Rhabdovirus in dogs and cats, will pass through cuts and abrasions or by a bite. Is carried in saliva	Hydrophobia, malaise, fever, difficulty in breathing, salivation and painful muscle spasms in throat. Convulsions and death follow. Injection of rabies vaccine and antiserum may prevent the disease from developing. Notifiable – police must be contacted immediately. Humans can be vaccinated by initial course and regular boosters
Ringworm	Dermatophytes: *Microsporum*, *Trichophyton* and *Epidermophyton* passed by direct contact with dogs, cats, rabbits or guinea-pigs	Circular lesions causing intense irritation. Treated by antifungal agents taken orally or locally
Salmonellosis	Gram-negative bacteria *Salmonella* spp. inhabit intestines of animals and man	Food poisoning, gastroenteritis and septicaemia
Sarcoptic mange	Burrowing mites *Sarcoptes scabiei* var. *canis*. Spread by direct contact with infected dogs. Foxes are a possible source	In humans the lesions are small and self-limiting. A separate type of *Sarcoptes* causes scabies in humans
Toxocara canis and *T. cati*	Nematode found in dogs and cats. Passed to children by them swallowing animal faeces	Toxocariasis or 'visceral larval migrans'. Larvae migrate through body and can cause blindness if they come to rest in retina
Toxoplasmosis	Protozoal parasite *Toxoplasma gondii* affecting mammals and birds. Passed to humans by eating infected meat or accidentally swallowing sporulated oocysts from cat faeces	Flu-like symptoms and malaise, can lead to blindness, brain defects and death. In pregnant women can result in abortion or foetal abnormalities
Tularaemia	*Pasteurella tularensis*, from hares and rabbits	Slow fever and weight loss

Appendix 5:
Biological data of smaller pets

Type of pet	*Average life expectancy*	*Age at maturity*	*Size of litter*	*Age at weaning*	*Body temperature (°C)*
Rabbit	6–8 years	3 months +	2–7 young	6 weeks	38.5
Guinea-pig	4–7 years	4–10 weeks	2–6 young	3–3.5 weeks	38–39
Rat	3 years	6 weeks +	6–12 young	21 days +	38
Mouse	1–2.5 years	3–4 weeks	5–7 young	18 days +	37.5
Gerbil	1.5–2.5 years	10–12 weeks	3–6 young	21–28 days	38
Hamster	1.5–2 years	6–10 weeks	3–7 young	21–28 days	37–38
Chinchilla	10–15 years	8 months	1–4 young	6–8 weeks	38–39
Ferret	5–7 years	6–9 months	2–10 young	8 weeks	38.8

Information on caring for smaller animals

Type of pet	*Amount of care needed*	*Special needs*
Rabbits and guinea-pigs	Roomy hutch and outside run. Hay, straw commercial food and vegetables. Fresh water always available	Keep dry. Clean out once weekly. Watch for diarrhoea and fly-strike. Clip nails and teeth. Myxomatosis vaccine available. Enjoy company
Rats and mice	Roomy cage, sawdust or shredded paper. Commercial diet, vegetables, fruit and seeds. Fresh water always available	Clean out once a week. Handle carefully
Gerbils and hamsters	As for rats and mice. Hygiene is important	As for rats and mice. Watch for wet-tail in hamsters
Chinchillas	Large cage with ledges and dust-bath. Commercial pellet diet, hay, fruit, vegetables and seeds. Fresh water always available	Clean out regularly. Best kept in pairs. Long lived when well cared for
Ferrets	As for rabbits and guinea-pigs. Eat meat, eggs and milk. Can buy frozen carcasses. Fresh water always available	Need lots of attention and exercise. Clean out regularly. Distemper vaccine available, but care needed with dosages

Appendix 5: *(continued)*

Type of pet	*Amount of care needed*	*Special needs*
Birds (e.g. budgies, canaries, parrots)	Roomy cage, toys to prevent boredom. Commercial seed diet, fruit, vegetables, grit, cuttlefish, cheese and bread. Fresh water always available	Clean out weekly. Handle carefully. Beak and claws need clipping. Parrots enjoy lots of company. Wing exercise if appropriate to the species
Reptiles/ amphibians	Adequate space in glass tanks with gravel/sand. Frozen carcasses, fish, crickets, locusts, fruit and vegetables. Fresh water always available	Temperature, humidity and lighting important. Good hygiene also essential. Research further into preferred species
Fish	Roomy glass tank or aquarium with gravel, ornaments and plants. Commercial food	Clean out weekly. Filters needed for large tanks. Research further into preferred types of fish, especially tropical fish
Invertebrates	Roomy tanks with leaves, foliage, fruit and vegetables. Spiders will need insects, etc	Tropical temperatures. Research further into specific needs of your preferred species

Appendix 6:
Obstetrical information for different species

Species	*Gestation period (days)*	*Other information*
Dog	63	Breeding season continuous. Two oestrus cycles each year
Cat	63	Induced ovulator. Oestrus cycle every 14 days. Seasonally polyoestrus (Feb.–Sept.)
Rabbit	31–32	Induced ovulator. Irregular oestrus cycle. Continuous breeding season but less active in winter
Guinea-pig	59–72	Continuous breeding season. Oestrus cycle every 13–20 days
Hamster	15–21	Continuous breeding season. Polyoestrus all year round
Gerbil	24	Continuous breeding season. Oestrus cycle every 4–6 days
Rat	21–23	Continuous breeding season. Oestrus cycle occurs for 12 hours every 4 days

Appendix 7:

Mathematical formulae for use in veterinary nursing

Converting °F to °C	°C = (°F −32) × 5/9
Radiography:	
New mAs with a grid	mAs normally used × grid factor
New mAs with new FFD* (inverse square law)	Old mAs × new FFD^2/old FFD^2
New mAs with non-screen film	Old mAs (using screen film) × screen factor or intensification factor
If kV increased by 10	mAs halved, to keep exposure the same
If kV decreased by 10	mAs doubled, to keep exposure the same
Surgical:	
Anaesthetic flow rate	Minute volume × circuit factor
Fluid deficits	% dehydration × weight (kg) × 10
Percentage solution, e.g. 1 in 100 = 1%	5 g thiopentone in 200 ml water = $2\frac{1}{2}$%

*FFD = film-focal distance

Converting body weight in kilograms and pounds into body surface area in metres squared

kg	*lbs*	*m^2*	*kg*	*lbs*	*m^2*
2	4.4	0.15	28	61.6	0.92
4	8.8	0.25	30	66.0	0.96
6	13.2	0.33	32	70.4	1.01
8	17.6	0.40	34	74.8	1.05
10	22.0	0.46	36	79.2	1.09
12	26.4	0.52	38	83.6	1.13
14	30.8	0.58	40	88.0	1.17
16	35.2	0.63	42	92.4	1.21
18	39.6	0.69	44	96.8	1.25
20	44.0	0.74	46	101.2	1.28
22	48.4	0.78	48	105.6	1.32
24	52.8	0.83	50	110.0	1.36
26	57.2	0.88			

Appendix 8:
Infectious diseases of dogs and cats

Disease	*Causative agent*	*Incubation period*
Canine:		
Canine distemper	Morbillivirus	7–12 days
Infectious canine hepatitis (ICH)	Canine adenovirus 1 (CAV-1)	5–9 days
Leptospirosis	Gram-negative bacteria, *L. canicola* and *L. icterohaemorrhagiae*	5–7 days
Canine contagious respiratory disease (CCRD)	CAV-1, CAV-2, canine parainfluenza virus (CPIV), canine herpes virus (CHV), reovirus	5–7 days
Parvovirus	Canine parvovirus virus 1 and 2 (CPV-1, CPV-2)	3–5 days
Rabies	Rhabdovirus	2 weeks to 4 months
Feline:		
Feline panleukopenia	Parvovirus	4–5 days
Feline upper respiratory tract disease (FURD)	Feline calici virus (FCV), feline herpes virus 1 (FHV-1)	2–10 days
Feline infectious peritonitis (FIP)	Coronavirus	Months
Feline pneumonitis	*Chlamydia psittaci*	4–10 days
Feline leukaemia virus	Retrovirus	Months/years
Feline immunodeficiency virus (FIV)	RNA retrovirus	Months/years

Appendix 9:
Current vaccination schedules for dogs and cats

Disease	*Type of vaccine*	*Schedule*
Canine:		
Canine distemper	Modified live vaccine	First vaccine from 6 weeks of age, second dose at 12 weeks. Boosted annually or every other year
Infectious canine hepatitis (ICH)	Live CAV-2 (canine adenovirus 2) vaccine	As for canine distemper
Canine leptospirosis	Killed sero-types of *L. canicola* and *L. icterohaemorrhagiae*	As for canine distemper. Annual boosting essential as immunity short-lived
Canine parvovirus	Live vaccine	As for canine distemper. Booster at 16–20 weeks now less necessary as vaccines have been improved
Canine contagious respiratory disease (CCRD)	Live vaccines available against *Bordetella bronchiseptica*, canine adenovirus (CAV) and canine parainfluenza virus (CPIV)	CPIV as for canine distemper. *Bordetella* vaccine given intranasally, booster every 6 months. Ideally give 10–14 days prior to kennelling
Rabies	Inactivated vaccine	Initial vaccination involves a single injection from 3–4 months, and regular boosters
Feline:		
Feline panleukopenia	Killed and modified live vaccines available	Initial vaccine from 6 weeks, second injection at 12 weeks, booster annually
Feline upper respiratory disease (FURD)	Injectable and intranasal vaccines available. Intranasal is modified live vaccine. Dead vaccine used in pregnant queens	Initial vaccine includes two injections at 9 and 12 weeks. Intranasal protection achieved within 5 days. Occasionally mild signs of the disease will follow. Booster annually
Feline pneumonitis (*Chlamydia*)	Modified live vaccine. Not for use in pregnant queens	Initial course starts at 9 weeks, second given 3–4 weeks later. Booster annually
Feline leukaemia virus (FeLV)	Genetically engineered vaccine	Initial course of two injections given 2–3 weeks apart. Booster annually. Ideally test cats for the disease before vaccinating

Appendix 10:

Average weights for common breeds of dog

Breed	*Weight (kg)*	*Weight (lb)*	*Breed*	*Weight (kg)*	*Weight (lb)*	*Breed*	*Weight (kg)*	*Weight (lb)*
Afghan hound	22–27	48.5–59.5	Deerhound	30–47	66.1–103.6	Poodle (toy)	4–5	8.8–11
Airedale terrier	21–24	46.3–52.9	Dobermann	33–38	72.7–83.7	Poodle (miniature)	5–7	11–15.4
Alaskan malamute	44–48	97–105.8	English setter	27–29	59.5–63.9	Poodle (standard)	25–40	55.1–88.1
Anatolian shepherd dog	54–57	119–125.6	Flat coat retriever	29–30	63.9–66.1	Pug	5–8	11–17.6
Basenji	9–11	19.8–24.2	German shepherd	29–37	63.9–81.5	Pyrenean mountain dog	40–60	88.1–132.2
Bassett hound	19–22	41.8–48.5	German short-haired pointer	24–30	52.9–66.1	Rhodesian ridgeback	32–37	70.5–81.5
Beagle	9–14	19.8–30.8	Golden retriever	29–34	63.9–74.9	Rough collie	18–30	39.6–66.1
Bearded collie	20–22	44–48.5	Great Dane	45–62	99.2–136.6	Rottweiler	38–50	83.7–110.2
Bedlington terrier	9–10	19.8–22	Greyhound	23–36	50.7–79.3	Saint Bernard	68–75	149.9–165.3
Bernese mountain dog	50–60	110.2–132.2	Hovawart	30–35	66.1–77.1	Saluki	19–24	41.8–52.9
Bichon frise	4–9	8.8–19.8	Hungarian vizsla	22–30	48.5–66.1	Samoyed	20–30	44–66.1
Bloodhound	40–55	88.1–121.2	Irish setter	26–31	57.3–68.3	Schnauzer (miniature)	4–8	8.8–17.6
Border collie	19–24	41.8–52.9	Irish terrier	11–12	24.2–26.4	Schnauzer (standard)	13–18	28.6–39.6
Border terrier	5–7	11–15.4	Irish wolfhound	50–70	110.2–154.3	Schnauzer (giant)	30–40	66.1–132.2

Borzoi	34–41	74.9–90.3	Italian greyhound	2–4	4.4–8.8	Scottish terrier	7–10	15.4–22
Boston terrier	8–11	17.6–24.2	Jack Russell terrier	5–8	11–17.6	Sealyham terrier	8–10	17.6–22
Boxer	26–31	57.3–68.3	Japanese akita	45–55	99.2–121.2	Shar Pei	15–22	33–48.5
Briard	34–39	74.9–85.9	Keeshund	18–20	39.6–44	Shetland sheepdog	8–13	17.6–28.6
Bulldog	22–25	48.5–55.1	King Charles spaniel	4–6	8.8–13.2	Shih Tzu	5–9	11–19.8
Bullmastiff	45–55	99.2–121.2	Labrador retriever	28–31	61.7–68.3	Siberian husky	15–25	33–55.1
Bull terrier	20–30	44–66.1	Lakeland terrier	7–8	15.4–17.6	Springer spaniel (English/Welsh)	18–25	39.6–55.1
Cairn terrier	5–7	11–15.4	Lhasa apso	5–8	11–17.6	Staffordshire bull terrier	13–15	28.6–33
Cavalier King Charles spaniel	5–7	11–15.4	Mastiff	67–78	147.7–171.9	Tibetan spaniel	5–7	11–15.4
Chihuahua	1–3	2.2–6.6	Newfoundland	52–67	114.6–147.7	Tibetan terrier	8–13	17.6–28.6
Chow chow	25–27	55.1–59.5	Norfolk terrier	5–7	11–15.4	Weimeraner	22–27	48.5–59.5
Clumber spaniel	29–36	63.9–79.3	Norwich terrier	5–7	11–15.4	Welsh corgi	10–12	22–26.4
Cocker spaniel	12–14	26.4–30.8	Old English sheepdog	29–37	63.9–81.5	West Highland white terrier	7–9	15.4–19.8
Curly coat retriever	32–35	70.5–77.1	Papillon	2–3	4.4–6.6	Whippet	10–12	22–26.4
Dachshund	4–10	8.8–22	Pekinese	4–6	8.8–13.2	Yorkshire terrier	1–3	2.2–6.6
Dalmation	25–27	55.1–59.5	Pomeranian	2–3	4.4–6.6			

Appendix 11:
Anaesthetic factors for dogs and cats

Essential data *Species*	*Resp. rate (breaths/min)*	*Tidal volume (ml/kg)*	*Minute volume (ml/kg/min)*	*O_2 consumption (ml/kg/min)*
Canine >30 kg	15.0–20.0	12.0–15.0	150–250	5.8
Canine <30 kg	20.0–30.0	16.0–20.0	200–300	6.2
Feline	20.0–30.0	7.0–9.0	180–380	7.3

Appendix 12:
Gas cylinder colour coding (UK only)

Name of gas	*Symbol*	*Colour of cylinder body*	*Colour of valve where different from body*
Oxygen	O_2	Black	White
Nitrous oxide	N_2O	Blue	–
Cyclopropane	C_3H_6	Orange	–
Carbon dioxide	CO_2	Grey	–
Ethylene	C_2H_4	Violet	–
Nitrogen	N_2	Grey	Black
Oxygen and carbon dioxide mixture	O_2+CO_2	Black	White and grey
Oxygen and helium mixture	O_2+He	Black	White and brown
Oxygen and nitrous oxide mixture	O_2+N_2O	Blue	Blue and black
Air, medical	AIR	Grey	White and black

Appendix 13:
Dog breeds and coat colours

Colour	*Breeds*
Any colour	Afghan, Border collie, Borzoi, Bulldog, Chinese crested dog, Chihuahua, Cocker spaniel, Dachshund, German shepherd, Japanese akita, Lowchen, Pekinese, Pomeranian, Shih-tzu, Siberian husky, Tibetan spaniel, Tibetan terrier (except liver and chocolate), Whippet
Any bicolour	English foxhound, Greyhound, Lhasa apso, Papillon, Staffordshire bull terrier
Any tricolour	Brittany, English bull terrier, English foxhound, English pointer, English setter, Otterhound, Rough collie, Shetland sheepdog, Staffordshire bull terrier
Apricot	Poodle, Pug
Black	Affenpinscher, American cocker spaniel, Bearded collie, Belgian shepherd dog, Bouvier de Flandres, Briard, Cairn terrier, Chow chow, Curly coat retriever, Dobermann, English bull terrier, English pointer, Field spaniel, Flat coat retriever, German short-haired pointer, Great Dane, Greyhound, Griffon Bruxellois, Hungarian puli, Irish wolfhound, Italian greyhound, Labrador retriever, Lakeland terrier, Lhasa apso, Norwegian buhund, Poodle, Pug, Schipperke, Schnauzer, Scottish terrier, Skye terrier, Staffordshire bull terrier
Black and grey	Keeshund, Miniature schnauzer
Black and tan	Airedale terrier, American cocker spaniel, Bloodhound, Cavalier King Charles spaniel, Dobermann, English toy terrier, Gordon setter, Griffon Bruxellois, King Charles spaniel, Lakeland terrier, Manchester terrier, Miniature pinscher, Norfolk terrier, Norwich terrier, Rottweiler, Saluki, Segugio Italiano, Shetland sheepdog, Smooth fox terrier, Welsh terrier, Yorkshire terrier
Black and white	Basenji, Bearded collie, Boston terrier, Brittany, English pointer, English setter, English springer spaniel, German short haired pointer, German wire haired pointer, Grand basset griffon vendeen, Japanese chin, Large munsterlander, Newfoundland, Shetland sheepdog, Wire fox terrier
Black, white and tan	Basenji, Basset griffon vendeen, Basset hound, Beagle, Bernese mountain dog, Cavalier King Charles spaniel, English Springer spaniel, King Charles spaniel, Saluki, Wire fox terrier
Blenheim	Cavalier King Charles spaniel, King Charles spaniel
Blue	Bearded collie, Bedlington terrier, Chow chow, Dobermann, Glen of Imaal terrier, Great Dane, Greyhound, Italian Greyhound, Kerry blue terrier, Lakeland terrier, Miniature pinscher, Old English sheepdog, Poodle, Staffordshire bull terrier

Appendix 13: (*continued*)

Colour	*Breeds*
Blue merle	Collie, Shetland sheepdog
Blue and tan	Australian terrier, Border terrier, Lakeland terrier, Yorkshire terrier
Blue and white	Italian greyhound, Old English sheepdog
Brindle	Boxer, bullmastiff, Deerhound, English bull terrier, French bulldog, Glen of Imaal terrier, Great Dane, Greyhound, Irish Wolfhound, Scottish terrier, Staffordshire bull terrier
Brindle and white	Boston terrier, St. Bernard
Brown	Bearded collie, Dobermann, Lhasa apso, Poodle
Chocolate	Labrador retriever, Miniature pinscher, Dobermann
Chocolate and white	Newfoundland
Cream	Cairn terrier, Chow chow, Golden retriever, Italian greyhound, Poodle, Saluki, Samoyed, Skye terrier
Fallow	Greyhound
Fawn	Bearded collie, Belgian shepherd dog, Bouvier de Flandres, Boxer, Briard, Bullmastiff, Chow chow, Dobermann, English bull terrier, French bulldog, Great Dane, Greyhound, Ibizan, Irish wolfhound, Italian greyhound, Mastiff, Saluki, Segugio Italiano, Skye terrier, Staffordshire bull terrier
Gold	Golden retriever, Hungarian vizsla, Lhasa apso, Sussex spaniel
Grey	Bearded collie, Belgian Shepherd Dog, Briard, Cairn terrier, Deerhound, Grand Basset Griffon Vendeen, Hungarian Puli, Irish Wolfhound, Norwegian Elkhound, Old English sheepdog, Skye terrier
Grey and white	Italian greyhound, Old English sheepdog, Pyrenean mountain dog, Swedish valhund
Grizzle	Airedale terrier, Lhasa apso, Norfolk terrier, Norwich terrier, Old English sheepdog, Otterhound, Saluki
Grizzle and tan	Border terrier, Welsh terrier
Harlequin	Dalmatian, Great Dane
Honey	Lhasa apso
Lemon	English pointer
Lemon and white	Basset hound, Clumber spaniel, English pointer, English setter, Maltese terrier, Otterhound, Pyrenean mountain dog
Liver	Bedlington terrier, Curly coat retriever, English pointer, Field spaniel, Flat coat retriever, German short haired pointer, German Wire pointer, Irish Water spaniel

Appendix 13: (*continued*)

Colour	*Breeds*
Liver and tan	Bedlington terrier, Bloodhound
Liver and white	Brittany, Dalmatian, English setter, English springer spaniel, English pointer, German short haired pointer, German wire haired pointer
Mustard	Dandie dinmont
Orange	English pointer, Otterhound
Orange and white	Basset griffon vendeen, Brittany, Clumber spaniel, English pointer, Italian spinone, St. Bernard
Pepper	Dandie dinmont, Schnauzer
Red	Belgian shepherd dog, Bloodhound, Border terrier, Bullmastiff, Cairn terrier, Chow chow, Deerhound, English bull terrier, Finnish spitz, Greyhound, Griffon Bruxellois, Ibizan, Irish setter, Irish terrier, Irish wolfhound, Italian greyhound, King Charles spaniel, Lakeland terrier, Miniature pinscher, Norfolk terrier, Norwegian buhund, Norwich terrier, Saluki, Staffordshire bull terrier, Vizsla
Red and white	Basenji, Irish setter, Italian greyhound, Japanese Chin, Swedish valhund, Welsh springer spaniel
Ruby	Cavalier King Charles spaniel
Silver	Poodle, Pug, Weimeraner
Tan	Chesapeake Bay retriever, Pharoah hound
Tan and white	Grand basset griffon vendeen, Smooth fox terrier, Wire fox terrier
Wheaten	Border terrier, Cairn terrier, Glen of Imaal terrier, Irish terrier, Irish wolfhound, Lakeland terrier, Norfolk terrier, Norwegian buhund, Norwich terrier, Rhodesian ridgeback, Scottish terrier, Soft coated wheaten terrier
White	Basset griffon vendeen, Bichon frise, Chow chow, English bull terrier, Greyhound, Ibizan, Irish wolfhound, Italian spinone, Japanese spitz, Lhasa apso, Poodle, Pyrenean mountain dog, Samoyed, Sealyham terrier, Smooth fox terrier, Staffordshire bull terrier, West Highland white terrier, Wire fox terrier
Yellow	Deerhound, Labrador retriever

Appendix 14:
Cat breeds and coat colours

Breed	*Coat colours*
Short hair:	
Abyssinian	Ruddy (usual), Red, Blue
American Short Hair	White, Black, Blue, Red, Cream, Chinchilla, Shaded silver, Shell cameo (red chinchilla), Shaded cameo (red shaded), Black smoke, Blue smoke, Cameo smoke (red smoke), Classic tabby, Mackerel tabby, Patched tabby, Brown patched tabby, Blue patched tabby, Silver patched tabby, Silver tabby, Red tabby, Brown tabby, Blue tabby, Cream tabby, Cameo tabby, Tortoiseshell, Calico, Dilute calico, Blue-cream, Bi-colour (e.g. black and white)
American Wire Hair	As for American short hair excluding Patched tabby, Brown patched tabby, Blue patched tabby, Silver patched tabby
Bombay	Black
British Short Hair	Blue-eyed white, Orange-eyed white, Odd-eyed white, Black, Blue, Cream, Blue-cream, Silver tabby, Red tabby, Brown tabby, Mackerel tabby, Black smoke, Blue smoke, Spotted, Tortoiseshell, Tortoiseshell and white, Bi-colour
Burmese	Brown, Blue, Chocolate, Lilac, Red, Brown (normal), Tortoiseshell, Cream, Blue tortie, Chocolate tortie, Lilac tortie (lilac-cream)
Colourpoint Short Hair	Red point, Cream point, Seal Lynx point, Chocolate Lynx point, Blue Lynx point, Lilac Lynx point, Red Lynx point, Seal-tortie point, Chocolate-cream point, Blue-cream point, Lilac-cream point
Exotic Short Hair	As for American short hair
Eygyptian Mau	Silver, Bronze, Smoke
Foreign Short Hair	Lilac, White, Black
Havana Brown	Brown
Japanese Bobtail	White, Black, Red, Black and white, Red and white, Mi-ke (tri-colour), Tortoiseshell
Korat	Silver-blue
Manx	As for American short hair excluding Shell cameo, Shaded cameo, Cameo smoke, Cameo tabby

Appendix 14: (*continued*)

Breed	*Coat colours*
Oriental Short Hair	White, Ebony, Blue, Chestnut, Lavender, Red, Cream, Silver, Cameo, Ebony smoke, Blue smoke, Chestnut smoke, Lavender smoke, Cameo (red) smoke, Classic tabby, Mackerel tabby, Spotted tabby, Ticked tabby, Ebony tabby, Blue tabby, Chestnut tabby, Lavender tabby, Red tabby, Cream tabby, Silver tabby, Cameo tabby, Tortoiseshell, Blue-cream, Chestnut tortie, Lavender-cream
Oriental Spotted Tabby	Brown, Blue, Chocolate, Lilac, Red, Cream
Rex (Cornish/Devon)	As for Manx
Russian Blue	Blue
Scottish Fold	As for American wire hair
Siamese	Seal point, Chocolate point, Blue point, Lilac point, Tabby point, Tortie point, Red point, Cream point.
Somali	Ruddy/Red
Long hair:	
Balinese	Seal point, Blue point, Chocolate point, Lilac point
Birman	As for Balinese
Himalayan/Colourpoint Long Hair	Seal point, Chocolate point, Blue point, Lilac point, Flame point, Tortie point, Blue-cream point, Chocolate solid colour, Lilac solid colour
Maine Coon	White, Black, Blue, Red, Cream, Chinchilla, Shaded silver, Shell cameo (red chinchilla), Shaded cameo (red shaded), Black smoke, Blue smoke, Cameo smoke (red smoke), Classic tabby, Mackerel tabby, Silver tabby, Red tabby, Brown tabby, Blue tabby, Cream tabby, Cameo tabby, Tabby and white, Tortoiseshell, Tortie and white, Calico, Dilute calico, Blue-cream, Bi-colour
Persian	As for Maine Coon including Patched tabby, Brown patched taby, Blue patched tabby, Silver patched tabby, Chinchilla golden, Shaded golden, Shell tortie, Shaded tortie, Smoke tortie, Lilac, Lilac-cream, Persian van bi-colour, Peke-face red, Peke-face red tabby, Pewter, Chocolate, Chocolate tortie, but excluding Tortie and white and Tabby and white
Turkish Angora	White, Black, Blue, Black smoke, Blue smoke, Classic tabby, Mackerel tabby, Silver tabby, Red tabby, Brown tabby, Blue tabby, Calico, Bi-colour

Appendix 15:
Veterinary qualifications: interpretation of letters after names

BSc: Bachelor of Science, most universities award a non veterinary BSc
BSc (Vet Sci): Bachelor of Veterinary Science (London)
BVBiol: Bachelor of Veterinary Biology
BVetMed: Bachelor of Veterinary Medicine, a London degree
BVMS: Bachelor of Veterinary Medicine and Surgery, a Glasgow degree
BVM&S: Bachelor of Veterinary Medicine & Surgery, an Edinburgh degree
BVSc: Bachelor of Veterinary Science, Bristol, Liverpool, overseas degrees
CertBR: Certificate in Bovine Reproduction (RCVS)
CertCHP: Certificate in Cattle Health and Reproduction (RCVS)
CertEM (IntMed): Certificate in Equine Medicine (Internal Medicine) (RCVS)
CertEO: Certificate in Equine Orthopaedics (RCVS)
CertEP: Certificate in Equine Practice (RCVS)
CertES (Orth): Certificate in Equine Surgery (Orthopaedics) (RCVS)
CertES (Soft Tissue): Certificate in Equine Surgery (Soft Tissue) (RCVS)
CertESM: Certificate in Equine Stud Medicine (RCVS)
CertFHP: Certificate in Fish Health and Production (RCVS)
CertLAS: Certificate in Laboratory Animal Science (RCVS)
CertPM: Certificate in Pig Medicine (RCVS)
CertPMP: Certificate in Poultry Medicine and Production (RCVS)
CertSAC: Certificate in Small Animal Cardiology (RCVS)
CertSAD: Certificate in Small Animal Dermatology (RCVS)
CertSAM: Certificate in Small Animal Medicine (RCVS)
CertSAO: Certificate in Small Animal Orthopaedics (RCVS)
CertSAS: Certificate in Small Animal Surgery (RCVS)
CertSHP: Certificate in Sheep Health and Production (RCVS)
CertVA: Certificate in Veterinary Anaesthesia (RCVS)
CertVC: Certificate in Veterinary Cardiology (RCVS)
CertVD: Certificate in Veterinary Dermatology (RCVS)
CertVOphthal: Certificate in Veterinary Ophthamology (RCVS)
CertVPH (MH): Certificate in Veterinary Public Health (Meat Hygiene) (RCVS)
CertVR: Certificate in Veterinary Radiology (RCVS)
CertWel: Certificate in Animal Welfare Science, Ethics and Law (RCVS)
CertZooMed: Certificate in Zoological Medicine (RCVS)
DPM: Diploma in Pig Medicine (RCVS)

Appendix 15: (*continued*)

DPMP: Diploma in Poultry Medicine and Production (RCVS)
DipRCPath: Diploma Royal College of Pathologists
DSHP: Diploma in Sheep Health and Production (RCVS)
DSAM: Diploma in Small Animal Medicine (RCVS)
DSAO: Diploma in Small Animal Orthopaedics (RCVS)
DSAS: Diploma in Small Animal Surgery (RCVS)
Dip (AVNSurg) Advanced nursing diploma (RCVS)
DipToxRC Path: Diploma in Toxicology of the Royal College of Pathologists
DiplEMVT: Diploma in Tropical Veterinary Medicine and Animal Husbandry
DipVetMed: Diploma in Large Animal Medicine
DVC: Diploma in Veterinary Cardiology (RCVS)
DVD: Diploma in Veterinary Dermatology (RCVS)
DVOphthal: Diploma in Veterinary Ophthamology (RCVS)
DipVetPath: Diploma in Veterinary Pathology
DVPH (MH): Diploma in Veterinary Public Health (Meat Hygiene) (RCVS)
DPVM: Diploma in Preventive Veterinary Medicine
DSc: Doctor of Science
DTVM: Diploma in Veterinary Tropical Medicine (Edinburgh University)
DVA: Diploma in Veterinary Anaesthesia (RCVS)
DVM: Doctor of Veterinary Medicine
DVetMed: Doctor of Veterinary Medicine (London)
DVM & S: Doctor of Veterinary Medicine and Surgery
DVR: Diploma in Veterinary Radiology (RCVS)
DVRep: Diploma in Veterinary Reproduction (RCVS)
DVSc: Doctor of Veterinary Science
DVSM: Diploma in Veterinary State Medicine (RCVS)
FRCVS: Fellow of the Royal College of Veterinary Surgeons
FPH: Fellow in Poultry Husbandry
DAP & E: Diploma in Applied Parasitology and Entomology
DBR: Diploma in Bovine Reproduction (University of Liverpool)
DCHP: Diploma in Cattle Health and Production (RCVS)
DEO: Diploma in Equine Orthopaedics (RCVS)
DER: Diploma in Equine Reproduction (Liverpool)
DESM: Diploma in Equine Orthopaedics (RCVS)
DESTS: Diploma in Equine Soft Tissue Surgery (RCVS)
DipAH: Diploma in Animal Health

Appendix 15: (*continued*)

DipAnGen: Diploma in Animal Genetics
DipBact: Diploma in Bacteriology
DipPar: Diploma in Parasitology
DLAS: Diploma in Laboratory Animal Science (RCVS)
FRAgS: Fellow of the Royal Agricultural Societies
FRCPath: Fellow of the Royal College of Pathologists 'UK'
GVSc Graduate in Veterinary Science
HonAssocRCVS: Honorary Associate of the RCVS
MAnimSc: Master of Veterinary Medicine
MRCVS: Member of the RCVS
MVB: Bachelor of Veterinary Medicine Dublin, Ireland
MVM: Master of Veterinary Medicine
MVetMed: Master of Veterinary Medicine (London)
MVSc: Master of Veterinary Science
NDA: National Diploma in Agriculture
NDD: National Diploma in Dairying
NDP: National Diploma in Poultry
PhD: Doctor of Philosophy (all universities, higher degree)
QHVS: Queen's Honorary Veterinary Surgeon
VetMB: Bachelor of Veterinary Medicine (Cambridge)

Appendix 16:
Useful addresses, telephone and fax numbers

Animal Health Trust, PO Box 5, Newmarket, Suffolk CB8 7DW.
Tel: 01638 661111; Fax: 01638 665789.

Blue Cross, 1 High Street, Victoria, London SW1V 1QQ. Tel: 0171 834 5556;
Fax: 0171 821 9083.

British Small Animal Veterinary Associaton (BSAVA), Kingsley House, Church Lane, Shurdington, Cheltenham, Gloucestershire Cl51 5TQ. Tel: 01242 862994;
Fax: 01242 863009.

British Veterinary Association (BVA), 7 Mansfield Street, London W1M 0AT.
Tel: 0171 636 6541; Fax: 0171 436 2970.

British Veterinary Nursing Association (BVNA), Level 15, Terminus House, Terminus Street, Harlow CM20 1XA. Tel: 01279 450 467;
Fax: 01279 420866.

Cats Protection League, 17 Kings Road, Horsham, West Sussex RH13 5PN.
Tel: 01403 221900; Fax: 01403 218414.

Dogs For The Disabled (DfD), The Old Vicarage, London Road, Ryton-On-Dunsmore, Coventry CV8 3ER. Tel: 01203 302050; Fax: 01203 302055.

European College of Veterinary Surgeons, Veterinar-Chirurgische Klinik, Winterhurer Strasse 260, CH-8057, Zurich, Switzerland. Tel: +41 1 365 1456;
Fax: +41 1 313 0384.

Feline Advisory Bureau (FAB), Taeselbury, High Street, Tisbury, Salisbury, Wiltshire SP3 6LD. Tel: 01747 871872; Fax: 01747 871873.

Governing Council of the Cat Fancy (GCCF), 4–6 Penel Orlieu, Bridgwater, Somerset. Tel: 01278 427575

Guide Dogs For The Blind Association (GDBA), Head Office, Hillfields, Burghfield Common, Reading, Berkshire RG7 3YG. Tel: 01189 835555;
Fax: 01189 835433.

International Zoo Veterinary Group, Keithley Business Centre, South Street, Keithley, West Yorks BD21 1AG. Tel: 01535 692000.

Irish Veterinary Association (IVA), 53 Lansdowne Road, Ballsbridge, Dublin 4, Ireland. Tel: +353 1 668 5263; Fax: +353 1 660 4345.

ISPCA (for Ireland), 300 Lower Rathmines Road, Dublin 6, Ireland.
Tel: +353 1 497 7874.

Ministry of Agriculture, Fisheries And Food (MAFF), East Block, 10 Whitehall Place, London SW1A 2HH. Tel: 0171 270 8791.

National Canine Defence League, 17 Wakley Street, London EC1V 7LT.
Tel: 0171 837 0006; Fax: 0171 833 2530.

National Fox Welfare Society, 32 Bradfield Close, Rushden, Northamptonshire NN10 0EP Tel: 01933 411996; Fax: 01933 411996.

National Welfare Animal Trust, Tyler's Way, Watford-By-Pass, Watford WD2 8HQ. Tel: 0181 950 8215; Fax: 0181 420 4454.

People's Dispensary for Sick Animals (PDSA), Head Office, Chapel Way, Priorslee, Telford, Shropshire TF2 9PQ. Tel: 01952 290999; Fax: 01952 291035.

Royal College Of Veterinary Surgeons (RCVS), Belgravia House, 62–64 Horseferry Road, London SW1P 2AF. Tel: 0171 222 2001; Fax: 0171 222 2004.

RSPCA Head Office, Causeway, Horsham, West Sussex RH12 1HG. Tel: 01403 264181; Fax: 01403 261048.

Royal Veterinary College (RVC), Hawkshead Campus, Hawkshead Lane, North Mymms, Hatfield, Hertfordshire AL9 7TA. Tel: 01707 666333; Fax: 01707 652090.

SSPCA, Braehead Mains, 603 Queensferry Road, Edinburgh EH4 6EA. Tel: 0131 339 0222; Fax: 0131 339 4777.

St Tiggywinkle's Wildlife Hospital, Aston Road, Haddenham, Aylesbury, Buckinghamshire HP17 8AF. Tel: 01844 292292; Fax: 01844 292640.

Society for the Protection of Animals Abroad, 15 Buckingham Gate, London SW1E 6LB. Tel: 0171 828 0997; Fax: 0171 630 5776.

The British Horse Society (BHS), Main Offices, Stoneleigh Park, Warwickshire CV8 2LR. Tel: 01203 696697; Fax: 01203 692351.

Pet Log (database for microchip numbers), PO Box 2037, Clarges Street, London W1A 1GP. Telephone number for reporting a lost animal: 01733 342266 (24 hours).

The Kennel Club, 15 Clarges Street, Piccadilly, London W1Y 8AB. Tel: 0171 493 6651; Fax: 0171 518 1058.

University of Bristol, Department of Veterinary Science, Langford House, Langford, Bristol B540 5DU. Tel: 0117 9289280; Fax: 0117 9289505.

University of Cambridge, Department of Clinical Veterinary Medicine, Madingley Road, Cambridge CB3 0ES. Tel: 01223 337600; Fax: 01223 337610.

University College Dublin, Faculty of Veterinary Medicine, Ballsbridge, Dublin 4, Ireland. Tel: +353 1 668 7988; Fax: +353 1 668 7878.

University of Edinburgh, Royal (Dick) School of Veterinary Studies, Summerhall, Edinburgh EH9 1QH. Tel: 0131 650 1000; Fax: 0131 650 6585.

University of Glasgow Veterinary School, Bearsden Road, Bearsden, Glasgow G61 1QH. Tel: 0141 339 8855; Fax: 0141 942 7215.

Appendix 16: (*continued*)

University of Liverpool, Faculty of Veterinary Science, Liverpool L69 3BX.
Tel: 0151 794 4281; Fax: 0151 794 4279.

USPCA (N Ireland), Unit 4, Boucher Business Centre, Apollo Road,
Belfast
BT12 6HP, N. Ireland. Tel: 0990 134329; Fax: 01232 381991.

Veterinary Defence Society, 4 Haig Court, Parkgate Industrial Estate, Knutsford, Cheshire WA16 8XZ. Tel: 01565 652737; Fax: 01565 751079.

Veterinary Practice Management Association, 23 Buckingham Road, Shoreham-By-Sea, West Sussex BN43 5UA. Tel: 01273 463022; Fax: 01273 464431.

Wildlife Licensing and Registration Dept., Department of the Environment, Room 822, Houlton Street, Bristol. Tel. 0117 9878120.

Wildlife Information Network, Royal Veterinary College, Royal College Street, London NW1 0TU. Tel: 0171 388 7003; Fax: 0171 3887110.

Wood Green Animal Shelter, Kings Bush Farm, Godmanchester, Huntingdon, Cambridgeshire PE18 8LJ. Tel: 01480 830014; Fax: 01480 830566.

World Society For The Protection Of Animals (WSPCA), 2 Langley Lane, London SW8 1TJ. Tel: 0171 793 0540; Fax: 0171 793 0208.

World Veterinary Association, Rosenlunds Alle 8, DK-2720 Vanlose, Denmark. Tel: +45 3 871 0156; Fax: +45 3 871 0322.

Zoology Institute of Regents Park, London NW1Y 4RY. Tel: 0171 722 3333; Fax: 0171 586 2870.

Further details of the Veterinary Poison Information Service are available from the National Poisons Information Service (NPIS), Medical Toxicology Unit, Avonley Road, London SE14 5ER. Tel: 0171 635 9195, or NPIS (Leeds), The General Infirmary, Great George Street, Leeds LS1 3EX. Tel: 0113 243 0715.